Management of Early Progressive Corneal Ectasia

Cosimo Mazzotta • Frederik Raiskup
Stefano Baiocchi • Giuliano Scarcelli
Marc D. Friedman • Claudio Traversi

Management of Early Progressive Corneal Ectasia

Accelerated Crosslinking Principles

Springer

Cosimo Mazzotta
Ophthalmology Speciality School Siena University and Siena Crosslinking Center
Siena
Italy

Stefano Baiocchi
Ophthalmology Speciality School Siena University
Siena
Italy

Marc D. Friedman
Avedro
Waltham, Massachusetts
USA

Frederik Raiskup
Department of Ophthalmology Carl Gustav Carus University
Dresden
Germany

Giuliano Scarcelli
Department of Bioengineering University of Maryland
College Park, Maryland
USA

Claudio Traversi
Ophthalmology Speciality School Siena University
Siena
Italy

ISBN 978-3-319-61136-5 ISBN 978-3-319-61137-2 (eBook)
DOI 10.1007/978-3-319-61137-2

Library of Congress Control Number: 2017952041

Printed on acid-free paper

This Springer imprint is published by Springer Nature
The registered company is Springer International Publishing AG
The registered company address is: Gewerbestrasse 11, 6330 Cham, Switzerland

To Paola, Martina, Giulia and Lucia and to all Authors' Families

Preface

For the last 10 years the advent of Riboflavin-UV-A-induced crosslinking (CXL) has drastically modified the natural history of Keratoconus and secondary corneal ectasia therapy. The number of corneal transplants for Keratoconus has notably reduced over a 30% drop in the last 5 years. Potentially correct and early use of CXL, at an early stage, can lead to its annulment in the next 5–10 years with notable savings for the health care system, of expenses for patients, and above all, radically improving patient quality of life which for years had been the "*sword of Damocles*" of surgery. This ambitious goal is possible if ophthalmologists pay ever more attention to timely diagnosis and early treatment, especially in the paediatric age. Early identification of Keratoconus is the fundamental stage in this "*ideal path*". The Scheimpflug cameras and new partial optical coherence light-based (OCT) tomographers available in the clinical practice allow us to "*surprise*" the illness at its onset. One can, at this point, hypothesize a treatment that immediately stabilizes the pathological process, impeding its evolution, and most importantly stabilizing the cornea when the refractive defect is still modest and correctable, without difficulties with spectacles or contact lenses. Over 10 years have passed since the effective introduction of corneal CXL therapy, and the Dresden protocol remains the most important point of reference because it is the most studied and the most used, as well as the protocol with the most valued clinical results and longest follow-up. The fields of application have rapidly stretched from keratoconus to iatrogenic secondary ectasias, especially post-Lasik, with excellent results and more recently extended to the treatment of therapy-resistant infectious keratitis. Nonetheless, the conventional CXL (C-CXL) protocol has shown some limits: the excessive duration (1 h), the need to remove the epithelium, post-operative pain, risk of infection, haze development (stromal wound healing complications), endothelial risks for thin corneas and long waiting lists. Recently, thanks to the principles articulated in the Bunsen-Roscoe law, accelerated crosslinking treatments (A-CXL) have emerged with the objective of shortening the procedure, maintaining efficiency. Some of these proposals are proving to be valid alternatives of the conventional CXL protocol, while other techniques such as super-fast A-CXL, trans-epithelial and iontophoresis-assisted CXL (I-CXL) have shown notable limits and are thus to be modified and evaluated in the long term, large number of cases and different age groups. Another challenging chapter is the attempt to combine treatments of improving the aberrometric and refractive defect induced by Keratoconus. This is a dream for all patients who are intolerant of contact lenses: stopping Keratoconus progression and simultaneously improving the visual acuity without the necessity of resorting to corneal transplants. The so-called "*Crosslinking plus*" is already a reality for selected cases, reserved for patients with scarce visual acuity and intolerant to contact lenses, who are usually candidates for lamellar keratoplasty. The existence of clinical and instrumental parameters permits these people to attempt a stabilizing approach associated with contemporary refractive empowerment or postponement before thinking about replacement surgery. The ball is rolling, but adjustments are necessary for patient ease and repetitive, satisfying results. Crosslinking is a therapy that has changed the story of Keratoconus all over the world, and it is in continuous evolution. Accelerated CXL procedures illustrated in the book will be the leading part of the future crosslinking revolution.

Acknowledgements

Special Thanks To
Prof. Gian Marco Tosi, Head of the Ophthalmology Unit, Department of Medicine, Surgery and Neurosciences of Siena University, IT

Prof. Ennio Polito, Head of the Post-Graduate Ophthalmology School of Siena University, IT

and to

Prof. Eberhard Spoerl, Ph.D., Dresden Technical University, GE
Dr. Joshua N. Webb, Ph.D., University of Maryland, USA
Dr. Robert Herber, Dresden Technical University, GE
Dr. Janine Lenk, Dresden Technical University, GE
Dr. Miguel Rechichi, M.D., Ph.D., Eye Center, Catanzaro, IT
Dr. Mario Fruschelli, Ophthalmology Unit, Siena University, IT
Dr. Maria Margherita De Santi, Dept. Human Pathology, Siena University, IT
Dr. Pietro Rosetta, Humanitas University, Milan, IT
*Dr. Yulia Litasova, Siena University, IT
*Dr. Fiorella Fusco, Siena University, IT
*Dr. Pierfrancesco Mellace, Siena University, IT
*Dr. Simone Alex Bagaglia, Siena University, IT
*Dr. Maria Eugenia Latronico, Siena University, IT
*Dr. Gennaro Chimenti, Siena University, IT
*Dr. Marco Capozzoli, Siena University, IT
*Dr. Francesco Rana, Siena University, IT
*Dr. Stefano Fazio, Siena University, IT
*Dr. Tommaso Bacci, Siena University, IT
*Dr. Francesco Martino, Siena University, IT
*Dr. Giulia Esposti, Siena University, IT
*Dr. Maria Sole Polito, Post-Graduate Ophthalmology School, Turin University, IT
*Dr. Antonio Tarantello, Siena University, IT
*Dr. Pietro Mittica, Siena University, IT
*Dr. Giulia Cratocci, Siena University, IT
+Dr. Giovanni Neri, Siena University, IT
*Post-Graduate Ophthalmology School, Siena University, IT
Mrs. Jennifer Berkeley for English editing of the Book

Contents

1 Principles of Accelerated Corneal Collagen Cross-Linking

1.1 Introduction

Prior to the advent of the corneal collagen cross-linking procedure, no conservative treatment for corneal ectasia existed, with 20% of keratoconus patients progressing to eventually require penetrating keratoplasty [1].

Collagen cross-linking in the cornea as a treatment for ectasia was the breakthrough of Theo Seiler, MD, PhD, a professor of ophthalmology at Dresden Technical University, Germany at the time of the discovery. As he has told the story many times, Professor Seiler had his moment of inspiration in a dental chair, when he learned that UV light is used to harden dental fillings through the induction of cross-links. If the natural increase in non-enzymatic cross-linking that occurred with age led to increased corneal strength, could a physical means of inducing cross-linking be used to stabilize keratoconus? This initiated his first investigation to determine "*whether the elastic modulus of corneal tissue can be increased by cross-links of collagen fibrils induces by UV irradiation of the cornea*" [2].

Cross-linking was developed as a method of stabilizing the structurally weak corneas of patients with keratoconus, and has not only revolutionized the treatment of ectatic disorders, but has also become a platform technology including accelerated crosslinking (ACXL) with numerous additional clinical applications.

1.2 Corneal Structure and Ectasia Pathophysiology

The structure of the cornea, interacting with the forces applied to it (predominantly, intra-ocular pressure and gravity) help define the shape of the cornea. Thus, the cornea can maintain a reasonably constant shape and corneal curvature due to the tensile strength of the stromal collagen fibrils. The orderly structure of the cornea, and particularly the orientation of the stromal collagen fibrils, enables light to pass through it with minimal disruption or scatter [3–6].

C. Mazzotta et al., *Management of Early Progressive Corneal Ectasia*,
DOI 10.1007/978-3-319-61137-2_1

The corneal stroma is composed mainly of collagen, proteoglycans and water. The lamellar organization of the collagen fibrils which make up the corneal stroma is the primary source of the biomechanical strength of the cornea, and is regulated by interaction with proteoglycans [7]. The precise arrangement of the stromal collagen lamellae is critical for maintaining ocular transparency and is thought to be responsible for the corneal shape [7, 8]. Stromal collagen lamellae run in bands across the cornea in a limbus to limbus orientation. Deeper lamellae tend to run parallel to one another, whereas anterior lamellae are more intertwined and insert into the anterior limiting lamina (Bowman's membrane) [7, 9].

Individual stromal collagen fibrils are composed of units of tropocollagen, each containing three protein chains wound together in a helical pattern [10]. Each triple helical tropocollagen molecule is nominally 300 nm long, 1.5 nm in diameter, and held together by interpeptide hydrogen bonds [11–13]. Multiple tropocollagen units are assembled into microfibrils that are natively cross-linked to form the individual collagen fibrils [11, 12]. In the normal eye, the corneal collagen fibrils lie in orthogonal sheets that are parallel to each other and to the plane of the cornea, forming about 200 lamellae and comprising the extracellular matrix of the corneal stroma [14]. The collagen lamellae also exist in two preferred orthogonal orientations, with collagen preferentially aligned uniformly in the vertical and horizontal medians throughout most of the central 7 mm of the cornea [15].

There are regional differences in the arrangement of the collagen lamellae. In the anterior one third of the stroma, collagen lamellae are thin (about 0.2–1.2 μm thick and 0.5–30 μm wide), run obliquely to the corneal surface, and sometimes split into two to three sublayers that branch and become interwoven [16]. In the posterior stroma, collagen lamellae tend to be arranged parallel to the surface and are thicker (about 1.0–2.5 μm thick and 100–250 μm wide) [16]. Additional anchoring collagen lamellae in the periphery also contribute to the increased peripheral thickness. In the periphery, the collagen fibrils weave into the limbal collagen imparting considerable biomechanical strength [15, 17] (Fig. 1.1).

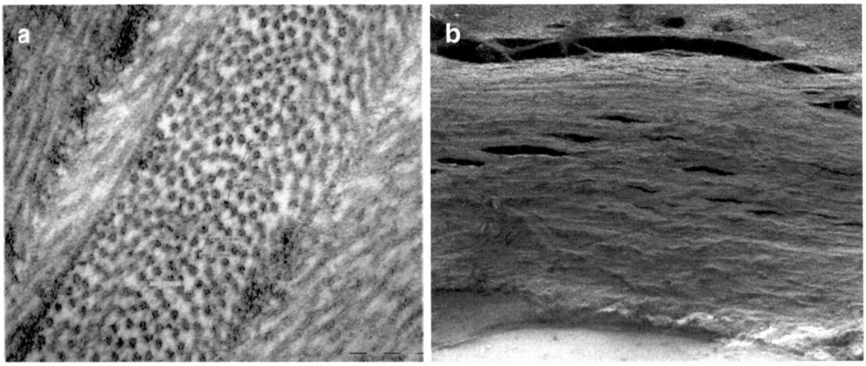

Fig. 1.1 Photomicrograph of collagen fibrils uranyl acetate-lead citrate 89.000X. Orthogonal arrangement of corneal collagen lamellae in the anterior stiff stroma (**a**). Parallel lamellar arrangement of the posterior (weak) stroma (**b**). TEM Philips EM 208S ultra-thin sections photomycrograph

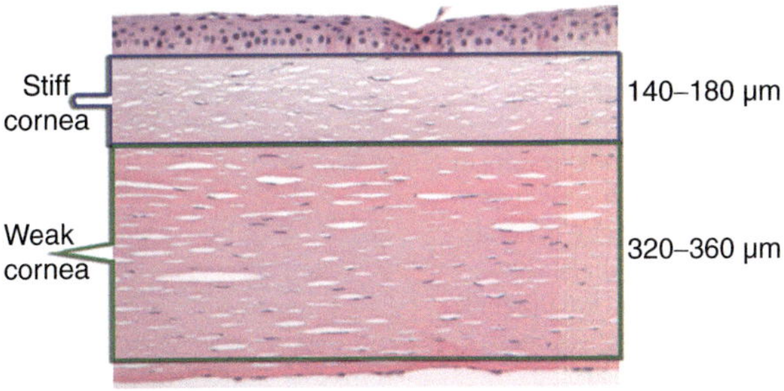

Fig. 1.2 Corneal lamellar organization divide the stroma into a superior biomechanically resistant portion (stiff cornea) and an intermediate-deep weak portion beyond 180 µm

Unlike other collagen connective tissues, the corneal collagen fibrils must maintain uniform spacing to allow light to pass with minimal scattering [3]. The spacing is influenced by proteoglycans, which are protein molecules from which glycosaminoglycan molecules extend in a bristle-like fashion [18].

The cornea's mechanical strength is primarily derived from Bowman's membrane and the anterior third of the corneal stroma because the fibers in these layers are the most interwoven making its biomechanical properties decidedly stiffer [7, 9] (Fig. 1.2).

1.2.1 Keratoconic Microstructure

The term corneal ectasia encompasses a group of disorders that share a common characteristic: progressive stromal thinning and loss of structural integrity resulting in corneal shape change, most typically inferior steepening [19, 20]. This corneal biomechanical weakness may be congenital, as in the case of keratoconus or pellucid marginal degeneration, or iatrogenic, as in the case of post-LASIK ectasia. The corneal thinning that occurs in keratoconic tissue appears to be due to the redistribution of the collagen fibrils [20]. In a normal cornea, approximately two thirds of the lamellae are oriented in a 45° sector around the vertical and horizontal meridian, with the remaining third oriented in the oblique sector between, Fig. 1.1 [21, 22]. This orthogonal arrangement is found to be absent over the area of an apical scar in keratoconus [21]. Meek et al. has demonstrated that a breakdown of cohesive strength of collagen-proteoglycan links leads to shearing between, and possibly within, stromal collagen lamellae in corneas with keratoconus [19]. Shearing between lamellae results in a phenomenon known as "creep," whereby lamellar sliding and collagen reorganization are thought to result in corneal shape change and resulting ectasia [7] (Fig. 1.3).

More recently, Roberts and Dupps [23] proposed that the earliest initiating changes for keratoconus occur in the stroma's biomechanical properties leading to clinical disease progression. They postulated that the initial biomechanical modification is focal in nature, rather than a uniform global weakening, and that the focal reduction in elastic modulus precipitates a cycle of biomechanical decompensation. Asymmetry in these biomechanical properties initiate a repeating cycle of increased strain, stress redistribution, and subsequent focal steepening and

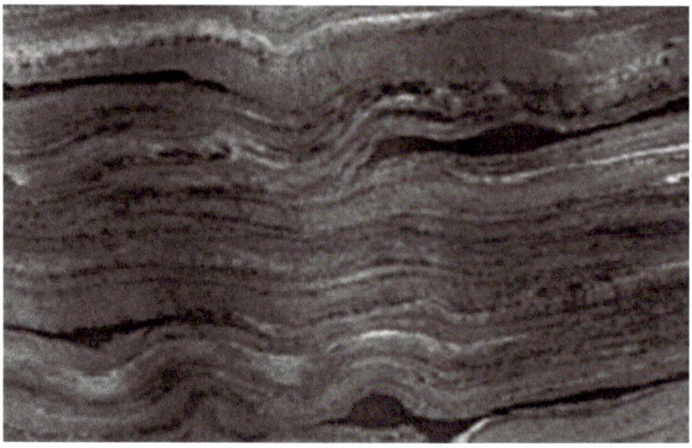

Fig. 1.3 Photomicrograph of collagen fibrils uranyl acetate-lead citrate 89.000X. Shearing between lamellae results in a phenomenon known as "creep," whereby lamellar sliding and collagen reorganization are thought to result in corneal shape change and resulting ectasia

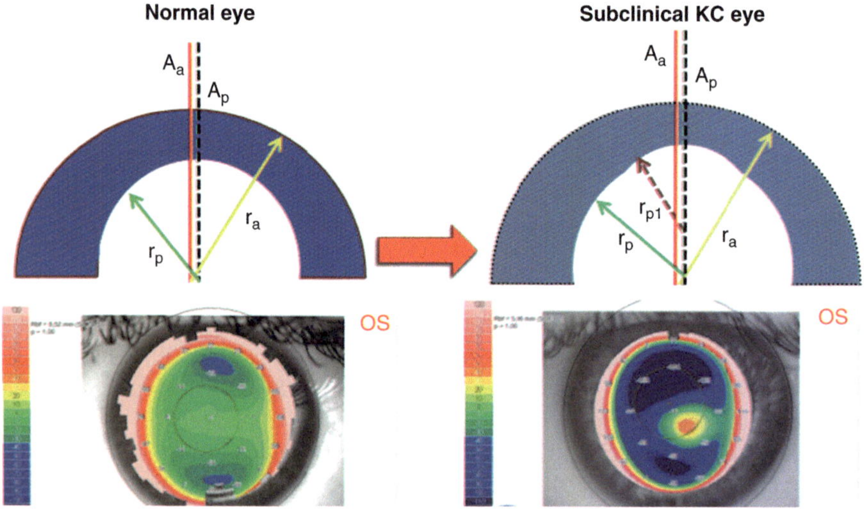

Fig. 1.4 The initial biomechanical modification driving to ectasia is focal in nature, rather than a uniform global weakening, and the focal reduction in elastic modulus generally starts in the infero-temporal region of the posterior corneal surface, precipitating a cycle of biomechanical decompensation

thinning. This is supported by Roy and Dupps [24] who showed through finite element analysis that steepening of Kmax is driven by elastic weakening. Scarcelli et al. utilizing Brillouin Microscopy verified both ex-vivo [25] and in-vivo [26] that the mechanical loss is primarily concentrated within the area of the keratoconic cone and that outside the cone, the mechanical properties of the stroma are comparable with that of healthy corneas. The causes of keratoconus and focal weakening remain unanswered but theories include genetic predisposition and eye-rubbing [23, 27–29] (Fig. 1.4).

1.2.2 Corneal Cross-Links

Keratoconus stabilizes with age [30]. Diagnosis and most rapid progression generally begin in puberty and continue throughout adolescence, arresting in the third or fourth decade of life. The stabilization of keratoconus with age [30], as well as the reduced incidence of post-LASIK ectasia in older patients [31] has provided indirect clinical evidence that the biomechanical properties of the human cornea change over time, which has been supported by laboratory research. Knox Cartwright, et al. describe a twofold increase in corneal stiffness between the ages of 20 and 100 years, demonstrated by a linear decrease in apical cornea displacement in response to change in intraocular pressure equivalent to that which occurs during the cardiac cycle [32].

Age-related increases in corneal stiffness have been attributed to the glycation induced cross-linking that occurs between or within stromal collagen lamellae as a result of the accumulation of non-enzymatic glycation end products over time [33, 34]. Similarly, it has been demonstrated that subjects with diabetes mellitus are significantly less susceptible to the development of keratoconus than non-diabetic subjects [35], attributed to greater corneal cross-linking induced through glycosylation and lysyl oxidase enzymatic activity resulting in greater corneal strength.

Corneal crosslinking using UVA light in combination with riboflavin induces extra covalent bonds. Exactly what molecules and where covalent bond formation is occurring in the stromal collagen microstructure is still not exactly known [19]. A thorough description of possible crosslinking scenarios is discussed by Hayes et al. [19]. The model describes the collagen fibrils, collagen molecules, and the bristle like hairs of the proteoglycan core proteins with their glycoaminoglycans. The possible sites include: (a) Within molecules (intramolecular), (b) Collagen molecular-collagen molecule at fibril surface (intermolecular), (c) Collagen molecule-collagen molecule at fibril surface (intermolecular), (d) Direct collagen fibril-collagen fibril (interfibrillar), (e) Proteoglycan-collagen molecule (fibril surface), (f) Within proteoglycan core proteins (intraproteoglycan), and (g) Proteoglycan core protein-proteoglycan core protein (interproteoglycan) [19]. They suggested that the covalent bonds formed during crosslinking occur predominately at the collagen fibril surface and in the protein network surrounding the collagen thereby stiffening the extracellular matrix. A simple analogy of this process would be likened to sugar coating a floppy piece of string in a glass of sugar water, the sugar coating causing the string to stiffen. They also concluded that "cross-links prevent the usual shrinkage associated with tissue dehydration during electron microscopy processing (which) may misleadingly appear larger in diameter than those in untreated corneas."

Exactly which molecules which are creating covalent crosslink bonds is still being investigated. McCall et al. [36] showed that carbonyl-based reactions dominated with minimal role of free amino groups for RFUVA cross-linking in the corneal stroma and suggested that these reactions may involve "histidine, hydroxyproline, hydroxylysine, tyrosine, and threonine." Brummer [37] discussed

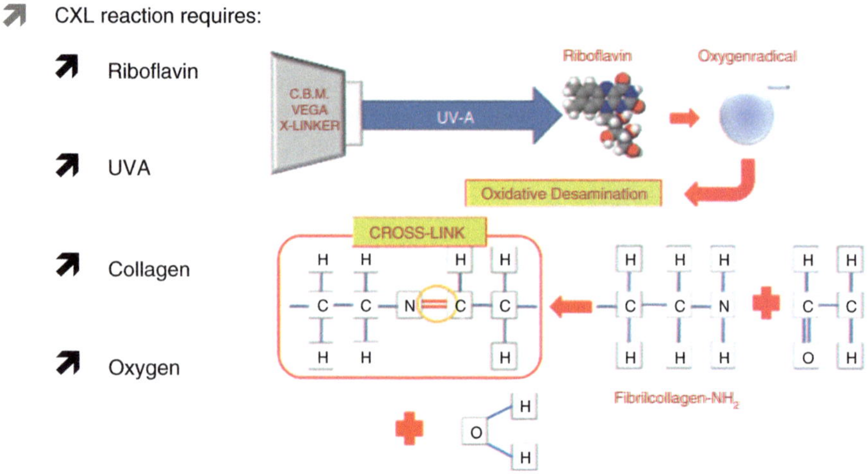

Fig. 1.5 Corneal crosslinking using UVA light in combination with riboflavin induces extra covalent bonds between and within collagen fibres and between collagen and proteoglycans

how these carbonyl-based reactions and advance glycation end products (AGEs) are involved in crosslinking formation and are similar to glycation in aging, diabetes, and cigarette smoking. Additionally, Zhang et al. [38] showed RFUVA causes crosslinking of collagen molecules among themselves and proteoglycan core proteins among themselves, together with limited linkages between collagen and keratocan, lumican, mimecan, and decorin. A table summarizing Zhang's results may be found in Meek and Hayes [39] (Fig. 1.5).

1.2.3 Standard Crosslinking and the "Dresden Protocol"

"We would emphasize that the in vitro-experiments reported here are intended to the first step in the direction of a conservative treatment of keratectasia" [1]. In this seminal paper, Spoerl, Huhle and Seiler performed the first series of experiments to determine whether the induction of crosslinks stiffened the cornea with riboflavin. They compared photochemical crosslinking with riboflavin using 365 and 436 nm light, 254 nm UV light only, sunlight and compared these with known chemical crosslinkers of glutaraldehyde and Karnovsky's solution utilizing uniaxial extensiometry. Their results demonstrated that corneal crosslinking and stiffening of the cornea was achievable with riboflavin in the presence of UVA light.

The group then investigated and developed many aspects of the science underlying corneal crosslinking. They began the search by measuring the dose response to various stiffening techniques of the cornea [40]. This was followed by a series of other studies which looked at keratocyte cytotoxicity [41], endothelial cytotoxicity in-vitro [42], endothelial cell damage in-vivo [43], stress-strain measurements of human and porcine corneas [44], collagen fiber diameter [45], thermomechanical Behavior [46], and resistance to enzymatic digestion [47] fully characterizing the safety and developing many of the methods for measuring crosslinking utilized today.

In 2003, Wollensak et al. [48] presented the results of the first clinical study of the use of riboflavin-5-phosphate and UVA light cross-linking as a treatment for progressive keratoconus. Twenty-three eyes of twenty-two patients with confirmed progressive keratoconus were treated in a prospective, non-randomized pilot study, with follow-up ranging from 3 to 47 months. The epithelium was mechanically debrided from the central 7 mm of the cornea of treated eyes. A solution of 0.1% riboflavin-5-phosphate and 20% dextran T-500 was applied 5 min before irradiation with 370 nm UV light, and every 5 min during irradiation. Irradiation was delivered using two UV diodes calibrated to an irradiance of 3 mW/cm^2 for 30 min, corresponding to a dose of 5.4 J/cm^2. In all cases, progression was stopped, as measured by change in maximum keratometry value (Kmax). In 16 of 22 eyes, reduction of Kmax was observed, with a mean flattening of 2.01 and of the refractive error of 1.14 diopters. In this first study, transient stromal edema was noted until re-epithelialization. No other complications were reported, and endothelial cell density remained unchanged from baseline.

The Dresden group achieved their 1998 goal as there have been numerous clinical studies utilizing the Dresden protocol (*See* Sect. 2.1) demonstrating stabilization of the cornea or continued flattening of Kmax with little to no long term side effects for the "conservative treatment of keratectasia". For over a decade it has been considered the standard of care for keratoconus and post Lasik ectasia across the world and was recently approved in the United States for both procedures [49].

The now more standardize "Dresden Protocol" has the main elements of de-epithelization of the corneal epithelium, a 30 min of pre-soak with 0.1% riboflavin-5-phosphate and 20% dextran T-500, followed by 30 min of 365 nm UVA light treatment at 3 mW/cm^2 for a total dose of 5.4 J/cm^2.

1.3 Accelerated Crosslinking, Photochemical Kinetic Principles

Although very effective, the Dresden protocol is a lengthy procedure and requires removal of the epithelium. In an effort to improve upon the Dresden protocol, newer technologies have emerged addressing these issues making the procedure more comfortable for patients and cost effective for hospitals [50]. The first of these technologies is accelerated crosslinking.

Accelerated cross-linking protocols follow one of the fundamental laws of photochemistry called the Bunsen-Roscoe Law of Reciprocity [51]. This law states that the photochemical biological effect is proportional to the total energy dose delivered regardless of the applied irradiance and time. Irradiance refers to the power per area delivered to the surface of the cornea. It is given in units of W/cm^2. The energy per area delivered to the surface of the cornea is the dose. Dose is given in units of J/cm^2. Irradiance and dose are related by the following equation:

$$\textit{Irradiance}\left(\textit{Watts/cm}^2\right) \times \textit{Time}(s) = \textit{Dose}\left(\textit{J/cm}^2\right)$$

The Dresden protocol uses 3 mW/cm^2 irradiation over 30 min, which delivers a 5.4 J/cm^2 dose.

$$\left(0.003\,W/cm^2\right) \times \left(1800\,s\right) = 5.4\,J/cm^2$$

To deliver an equivalent energy dose, an accelerated protocol using 30 mW/cm^2 irradiance requires only 3 min to achieve the same dose of 5.4 J/cm^2 obtained in 30 min of irradiation with 3 mW/cm^2 irradiance.

$$\left(0.030\,W/cm^2\right) \times \left(180\,s\right) = 5.4\,J/cm^2$$

Other accelerated protocols may be derived using this equation, and have been employed clinically up to 45 mW/cm^2 irradiation.

The Bunsen-Roscoe reciprocity law may hold if all other parameters are controlled. However, in the case of corneal cross-linking, there are many other factors beyond the UVA dose that contribute to the total amount and 3-dimensional distribution of cross-linking obtained in the cornea. Factors related to the clinical procedure include the beam profile and illumination pattern of the UVA delivery device, the concentration and diffusion rate of the formulation of the riboflavin used, the length of the riboflavin presoak time, the viscosity of the riboflavin film, as well as the presence and concentration of oxygen in the stromal tissue. Individual patient variability, including corneal structure and baseline corneal biomechanics may also influence the outcome of the procedure.

The first reported laboratory investigation and clinical use of accelerated cross-linking for bullous keratopathy was by Krueger [52] utilizing 15 mW/cm^2 for 7 min and a staged intrastromal delivery riboflavin. Krueger also retrospectively reported the first laboratory investigation of accelerated crosslinking [53] using a 370 nm UVA source they crosslinked porcine globes with irradiances of 2, 3, 9, and 15 mW/cm^2 continuously and 15 mW/cm^2 fractionated (with alternate cycles of 30 s "ON" and 30 s "OFF" exposure) for a total dose of 5.4 mJ/cm^2 and performed extensiometry to measure increases in stiffness. Their results showed no statistically significant differences between standard and higher irradiances.

Since that initial study, accelerated crosslinking has been extensively studied utilizing various methods for understanding and quantifying corneal crosslinking.

1.3.1 Laboratory Methods for Quantifying Crosslinking

While there is currently no direct method for measuring the exact amount and distribution of cross-links that occur in tissue, there are a number of methods available to indicate the relative efficacy of cross-linking procedures. These measures include theoretical modeling of the cross-linking process, mechanical techniques, such as extensiometry or inflation testing commonly used as measures of the change in stress-strain behavior of the cornea, Interferometry, OCT, Brillouin microscopy, the measure of oxygen consumption, as well chemical assessment through enzymatic digestion techniques. This information has been used to indirectly describe changes in the biomechanical properties of the cornea.

1.3.1.1 Interferometry

Interferometry is a family of optical techniques which uses the addition and subtraction of combined light waves to assess the properties of an object. It has been used to measure the biomechanical properties of the cornea using electronic speckle interferometry (ESPI) [32, 54] and low coherence optical tomography [55].

1.3.1.2 Stress-Strain Techniques: Extensiometry and Inflation Testing

Young's modulus, measured in Pascal, describes the resistance of a material to change in length, and is defined as the ratio of stress to strain. Stress refers to the force applied to a material per unit area, and strain refers to the change in length per unit of the original length. The Young's modulus of a material is a constant to a point of breakdown, after which the force applied exceeds the limit of proportionality and the material will no longer rebound from deformation.

The Young's modulus of a material may be obtained through tensile testing of the material, by applying a known force and measuring change using extensiometry techniques. In corneal tissue, extensiometry may be performed using a uniaxial method with a long strip of tissue, or by using corneal flaps [2, 32, 56]. Since corneal tissue is radially oriented, uniaxial strip extensiometry is a less accurate measure than a biaxial extensiometry due to lamellar disruption in one axis, leaving half the collagen fibers in an unknown state. Biaxial extensiometry has the benefit of measuring the collagen fibers in a manner more closely related to the forces they see in-vivo [57].

Corneal tissue used in bi-axial extensiometry may be full thickness, or separated into flaps of known thicknesses. The anterior and posterior cornea have different biomechanical behaviors, and different cross-linking techniques may create deeper or shallower cross-linking, it is therefore important that the thickness of the flap used in extensiometry be known. Commercially available biaxial extensometers use biorake attachments that allow for minimal and repeatable handling of the tissue. Each sample is lowered into a temperature controlled bath and stretched at a constant rate (μm/s) until sample failure.

Inflation testing is another method of obtaining the biomechanical properties of the cornea. An advantage to inflation testing is that the force is applied radially, which more closely mimics physiological conditions [58]. Inflation methods using whole globes were first used to test for ocular rigidity [59–64]. In other inflation studies, only the cornea with varying amounts of scleral ring are mounted to pressure chambers in a variety of configurations to allow their measurement [32, 54, 58]. As with extensiometry, it is critical that temperature and hydration are controlled as these affect the tissue biomechanics and the reproducibility of the results.

1.3.1.3 Tissue Preparation

In-vitro cross-linking is usually performed using human or various animal whole globes. Preconditioning of the globes is a first and necessary step in obtaining repeatable laboratory so tissue hydration is stabilized. Additionally, as corneal crosslinking is a photochemical process, variations in temperature can change the dynamics of the reaction and impacts the amount of cross-linking and the subsequent mechanical response of the tissue [65]. Therefore maintenance of physiologic temperature and hydration of the globes during experimental cross-linking is recommended in addition to maintaining the globes intraocular pressure. This helps to ensure the precision and accuracy of the experimental measurement.

1.3.1.4 Oxygen Monitoring

The use of oxygen monitoring may also function as a proxy for understanding the chemical kinetic mechanisms of corneal cross-linking [66]. In this method, oxygen levels are measured using an O_2 sensor. Drops of riboflavin solution are instilled onto corneas which are then exposed to 365 nm UVA under varying irradiance and temperature. Oxygen concentration in the cornea at a known depth is monitored during UVA illumination. The oxygen dynamics are then used to gather insight into the mechanisms of corneal cross-linking.

1.3.1.5 Chemical Digestion

The use of chemical digestion with enzymes for measuring corneal cross-linking was first performed by Spoerl et al. [47]. In this experiment, porcine corneas were irradiated at three different doses. The corneas were then trephined and allowed to digest in different enzymes. The resistance to enzymatic degradation was measured as a function of time, demonstrating that increased corneal cross-linking caused increased resistance to digestion. Enzymatic digestion has also been utilized to study corneal crosslinking several others [18, 67, 68].

Another enzymatic digestion method utilizes the enzyme papain in combination with spectrofluorometer analysis as a means to quantify the amount of cross-linking in porcine corneal flaps that have undergone various UVA-riboflavin based corneal cross-linking protocols [69]. This method ensures that the same amount of tissue is utilized minimizing corneal thickness variation often seen in uniaxial testing.

In this method, porcine globes are preconditioned as previously described and treated under various cross-linking protocols. Using a femtosecond laser, corneal flaps of various thicknesses are excised after cross-linking. The thicknesses of the corneal flaps are confirmed using ultrasonic pachymetry. To prepare for digestion, the corneal flaps are washed with distilled water 15 times to remove residual riboflavin, and dried in a vacuum until the weight change becomes less than 10%. Each flap is digested for 2.5 h at 65 °C with 2.5 units/mL of papain (from Papaya latex, Sigma) in 1 mL of papain buffer [1× PBS (pH 7.4), 2 mM L-cysteine and 2 mM EDTA]. Papain digests are centrifuged for 20 s at 2200 × G (Mini centrifuge 05-090-100, Fisher Scientific) and diluted 0.5 times with 1× PBS solution.

Fluorescence of the of the corneal flap digested solutions is measured with excitation of $\lambda ex = 360$ nm in a QM-40 Spectrofluorometer (Photon Technology Int., London, Ontario, Canada) with the emission fluorescence measured between 375 and 650 nm. Fluorescence of remaining riboflavin is subtracted out of the recorded fluorescence and normalized to untreated controls. The fluorescence at 450 nm is indicative of the amount of cross-linking in the corneal flap [70]. Using this technique, statistically significant results ($P < .05$) are observable for small variations in protocol. One significant advantage of this method is that multiple flaps can be excised from one cornea to analyze the amount of cross-linking at different depths.

1.3.2 Photochemical Kinetics of Corneal Crosslinking with Riboflavin and UVA Light

There is a large body of literature starting in the 1950s and 1960s, but especially from the 1990s and early 2000s with regard to its photochemical kinetic mechanisms of riboflavin chemistry. The initial hypothesis of the mechanism of UVA and riboflavin for mediated corneal cross-linking was that exposure of riboflavin to UVA light in an oxygenated environment causes the formation of singlet oxygen, which then acts on tissue to produce additional cross linked bonds [35, 71]. Current understanding suggests that the photochemical kinetic mechanisms involve both Type I and Type II photochemical kinetic mechanisms.

Much of this literature through analysis of the photochemical kinetics chemistry, observed tissue oxygen concentration and resultant cross-linking under varied treatment conditions suggests that ROS and especially the type I electron transfer kinetic mechanism are mostly responsible for creating crosslinks within the cornea and that reactive oxygen species (ROS) act as the predominant agent [66, 72, 73].

Several families of reactions underlie riboflavin cross-linking chemistry. Some of these reactions are UV mediated while others occur without UV light. Among these reaction paths, some mechanisms enhance the production of radical species that promote cross-linking, while others degrade riboflavin without creating cross-links. To optimize the clinical cross-linking process, it is important to understand these reactions, how they relate to one another and to environmental conditions.

Some of the major kinetic reactions involved in Type I and Type II mechanisms derived from the literature are shown in Fig. 1.6 [66, 72–85]. In the presence of light, riboflavin can exhibit photosensitizing properties reacting with a wide range of electron donating tissue sites (such as amines or amino acids) [35, 70, 76, 85, 86] through mixed Type I – Type II photochemical mechanisms [81].

The reaction diagram in Fig. 1.7 generally illustrates these major reactions and their interactions with each other. In the Type I mechanism, the sensitizer excited state generates radicals or radical ions, predominately ROS, which react with the tissue through hydrogen atoms or electron transfer. For the Type I crosslinking mechanism the first pathway in which radical Rf on its own creates crosslinks is a very minor contributor amount of crosslinks [72, 73]. The second pathway in which ROS and predominately hydroxyl radical create the majority of crosslinks is the major contributor to the process [72, 73]. In the Type II mechanism, the excited sensitizer reacts with oxygen to form singlet molecular oxygen. This energy transfer process although present has only a minor impact on the total amount of crosslinking produced during UV treatment [72, 73].

Common:

$Rf \rightarrow Rf_1^*$, I; (r1)

$Rf_1^* \rightarrow Rf$, $\kappa 1$; (r2)

$Rf_1^* \rightarrow Rf_3^*$, $\kappa 2$; (r3)

Type I:

$Rf_3^* + DH \rightarrow RfH' + D'$, $\kappa 3$; (r4)

$2RfH' \rightarrow Rf + RFH_2$, $\kappa 4$; (r5)

Type II:

$Rf_3^* + O_2 \rightarrow Rf + O_2^1$, $\kappa 5$; (r6)

$DH + O_2^1 \rightarrow D_{ox}$, $\kappa 6$; (r7)

$D_{ox} + DH \rightarrow D - D$, $\kappa 7$; **CXL** (r8)

Additional:

$Rf_3^* \rightarrow Rf$, $\kappa 8$; (r9)

$Rf_3^* + Rf \rightarrow 2RfH'$, $\kappa 9$; (r10)

$RfH_2 + O_2 \rightarrow RfH' + H^+ + O_2^-$, $\kappa 10$; (r11)

$RfH' + O_2 \rightarrow RF + H^+ + O_2^-$, $\kappa 11$; (r12)

$2\,RfH_2 + O_2^- \rightarrow 2\,RFH' + H_2O_2$, $\kappa 12$; (r13)

$2\,RFH' + O_2^- \rightarrow 2\,RF + H_2O_2$, $\kappa 13$; (r14)

$RFH' + H_2O_2 \rightarrow OH' + RF + H_2O_2$, $\kappa 14$; (r15)

$OH' + DH \rightarrow D' + H_2O$, $\kappa 15$; (r16)

$D' + D' \rightarrow D - D$, $\kappa 16$; **CXL** (r17)

$O_2^1 \rightarrow O_2$, $\kappa 18$; (r18)

$D' + RfH_2 \rightarrow RFH - DH$, $\kappa 19$; (r19)

Aggregation

$Rf + Rf \underset{\kappa_a^-}{\overset{\kappa_a^+}{\rightleftarrows}} A_1$, $\kappa_a = \kappa_a^+ / \kappa_a^-$ (r20)

$RfH_2 + RfH_2 \underset{\kappa_a^-}{\overset{\kappa_a^+}{\rightleftarrows}} A_2$, $\kappa_a = \kappa_a^+ / \kappa_a^-$ (r21)

$Rf + RfH_2 \underset{\kappa_b^-}{\overset{\kappa_b^+}{\rightleftarrows}} A_3$, $\kappa_b = \kappa_b^+ / \kappa_a^-$ (r22)

$Rf_1^* + A \rightarrow Rf + A$, κ_{1a} (r23)

$Rf_3^* + A \rightarrow Rf + A$, κ_{3a} (r24)

Peroxides

$2\,O_2^- \rightarrow O_2 + H_2O_2$, κ_{12} (r25)

$OH^* + CXL \rightarrow$ inert products, κ_{OH} (r26)

Fig. 1.6 Some of the major kinetic reactions involved in Type I and Type II mechanisms for riboflavin crosslinking

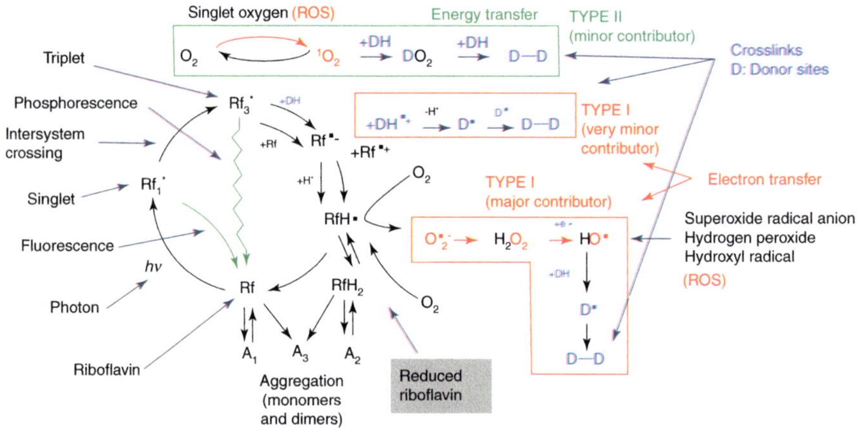

Fig. 1.7 Reaction diagram illustrating the major reactions involved in riboflavin crosslinking and their interactions with each other

The major reactions represented by the reaction diagram have been modeled utilizing finite element analysis [73, 84].

An important aspect of the photochemical kinetic theory and model is understanding how various concentrations of riboflavin affect the amount of crosslinking for concentrations typical for present CXL clinical protocols [84]. The total amount of riboflavin is made up of both riboflavin (Rf) and reduced riboflavin (RfH_2). It is not surprising that as the concentrations of single Rf and RfH_2 molecules (monomers) increases, there is a tendency for the molecules to stick or aggregate into dimers to create molecules of 2Rf, $2RfH_2$ and $RfRfH_2$. For a 0.1% solution, typically used for CXL, ~37% of total riboflavin is in dimers which increases to ~72% for a 0.5% solution [87].

An experiment [84] was performed measuring the amount of photobleaching of riboflavin under anaerobic conditions as a function of irradiated dose at both 3 and 30 mW/cm² for different initial concentrations of 0.01, 0.05, 0.1 and 0.5% and were shown to correlate with the theoretical model. The results are seen in Fig. 1.8.

These results and their correlations with the model implies that for more concentrated solutions, the fraction of dimers is higher (relative to monomers) and that these dimers quench both singlet and triplet forms of riboflavin that reduce the quantum yield of triplets and in turn, reduced riboflavin. This results in less efficient crosslinking as the concentration of riboflavin goes up. This was corroborated with

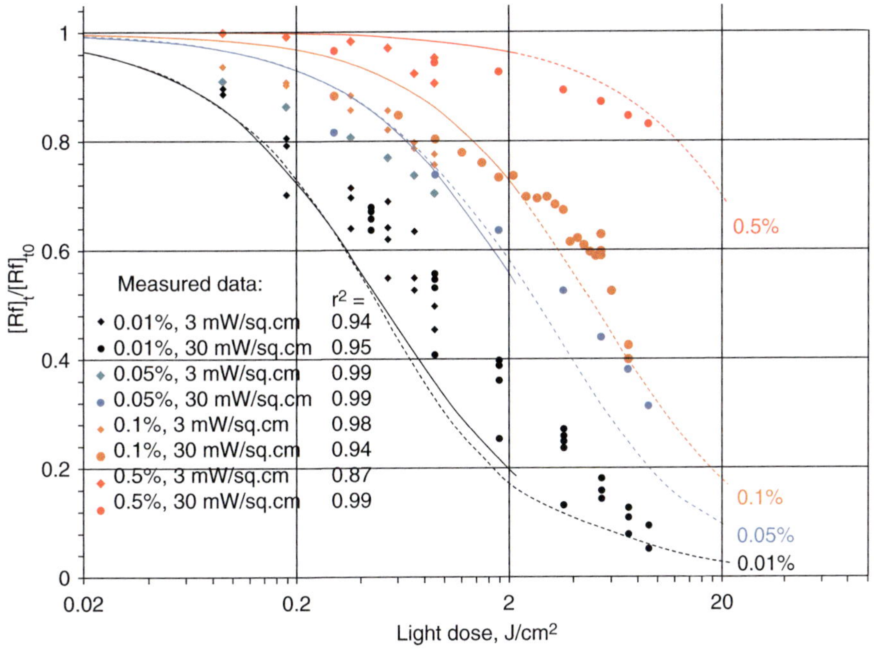

Fig. 1.8 Photobleaching of riboflavin as a function of irradiated dose for different initial concentrations of 0.01, 0.05, 0.1, and 0.5% and its theoretical modeling (3 mW/cm²—*solid lines* as modeled and diamonds as experimental points, 30 mW/cm²—*dashed lines* as modeled and circles as experimental points)

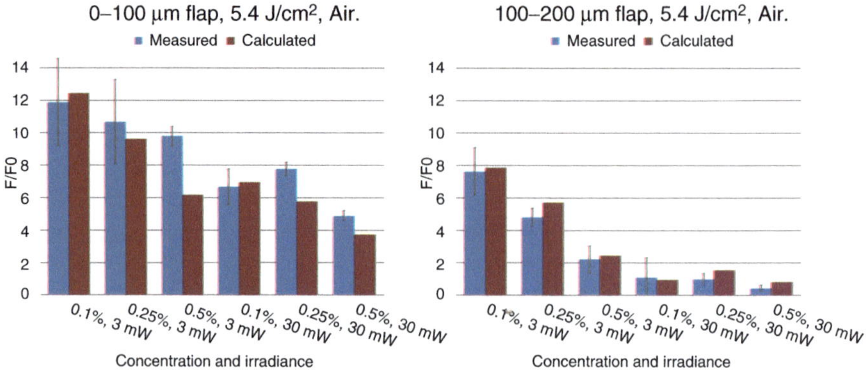

Fig. 1.9 Normalized fluorescence measuring the amount of crosslinking versus the theoretical model for riboflavin concentrations of 0.1, 0.25, and 0.5% and a dose of 5.4 J/cm^2 at 3 and 30 mW/cm^2 for the first and second 100 μm of a crosslinked porcine cornea in air

another experiment in which different concentrations of riboflavin (0.1, 0.25 and 0.5%) were utilized under the same conditions (3 and 30 mW/cm^2 irradiance; 5.4 J/cm^2 dose) to crosslink porcine corneas and the amounts of crosslinking were determined by the papain digestion method [73] (Fig. 1.9).

In the major reaction of crosslinking the radical form of riboflavin (RfH$^•$) creates superoxide radical anion ($O^•{}_2{}^-$) which converts to hydrogen peroxide (H_2O_2) and finally to hydroxyl radical (OH^-). Hydroxyl radical is the major ROS species that reacts with the donor sites of the collagen to create crosslinks. Additionally, Gorner [82] showed that in an anaerobic environment, riboflavin (Rf) is converted into reduced riboflavin (RfH_2). Reduced riboflavin is unique in that it is metastable and does not absorb UVA light. This is important as reduced riboflavin is converted back to the radical form of riboflavin (RfH$^•$) in the presence of oxygen. Therefore, reduced riboflavin consumes and utilizes oxygen as it becomes available competing for oxygen utilized for crosslinks.

This process may be illustrated through a time elapsed (log scale) analysis of the various concentrations of the major chemical reactants based on the model (Dresden Protocol). Beginning with Fig. 1.10a, a transition zone of reaction or phase front from the surface is established within the first 15–20 s where the anterior stroma has oxygen but the posterior stroma is depleted of oxygen [66]. In Fig. 1.10b, as the reaction proceeds 9–10 min, the concentration of crosslinks (blue line) begin to accumulate at the anterior surface, while the concentration of potential crosslinking sites decreases proportionality noting that two crosslinking or donor sites (black line) are required for every crosslink. In the posterior of the stroma, reduced riboflavin (red line) has accumulated and is modulating/governing the consumption of oxygen (green line). At 30 min into the reaction as illustrated in Fig. 1.10c, the reaction has propagated deeper into the tissue having established a transition zone or phase front where the anterior of the cornea is nearly saturated with crosslinks (blue line) and the crosslinking distribution follows the distribution of the oxygen (green line).

This analysis shows that as irradiance increases and the number of photons of light per time increases, the concentration of reduced riboflavin increases in the

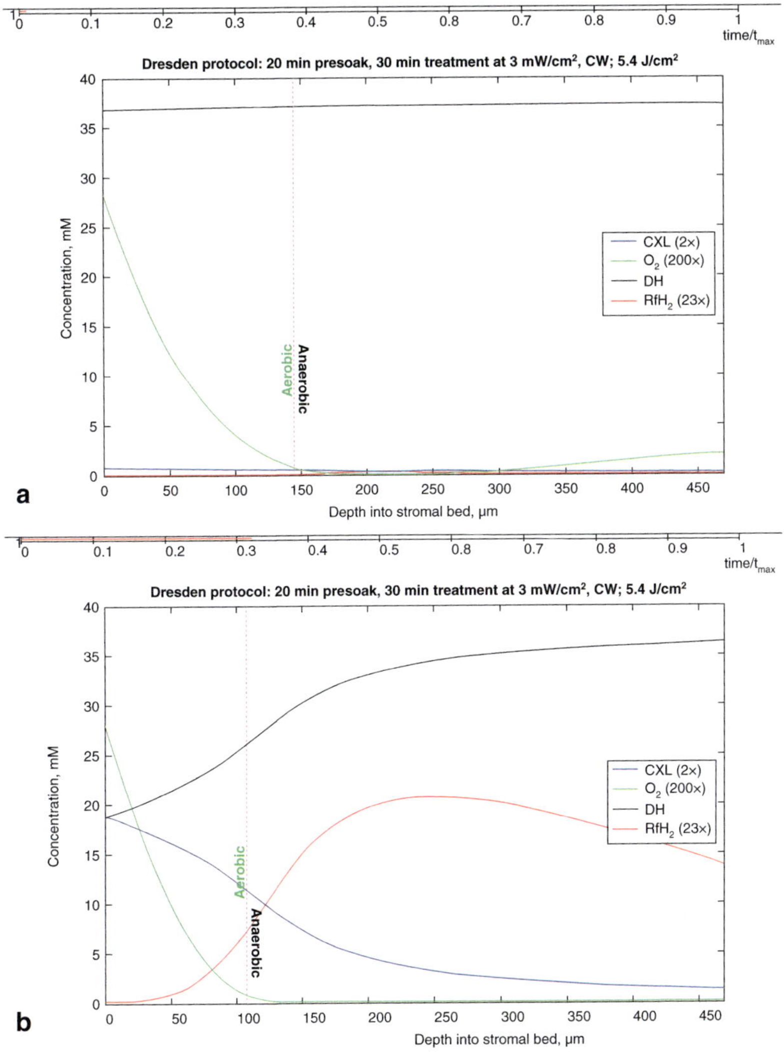

Fig. 1.10 (**a**) A time elapsed (log scale) analysis of the Dresden protocol illustrating the molar concentrations of potential crosslinking sites (DH), of crosslinks (CXL), oxygen (O_2), and reduced riboflavin (RfH_2), as a function of depth and time. A transition zone of reaction or phase front from the surface is established within the first 15–20 s where the anterior stroma has oxygen but the posterior stroma is depleted of oxygen. The reduced riboflavin (*red line*) has accumulated and is modulating/governing the consumption of oxygen (*green line*). (**b**) A time elapsed (log scale) analysis of the Dresden protocol illustrating the molar concentrations of potential crosslinking sites (DH), of crosslinks (CXL), oxygen (O_2), and reduced riboflavin (RfH_2), as a function of depth and time. As the reaction proceeds 9–10 min, the concentration of crosslinks (*blue line*) begin to accumulate at the anterior surface, while the concentration of potential crosslinking sites decreases proportionality noting that two crosslinking or donor sites (*black line*) are required for every crosslink. (**c**) A time elapsed (log scale) analysis of the Dresden protocol illustrating the molar concentrations of potential crosslinking sites (DH), of crosslinks (CXL), oxygen (O_2), and reduced riboflavin (RfH_2), as a function of depth and time. At 30 min, the reaction has propagated deeper into the tissue having established a transition zone or phase front where the anterior of the cornea is nearly saturated with crosslinks (*blue line*) and the crosslinking distribution follows the distribution of the oxygen (*green line*)

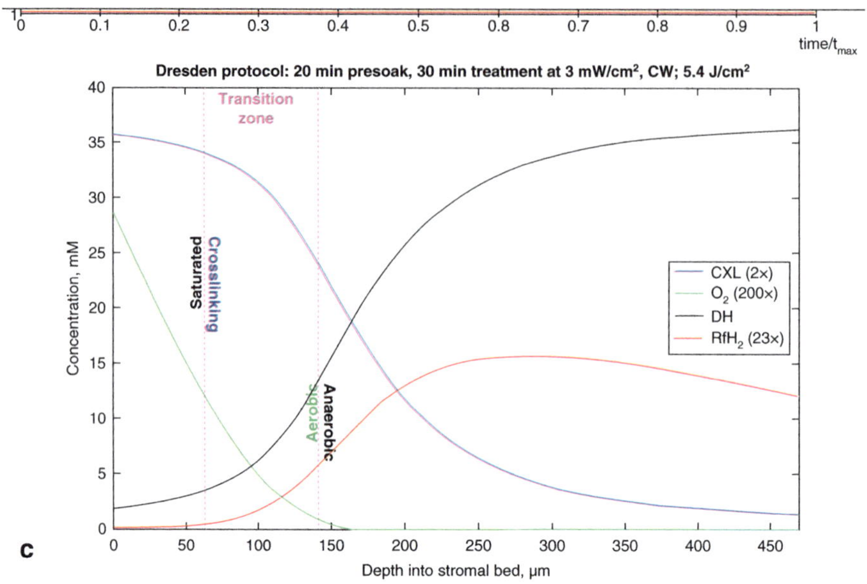

Fig. 1.10 (continued)

posterior side of the transition zone within the stroma. The increased concentration of reduced riboflavin in the posterior anaerobic stroma utilizes more oxygen and is the reason why crosslinking efficiency decreases as the irradiance increases under equivalent conditions. This can be modulated however with the introduction of oxygen as seen in Fig. 1.11.

In this experiment, irradiances of 3, 10, 15, 30, 45, 60, and 100 mW/cm^2, in both air and 100% oxygen environments were used to crosslink whole porcine globes using CW 365 nm UVA for a total dose of 5.4 J/cm^2 [73]. Two hundred micron flaps were taken and the papain digestion method [69] was utilized to analyze the relative amount of crosslinks. This was compared to the theoretical model [73]. The results show that the efficiency of crosslinking decreases with increasing irradiance and the addition of oxygen significantly boost the efficiency for high irradiance but reduces crosslinking efficiency at low irradiance as predicted. Reduced crosslinking efficiency is observed at low irradiance and is attributable to quenching of the reaction by having an overabundance of available oxygen.

This has clinical implications for the introduction of oxygen during crosslinking. As can be seen in Fig. 1.11, for accelerated crosslinking epi-off protocols *the addition of oxygen can greatly enhance higher irradiance crosslinking efficiency* (≥10 mW/cm^2), significantly reducing treatment time over standard crosslinking in air but inhibit the crosslinking efficiency for the standard protocol (3 mW/cm^2) making it undesirable to do so. For epithelium on or transepithelial protocols, crosslinking efficiency appears to be lower showing shallower lines of demarcation [88]. Low oxygen concentration and residual riboflavin absorption in the epithelium are two primary reasons for reduced crosslinking efficiency and the addition of oxygen may greatly enhance transepithelial protocols.

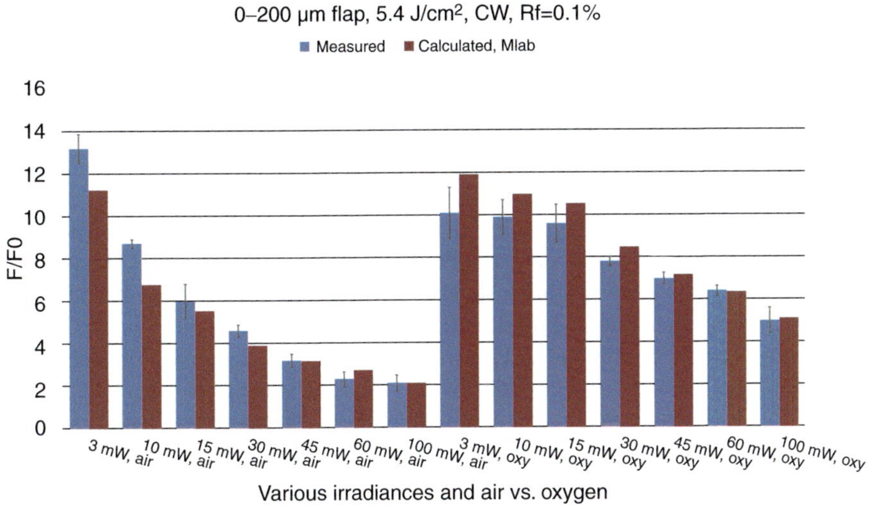

Fig. 1.11 Normalized fluorescence measuring the amount of crosslinking versus the theoretical model for irradiances of 3, 10, 15, 30, 45, 60, and 100 mW/cm², in both air and 100% oxygen for a total dose of 5.4 J/cm²

Fig. 1.12 Normalized fluorescence measuring the amount of crosslinking versus the theoretical model for continuous and pulsed light illumination both in air and oxygen at 30 mW/cm² of for a total dose of 7.2 J/cm²

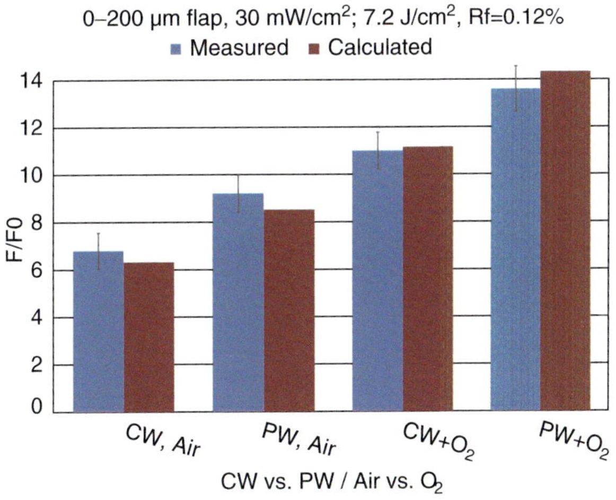

These oxygen/reduced riboflavin dynamics are illustrated again in a similar experiment crosslinking using porcine eyes, 0.1% riboflavin, 30 mW/cm², in air or oxygen with the UVA illumination either continuous wave (CW) or Pulsed (1 s on, 1 s off), Fig. 1.12. Crosslinking efficiency increases over standard crosslinking with pulsed light, oxygen, and pulsed light + oxygen as predicted by the model. Although it takes 2–3 min for full oxygen replenishment of the tissue at depth [66], in the transition zone along the phase front of the photochemical reaction as previously described, the 1 s off time produces less reduced riboflavin and allows more oxygen to accumulate in a microscopic manner along its leading edge during the off cycle of the pulse. Therefore, more total oxygen is available along the phase front of the reaction producing increased crosslinking efficiency.

The model also incorporates the concept of crosslinking saturation at the surface. An experiment was performed to establish anterior crosslinking saturation [73]. In this experiment porcine whole globes were crosslinked (0.1% riboflavin, 20 min soak, 3 mW/cm^2) with increasing exposure times of 7.5, 15, 30, 45, 120 and 150 min. Two hundred micron flaps were made with a femotosecond laser (Intralase, AMO). Extensiometry was performed using a biaxial extensometer (CellScale Biotester 5000, Waterloo, ON). Each sample was allowed to presoak in saline for 20 min before testing to allow complete hydration stability, lowered into a saline bath at 37 °C and stretched at a constant rate of 4 μm/s until sample failure. The output was fitted to the maximum slope for both X and Y. This was compared to the theoretical model where the area under the curve for a depth of 200 microns was calculated (Fig. 1.13a). Figure 1.13b, illustrates the relative correlation between the biomechanics and the model demonstrating the saturation effect of the anterior surface of the stroma.

In a study by Chai et al. [65], collagen fluorescence as a function of depth was measured using non-linear optical microscopy for crosslinked porcine corneas using 3 mW/cm^2 at 15 and 30 min for a total dose of 2.7 and 5.4 J/cm^2. The theory and model were then compared to this data [73]. As shown in the extensiometry experiment previously described, the 15 min dose does not saturate the anterior surface of the stroma with the 30 min showing a nearly doubling of fluorescence as both measured and predicted by the model seen in Fig. 1.14 demonstrating the distribution of corneal crosslinks as a function of depth for these two CXL protocols.

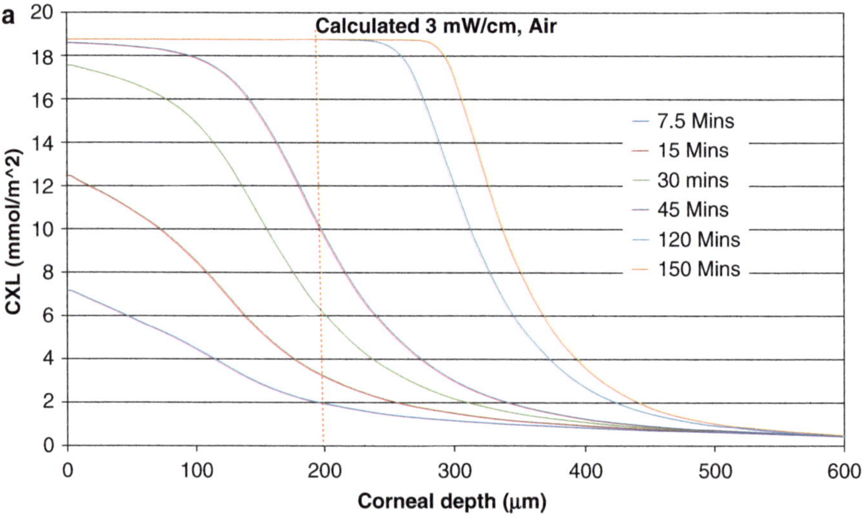

Fig. 1.13 (**a**) Theoretical crosslinking concentration as a function of depth for the Dresden protocol for illumination times of 7.5, 15, 30, 45, 120 and 150 min. The areas under the curves to a depth of 200 μm were calculated. (**b**) The maximum slope for both X and Y extensiometry of 200 μm corneal flaps versus the theoretical model for illumination times of 7.5, 15, 30, 45, 120 and 150 min. The relative correlation between the biomechanics and the model illustrate the crosslinking saturation effect of the anterior surface of the stroma

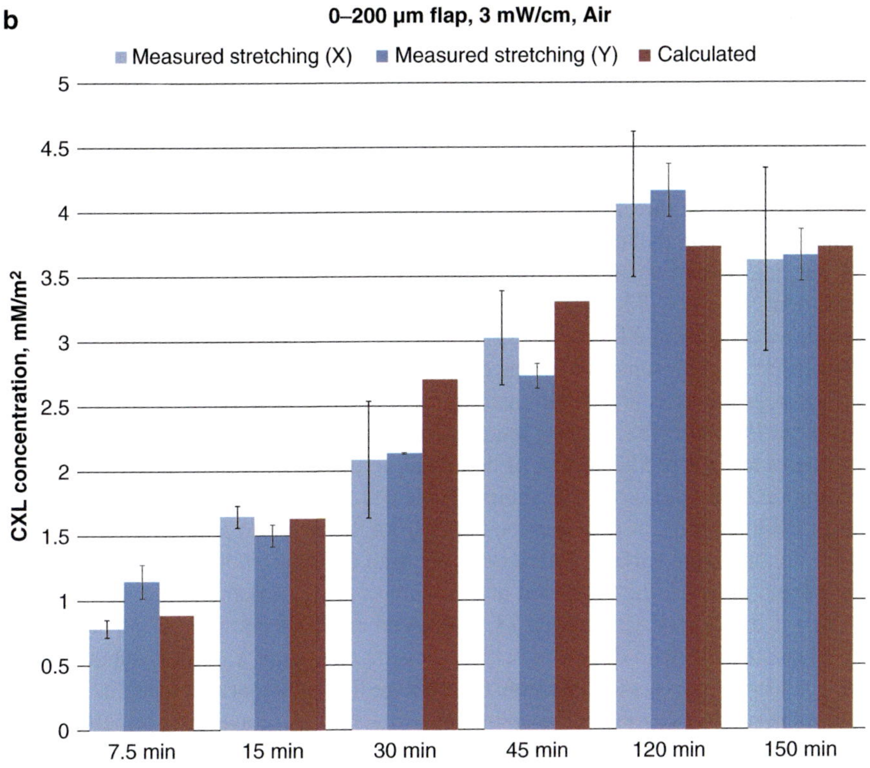

Fig. 1.13 (continued)

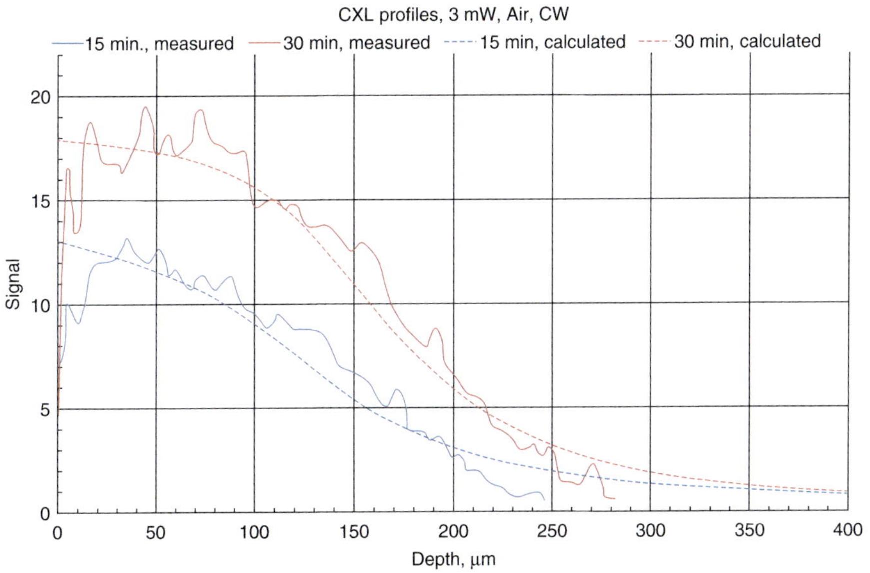

Fig. 1.14 Collagen fluorescence as a function of depth measured using non-linear optical microscopy [65] versus the theoretical model for crosslinked porcine corneas using the 3 mW/cm^2 at 15 and 30 min for a total dose of 2.7 and 5.4 J/cm^2

1.4 Clinical Correlation

As seen by experiment and the model, oxygen dynamics and irradiance can be modulated to achieve various amounts and distributions of crosslinking, Fig. 1.15a, b. The theory and model may also be correlate clinically. As discussed previously, the line of demarcation represents the depth of crosslinking and the tissues healing response to some threshold. If so, this threshold is related to some minimum concentration of ROS that causes enough damage to the tissue to elicit a tissue response as the line of demarcation is most visible approximately 1–3 months post CXL treatment. A study [73, 89] was undertaken in which the theoretical crosslinking profile was determined as a function of depth and a potential threshold crosslink concentration representative for the demarcation line was chosen using the Dresden protocol as the standard. Additional epithelium off crosslinking protocols chosen from the literature [88, 90–98] were calculated for their crosslinking distribution profiles and their predicted line of demarcation depths based on the crosslink concentration threshold were determined. Table 1.1 shows the results of the measured and calculated lines of demarcation depth from the reported protocols as measured from the epithelial surface. There is a very high correlation of the line of demarcation depth between the measured and calculated lines of demarcation with a slope of m = 1.03 and a R [2] value 0.73. The green circles seen in Fig. 1.16 are that of C. Mazzotta [88] who to ensure better precision an accuracy of their data used two independent observers to determine the average line of demarcation depth. All measurements were taken from the epithelial surface with the average epithelial thickness being 50 ± 10 μm. The lines of demarcation were evaluated on 44 eyes using conventional (3mw/cm^2), 10 eyes using continuous accelerated crosslinking at 30 mW/cm^2 and 10 eyes using pulsed light accelerated crosslinking (1 s on: 1 s off). The measured lines of demarcation depth were 350 ± 20 μm, 200 ± 20 μm, and 250 ± 20 μm respectively showing high correlation to the model.

As seen in Table 1.1, the reported standard deviations for this measurement are large, revealing variability of as much as 40% in depth of demarcation line depth for nominally equivalent clinical protocols. To evaluate what factors might contribute to this variability in clinical outcome, treatment parameters, including riboflavin formulation, illumination systems, UVA irradiance, and environmental conditions were simulated using the photochemical kinetic model to evaluate the impact of these parameters on cross-linking outcomes and their sensitivity to variation [99]. Riboflavin formulations when manufactured can vary from 0.1 to 0.16% in concentration lot to lot as specified by the manufacturer, had a −22 μm impact on the line of demarcation depth for increased concentration. The use of a thickening agent [100] left on the surface versus the use of saline impacted the line of demarcation depth by +22 μm. Individual device calibration impacted the line of demarcation depth by ±34 μm and center to edge variance of the device beam profiles impacted the line of demarcation depth by as much as ±51 μm. Altitude changes of 1600 m had a 5 μm in the line of demarcation depth difference because of lower partial pressures of oxygen in the air. The findings of this evaluation revealed that inconsistency and variation in surgical procedure, materials and equipment when added up, could

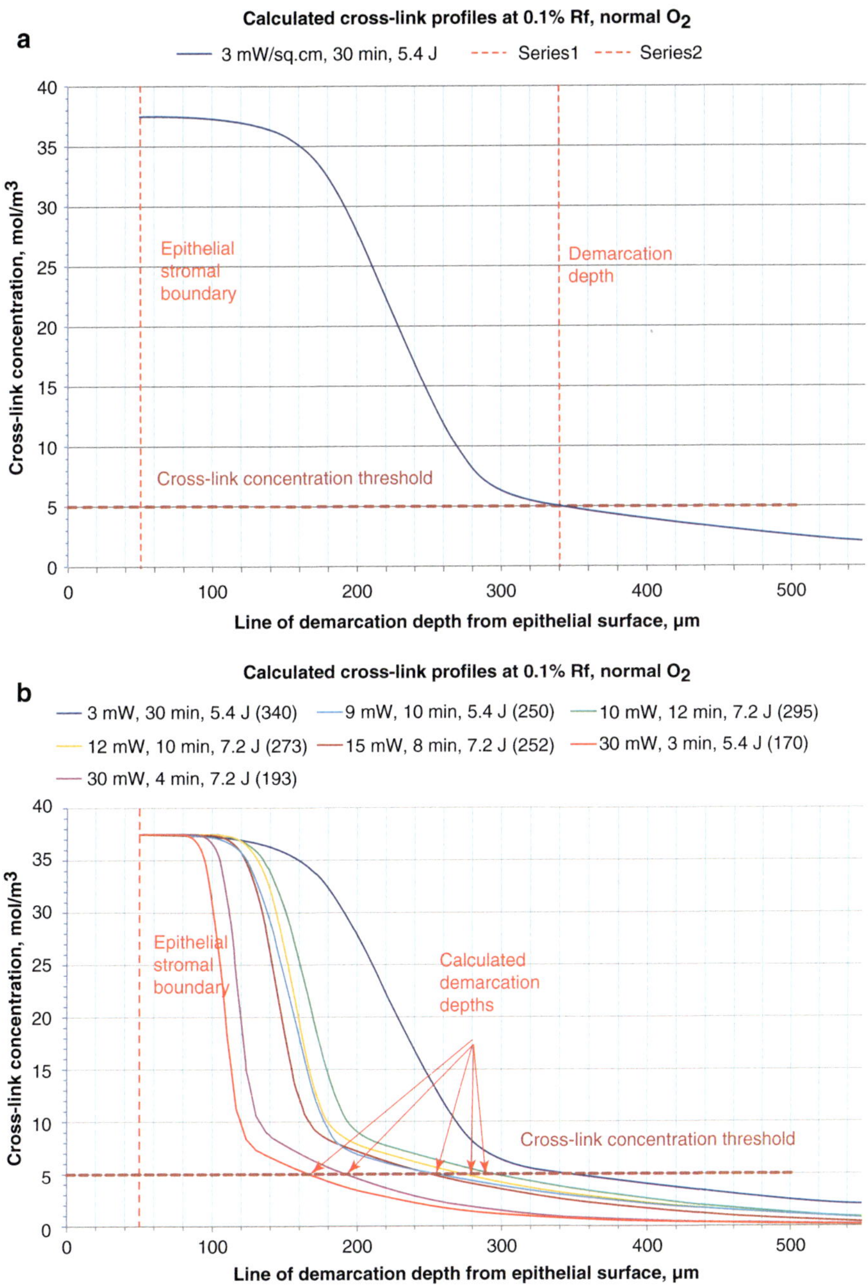

Fig. 1.15 (**a**) Determination of the potential crosslink concentration threshold representative for the demarcation line using the Dresden protocol as the standard. (**b**) Additional epithelium off crosslinking protocols chosen from the literature calculated for their crosslinking distribution profiles and their predicted line of demarcation depths based on the crosslink concentration threshold

Table 1.1 Measured and calculated lines of demarcation depth for various crosslinking protocols for keratoconus taken from the literature

Protocol				Results		
Presoak, min	UVA Irrad, mW/cm²	UVA time, min	Dose, J/cm²	Measured depth, μm	Calculated depth, new model, μm	References
30	3	30 CW	5.4	294.2 ± 51.2	352	Yam 2012
30	3	30 CW	5.4	350 ± 20	352	Mazzotta 2015
30	3	30 CW	5.4	341.8 ± 7.02	352	Tsakalis 2016
30	3	30 CW	5.4	350.78 ± 49.34	352	Kymionis 2013
30	3	30 CW	5.4	337 ± 46.46	352	Zygoura 2015
15	30	3 CW	5.4	140.4 ± 39.1	185	Fontana 2014
30	30	4 CW	7.2	200 ± 20	209	Mazzotta 2015
30	30	8 pulsed (1 s, 1 s)	7.2	250 ± 20	255	Mazzotta 2015
15	30	4 CW	7.2	153.85 ± 33.11	195	Fontana 2014
10	30	8 pulsed (1 s, 1 s)	7.2	213 ± 47	239	Fontana 2014
10	20	12 pulsed (1 s, 1 s)	7.2	233 ± 92	262	Fontana 2014
20	30	4 CW	7.2	160 ± 20	202	Mazzotta 2013, 2014
20	9	10 CW	5.4	288.46 ± 42.37	265	Kymionis 2013
20	18	5 CW	5.4	208.64 ± 18.41	219	Ozgurhan 2014
30	18	5 CW	5.4	240.37 ± 18.89	225	Ozgurhan 2014
30	18	7 CW	7.56	313.37 ± 48.85	245	Bikbova 2016
30	18	5 CW	5.4	223 ± 32	225	Kymionis 2015
30	9	14 CW	7.56	322.91 ± 48.28	296	Zygoura 2015
10	30	4 CW	7.2	159.88	195	Peyman 2016
10	30	8 pulsed (1 s, 1 s)	7.2	201.11	213	Peyman 2016

lead to variability in the depth of the corneal demarcation line potentially leading to variability in clinical outcomes as well. Although the correlation to clinical outcome especially for keratoconus has yet to be determined. The take home message of this study was that to achieve consistent lines of demarcation depths and potentially repeatable results, attention and consistency to seemingly minor details of surgical technique and clinical protocol matter.

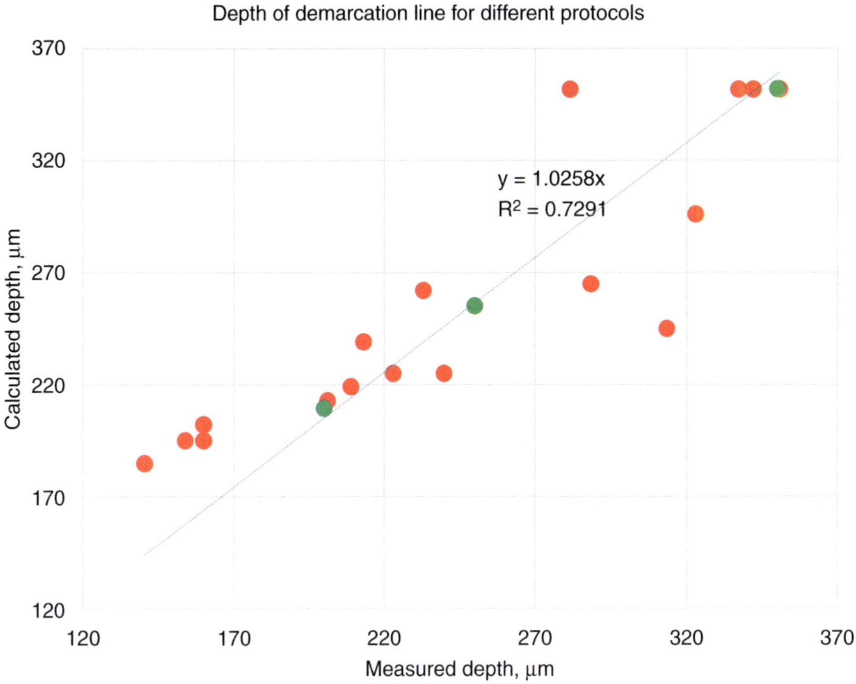

Fig. 1.16 Calculated versus measured line of demarcation depth for various protocols for the treatment of keratoconus

1.5 Accelerated Crosslinking Systems

There are several standard and accelerated crosslinking systems that have been commercialized. The first generation of systems perform standard crosslinking and are all fixed at 3 mW/cm^2 with Gaussian beam profiles. These systems include the "UVX-1000" (IROC Innocross, Zurich, Switzerland), the "Vega CBM" developed by Caporossi-Baiocchi and Mazzotta (OFTA Hi-Tech, C.S.O. Italy), and the "CCL Vario" (Peschke Meditrade) and are simple in design using multiple LED illumination without the use of a homogenizing optical element. Because of their calibration methodology, these initial systems deliver central energy exposures of up to 8.4 J/cm^2, Fig. 1.17.

Second generation accelerated systems included higher and variable irradiances, top hat beam profiles, variable spot sizes and specific features such as camera systems for viewing the eye. Top hat beam profiles allow for a more predictable and determined output of the device as they are more easily manufactured, calibrated and qualified. Average movement because of the eye's saccadic motions and drift during a crosslinking procedure, cause the average beam profile illuminating the

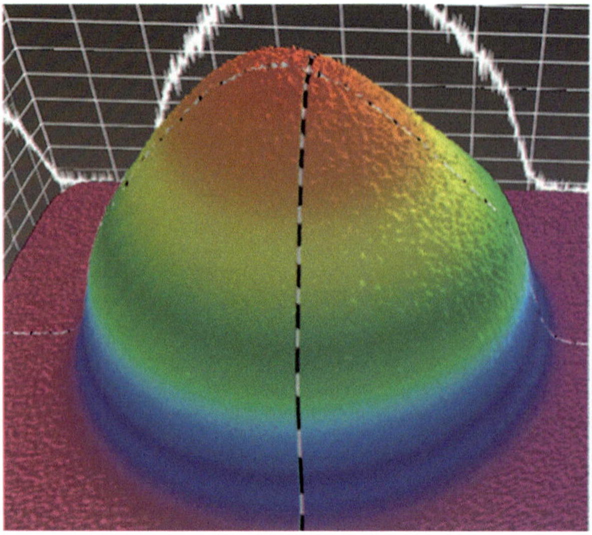

Annulus (mm)	Total surface exposure energy (J)
Central 2	8.4
2–4	6.5
4–6	5.9
6–7	5.9
7–9	5.0
9–11	3.7

Fig. 1.17 Measured beam profile of a multi-LED cross-linking device, demonstrating a Gaussian like energy distribution and central hot spot of approximately 8.4 J/cm^2 with application of nominal 5.4 J/cm^2 dose

eye Gaussian in nature, with more beam energy in the center than at the edges. These systems are being used for the newer applications of crosslinking including Lasik Xtra, PRK Xtra, Smile Xtra and PiXL. The first of these outside the USA was the KXL system (Avedro) which has variable CW or pulsed irradiance output from 3 to 45 mW/cm^2, a 9 mm flat top beam profile, and the ability to align and maintain alignment of the patient through remote control, Fig. 1.18. A second version has a camera for visualization of the eye. A similar FDA approved version of the device is available in the US but is fixed at the standard 3 mW/cm^2. LIGHTLink-CXL (Lightmed) is a similar system manufactured with these same second generation features.

A slight modification to the accelerated second Generation Systems includes the UVX-2000 which has an irradiance of 9 mW/cm^2 and "cosine fall-off" compensating beam profile. The purpose of this beam profile system is to correct for the change in irradiance caused by the changing projected area of the beam over the curvature of the eye. This system produces lines of demarcation depth with more consistent depth across the entire treatment zone. An example of the UVX-2000 beam profile is seen in Fig. 1.19.

The newest third generation accelerated systems have the ability to produce precise, patterned, topography-guided accelerated cross-linking, programmable and customizable illumination patterns, real-time eye tracking and significantly higher power outputs. The Mosaic™ System (Avedro, Waltham, USA) is the only currently available system in this category. The Mosaic™ System interfaces with the Pentacam Corneal Topographer and has an output up to 100 mW/cm^2 in either continuous or pulsed modes.

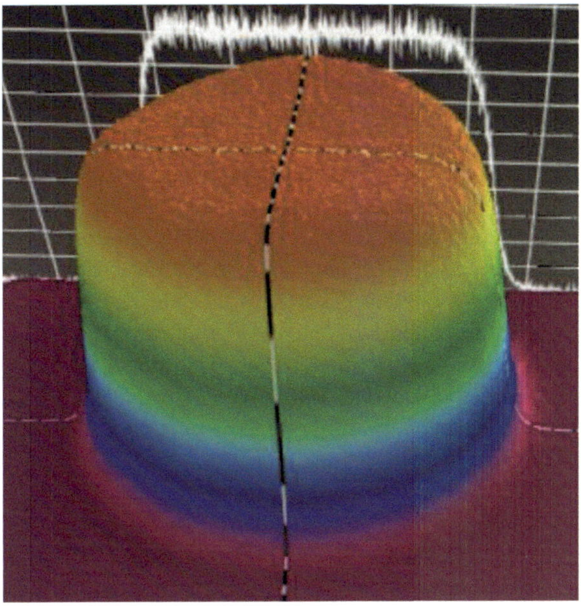

Fig. 1.18 Measured beam profile of a KXL device, demonstrating a 3% uniform top hat energy distribution with application of a nominal 5.4 J/cm^2 dose

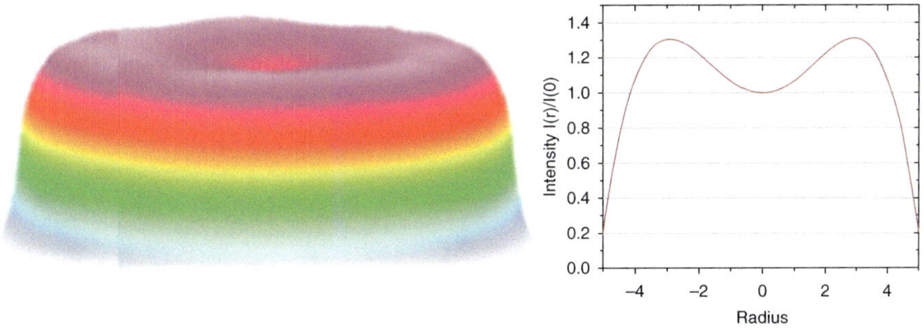

Fig. 1.19 Beam profile with inverse function

Another CXL medical device now available in the market is the "PXL Platinum 330"™ (Peschke Meditrade, Switzerland). which has an irradiance of 3-9-18 and 30 mW/cm^2, with top-hat beam profile, 50 ± 5 mm working distance from the corneal plane, continuous and pulsed-light, LASIK radiation mode and integrated infrared camera with integrated contact pachymeter.

1.6 Accelerated Crosslinking Applications

With the advent of higher irradiance systems several other applications for accelerated crosslinking have emerged. New procedures have been developed to prophylactically strengthen or stabilize corneas weakened by refractive surgery. These include

Lasik Xtra [101–104], PRK Xtra [105, 106] and Smile Xtra [107]. As crosslinking has a sterilizing effect due to the production of ROS, it is also being utilized for corneal melt and infectious keratitis. Most recently, accelerated crosslinking has been used for refractive correction through a technology called photorefractive intrastromal cross-linking (PiXL™) requiring specific UVA beam patterning. This procedure uses zone-specific cross-linking to induce a controlled corneal shape change for either focal treatment of ectatic disease or correction of refractive error [108].

Since the initial proof-of-concept pre-clinical and clinical trials, a finite element computer model for analysis of zonal cross-linking has been developed [23, 24, 108]. This modeling has been used to investigate ectatic disease and both myopic and astigmatic corrections, evaluating the impact of different shapes and sizes of zonal cross-linking applications. The model predicts that a circularly symmetric application will lead to central flattening and the application of a bow tie pattern will result in steepening on the axis of treatment, with slight flattening of the perpendicular axis [109].

Conclusion

Accelerated crosslinking and our understanding of it and its applications have rapidly developed since its initial inceptions for treating ectatic disease only. The future includes the development of new measurement modalities, crosslinking devices, riboflavin formulations, surface preparation techniques, the addition of supplemental oxygen, and the development of many new applications and protocols all with the continued goal of reducing overall treatment time and improving patient outcome and comfort.

References

1. Spoerl E, Huhle M, Seiler T. Induction of cross-links in corneal tissue. Exp Eye Res. 1998;66(1):97–103.
2. Seiler T, Spoerl E, Huhle M, Kamouna A. Conservative therapy of keratoconus by enhancement of collagen cross-links. Invest Ophthalmol Vis Sci. 1996;37:S1017.
3. Maurice DM. The structure and transparency of the cornea. J Physiol. 1957;136(2):263–86.
4. Hart RW, Farrell RA. Light scattering in the cornea. J Opt Soc Am. 1969;59(6):766–74.
5. Benedek GB. Theory of transparency of the eye. Appl Opt. 1971;10(3):459–73.
6. Twersky V. Transparency of pair-related, random distributions of small scatterers, with application to the cornea. J Opt Soc Am. 1975;65(5):524–30.
7. Meek KM. The cornea and sclera. Structure. Chapter 13. p. 359–96, 2008 from Collagen structure and mechanics (isbn:978-0-387-73905-2 (Print) 978-0-387-73906-9 (Online)).
8. Meek KM, Quantock AJ. The use of X-ray scattering techniques to determine corneal ultrastructure. Prog Retin Eye Res. 2001;20(1):95–137.
9. Winkler M, Chai D, Kriling S, Nien CJ, Brown DJ, Jester B, Juhasz T, Jester JV. Nonlinear optical macroscopic assessment of 3-D corneal collagen organization and axial biomechanics. Invest Ophthalmol Vis Sci. 2011;52(12):8818–27.
10. Pauling L, Corey RB. The structure of fibrous proteins of the collagen-gelatin group. Proc Natl Acad Sci U S A. 1951;37(5):272–81.
11. Ramachandran GN, Kartha G. Structure of collagen. Nature. 1954;174(4423):269–70.
12. Ramachandran GN, Kartha G. Structure of collagen. Nature. 1955;176(4482):593–5.

13. Baldwin SJ, Quigley AS, Clegg C, Kreplak L. Nanomechanical mapping of hydrated rat tail tendon collagen I fibrils. Biophys J. 2014;107(8):1794–801.
14. Aghamohammadzadeh H, Newton RH, Meek KM. X-ray scattering used to map the preferred collagen orientation in the human cornea and limbus. Structure (London, England: 1993). 2004;12(2):249–56.
15. Abahussin M, Hayes S, Knox Cartwright NE, Kamma-Lorger CS, Khan Y, Marshall J, Meek KM. 3D collagen orientation study of the human cornea using X-ray diffraction and femtosecond laser technology. Invest Ophthalmol Vis Sci. 2009;50(11):5159–64.
16. Fraser SA, Ting YH, Mallon KS, Wendt AE, Murphy CJ, Nealey PF. Sub-micron and nanoscale feature depth modulates alignment of stromal fibroblasts and corneal epithelial cells in serum-rich and serum-free media. J Biomed Mater Res A. 2008;86(3):725–35.
17. Holmes DF, Gilpin CJ, Baldock C, Ziese U, Koster J, Kadler KE. Corneal collagen fibril structure in three dimensions: structural insights into fibril assembly, mechanical properties, and tissue organization. Proc Natl Acad Sci U S A. 2001;98(13):7307–12.
18. Hayes S, Kamma-Lorger CS, Boote C, Young RD, Quantock AJ, Rost A, Khatib Y, Harris J, Yagi N, Terrill N, Meek KM. The effect of riboflavin/UVA collagen cross-linking therapy on the structure and hydrodynamic behaviour of the ungulate and rabbit corneal stroma. PLoS One. 2013;8(1):e52860.
19. Meek KM, Tuft SJ, Huang Y, Gill PS, Hayes S, Newton RH, Bron AJ. Changes in collagen orientation and distribution in keratoconus corneas. Invest Ophthalmol Vis Sci. 2005;46(6):1948–56.
20. Meek KM. Corneal shape supported by collagen organization. Presented at the 8th Annual CXL Congress. Geneva; Dec 2012.
21. Daxer A, Fratzl P. Collagen fibril orientation in the human corneal stroma and its implications in keratoconus. Invest Ophthalmol Vis Sci. 1997;38(1):121–9.
22. Newton RH, Meek KM. The integration of the corneal and limbal fibrils in the human eye. Biophys J. 1998;75(5):2508–12.
23. Roberts CJ, Dupps WJ. Biomechanics of corneal ectasia and biomechanical treatments. J Cataract Refract Surg. 2014;40:991–8.
24. Roy AS, Dupps WJ. Patient-specific computational modeling of keratoconus progression and differential responses to collagen cross-linking. Invest Ophthalmol Vis Sci. 2011;52(12):9174–87.
25. Scarcelli G, Besner S, Pineda R, Yun SH. Biomechanical characterization of keratoconus corneas ex vivo with Brillouin microscopy. Invest Ophthalmol Vis Sci. 2014;55(7):4490–5.
26. Scarcelli G, Besne S, Pineda R, Kalout P, Yun SH. In vivo biomechanical mapping of normal and keratoconic corneas. JAMA Ophthalmol. 2015;133(4):480–2.
27. Rabinowitz YS. Keratoconus. Surv Ophthalmol. 1998;42(4):297–319.
28. McMonnies CW. Abnormal rubbing and keratectasia. Eye Contact Lens. 2007;33(6 Pt 1):265–71.
29. Zadnik K, Barr JT, Edrington TB, Everett DF, Jameson M, McMahon TT, Shin JA, Sterling JL, Wagner H, Gordon MO. Baseline findings in the collaborative longitudinal evaluation of keratoconus (CLEK) study. Invest Ophthalmol Vis Sci. 1998;39(13):2537–46.
30. Ertan A, Muftuoglu O. Keratoconus clinical findings according to different age and gender groups. Cornea. 2008;27(10):1109–13.
31. Randleman JB, Woodward M, Lynn MJ, Stulting RD. Risk assessment for ectasia after corneal refractive surgery. Ophthalmology. 2008;115(1):37–50.
32. Knox Cartwright NE, Tyrer JR, Marshall J. Age-related differences in the elasticity of the human cornea. Invest Ophthalmol Vis Sci. 2011;52(7):4324–9.
33. Malik NS, Moss SJ, Ahmed N, Furth AJ, Wall RS, Meek KM. Ageing of the human corneal stroma: structural and biochemical changes. Biochim Biophys Acta. 1992;1138(3):222–8.
34. Daxer A, Misof K, Grabner B, Ettl A, Fratzl P. Collagen fibrils in the human corneal stroma: structure and aging. Invest Ophthalmol Vis Sci. 1998;39(3):644–8.
35. Seiler T, Huhle S, Spoerl E, Kunath H. Manifest diabetes and keratoconus: a retrospective case-control study. Graefes Arch Clin Exp Ophthalmol. 2000;238(10):822–5.

36. McCall AS, Kraft S, Edelhauser HF, Lundquist RR, Bradshaw HE, Dedeic Z, Dionne MJ, Clement EM, Conrad GW. Mechanisms of corneal tissue cross-linking in response to treatment with topical riboflavin and long-wavelength ultraviolet radiation (UVA). Invest Ophthalmol Vis Sci. 2010;51(1):129–38.
37. Brummer G, Littlechild S, McCall S, Zhang Y, Conrad GW. The role of nonenzymatic glycation and carbonyls in collagen cross-linking for the treatment of keratoconus. Invest Ophthalmol Vis Sci. 2011;52(9):6363–9.
38. Zhang Y, Mao X, Schwend T, Littlechild S, Conrad GW. Resistance of corneal RFUVA–cross-linked collagens and small leucine-rich proteoglycans to degradation by matrix metalloproteinases. Invest Ophthalmol Vis Sci. 2013;54(2):1014–25.
39. Meek KM, Hayes S. Corneal cross-linking—a review. Ophthalmic Physiol Opt. 2013;33(2):78–93.
40. Spoerl E, Seiler T. Techniques for stiffening the cornea. J Refract Surg. 1999;15(6):711–3.
41. Wollensak G, Spoerl E, Reber F, Seiler T. Keratocyte cytotoxicity of riboflavin/UVA-treatment in vitro. Eye (Lond). 2004;18(7):718–22.
42. Wollensak G, Spoerl E, Reber F, Pillunata L, Funk R. Corneal endothelial cytotoxicity of riboflavin/UVA treatment in vitro. Ophthalmic Res. 2003;35(6):324–8.
43. Wollensak G, Spoerl E, Wilsch M, Seiler T. Endothelial cell damage after riboflavin-ultraviolet-A treatment in the rabbit. J Cataract Refract Surg. 2003;29(9):1786–90.
44. Wollensak G, Spoerl E, Seiler T. Stress-strain measurements of human and porcine corneas after riboflavin-ultraviolet-A-induced cross-linking. J Cataract Refract Surg. 2003;29(9):1780–5.
45. Wollensak G, Wilsch M, Spoerl E, Seiler T. Collagen fiber diameter in the rabbit cornea after collagen crosslinking by riboflavin/UVA. Cornea. 2004;23(5):503–7.
46. Spoerl E, Wollensak G, Dittert D, Seiler T. Thermomechanical behavior of collagen-cross-linked porcine cornea. Ophthalmologica. 2004;218(2):136–40.
47. Spoerl E, Wollensak G, Seiler T. Increased resistance of crosslinked cornea against enzymatic digestion. Curr Eye Res. 2004;29(1):35–40.
48. Wollensak G, Spoerl E, Seiler T. Riboflavin/ultraviolet-a-induced collagen crosslinking for the treatment of keratoconus. Am J Ophthalmol. 2003;135(5):620–7.
49. NDA 203324: (Keratoconus Approved 4/15/16) (Ectasia Approved 7/15/16).
50. Kanellopoulos AJ. Long term results of a prospective randomized bilateral eye comparison trial of higher fluence, shorter duration ultraviolet A radiation, and riboflavin collagen cross linking for progressive keratoconus. Clin Ophthalmol. 2012;6:97–101.
51. Bunsen R, Roscoe H. Photochemische Untersuchungen, Poggendorff's Annalen; 1855.
52. Krueger RR, Ramos-Esteban JC, Kanellopoulos AJ. Staged intrastromal delivery of riboflavin with UVA cross-linking in advanced bullous keratopathy: laboratory investigation and first clinical case. J Refract Surg. 2008;24(7):S730–6.
53. Krueger RR, Herekar S, Spoerl E. First proposed efficacy study of high versus standard irradiance and fractionated riboflavin/ultraviolet a cross-linking with equivalent energy exposure. Eye Contact Lens. 2014;40(6):353–7.
54. Jaycock PD, Lobo L, Ibrahim J, Tyrer J, Marshall J. Interferometric technique to measure biomechanical changes in the cornea induced by refractive surgery. J Cataract Refract Surg. 2005;31(1):175–84.
55. Ford MR, Dupps WJ, Rollins AM, Roy AS, Hu Z. Method for optical coherence elastography of the cornea. J Biomed Opt. 2011;16(1):016005.
56. Kohlhaas M, Spoerl E, Schilde T, Unger G, Wittig C, Pillunat LE. Biomechanical evidence of the distribution of cross-links in corneas treated with riboflavin and ultraviolet A light. J Cataract Refract Surg. 2006;32(2):279–83.
57. Kanellopoulos AJ, Krueger RR, Asimellis G. Cross-linking and corneal imaging advances. Biomed Res Int. 2015;2015:306439.
58. Kling S, Remon L, Pérez-Escudero A, Merayo-Lloves J, Marcos S. Corneal biomechanical changes after collagen cross-linking from porcine eye inflation experiments. Invest Ophthalmol Vis Sci. 2010;51(8):3961–8.
59. Elsheikh A, Anderson K. Comparative study of corneal strip extensometry and inflation tests. J R Soc Interface. 2005;2(3):177–85.

60. Pallikaris IG, Kymionis GD, Ginis HS, Kounis GA, Tsilimbaris MK. Ocular rigidity in living human eyes. Invest Ophthalmol Vis Sci. 2005;46(2):409–14.
61. Asejczyk-Widlicka M, Pierscionek BK. The elasticity and rigidity of the outer coats of the eye. Br J Ophthalmol. 2008;92(10):1415–8.
62. Jue B, Maurice DM. The mechanical properties of the rabbit and human cornea. J Biomech. 1986;19(10):847–53.
63. Hjortdal JO. Regional elastic performance of the human cornea. J Biomech. 1996;29(7):931–42.
64. Cabrera Fernández D, Niazy AM, Kurtz RM, Djotyan GP, Juhasz T. Finite element analysis applied to cornea reshaping. J Biomed Opt. 2005;10(6):064018.
65. Chai D, Gaster RN, Roizenblatt R, Juhasz T, Brown DJ, Jester JV. Quantitative assessment of UVA-riboflavin corneal cross-linking using nonlinear optical microscopy. Invest Ophthalmol Vis Sci. 2011;52(7):4231–8.
66. Kamaev P, Friedman MD, Sherr E, Muller D. Photochemical kinetics of corneal cross-linking with riboflavin. Invest Ophthalmol Vis Sci. 2012;53(4):2360–7.
67. Aldahlawi NH, Hayes S, O'Brart DP, Meek KM. Standard versus accelerated riboflavin-ultraviolet corneal collagen crosslinking: resistance against enzymatic digestion. J Cataract Refract Surg. 2015;41(9):1989–96.
68. Aldahlawi NH, Hayes S, O'Brart DP, Akhbanbetova A, Littlechild SL, Meek KM. Enzymatic resistance of corneas crosslinked using riboflavin in conjunction with low energy, high energy, and pulsed UVA irradiation modes. Invest Ophthalmol Vis Sci. 2016;57(4):1547–52.
69. Rood-Ojalvo S, Kamaev P, Friedman M, Sherr E, Muller D. Papain digestion method for analysis of cross-linking in corneal flaps. ARVO. 2013;5280:C0199.
70. Verzijl N, DeGroot J, Oldehinkel E, BanK RA, Thorpe SR, Baynes JW, Bayliss MT, Bijlsma JW, Lafeber FP, Tekoppele JM. Age-related accumulation of Maillard reaction products in human articular cartilage collagen. Biochem J. 2000;350(Pt 2):381–7.
71. Zhang Y, Conrad AH, Conrad GW. Effects of ultraviolet-A and riboflavin on the interaction of collagen and proteoglycans during corneal cross-linking. J Biol Chem. 2011;286(15):13011–22.
72. Criado S, Ma'rtire D, Allegretti P, Furlong J, Bertolotti SG, La Falce E, Garcia NA. Singlet molecular oxygen generation and quenching by the antiglaucoma ophthalmic drugs, Timolol and Pindolol. Photochem Photobiol Sci. 2002;1(10):788–92.
73. Friedman M, Kamaev P, Eddington W, Smirnov M, Sherr E, Peterson S, Muller D. Photochemical reactions during CXL. CXL Congress. Boston; 2015.
74. Chace KV, Carubelli R, Nordquist RE, Rowsey JJ. Effect of oxygen free radicals on corneal collagen. Free Radic Res Commun. 1991;12–13(Pt 2):591–4.
75. Massey V. Activation of molecular oxygen by flavins and flavoproteins. J Biol Chem. 1994;269(36):22459–62.
76. Kato Y, Uchida K, Kawakishi S. Aggregation of collagen exposed to UVA in the presence of riboflavin: a plausible role of tyrosine modification. Photochem Photobiol. 1994;59(3):343–9.
77. Lu CY, Wang WF, Lin WZ, Han ZH, Yao SD, Lin NY. Generation and photosensitization properties of the oxidized radicals of riboflavin: a laser flash photolysis study. J Photochem Photobiol B Biol. 1999;52(1–3):111–6.
78. Görner H. Oxygen uptake after electron transfer from amines, amino acids and ascorbic acid to triplet flavins in air-saturated aqueous solution. J Photochem Photobiol B. 2007;87(2):73–80.
79. Lu C, Bucher G, Sander W. Photoinduced interactions between oxidized and reduced lipoic acid and Riboflavin (Vitamin B2). Phys Chem. 2004;5:47–56.
80. Ahmad I, Fasihullah Q, Noor A, Ansari IA, Ali QNM. Photolysis of riboflavin in aqueous solution: a kinetic study. Int J Pharm. 2004;280(1–2):199–208.
81. Flavins: photochemistry and photobiology. Comprehensive Series in Photochemical and Photobiological Sciences. In: Silva E, Edwards AM, editors. Santiago: P. Universidad Catolica de Chile; Cambridge: Royal Society of Chemistry; 2006. isbn:0-85404-331-4.
82. Görner H. Oxygen uptake induced by electron transfer from donors to the triplet state of methylene blue and xanthene dyes in air-saturated aqueous solution. Photochem Photobiol Sci. 2008;7(3):371–6.
83. Ahmed S. Effect of complexing agents on the photodegradation of riboflavin in aqueous solution. PhD Thesis. Karachi: Baqai Medical University; 2009.

84. Kamaev P, Smirnov M, Friedman M, Sherr E, Muller M. Aggregation and photoreduction in anaerobic solutions of flavin mononucleotide. J Photochem Photobiol A Chem. 2015;310:60–5.
85. Spikes JD, Shen HR, Kopecková P, Kopecek J. Photodynamic crosslinking of proteins. III. Kinetics of the FMN- and rose bengal-sensitized photooxidation and intermolecular crosslinking of model tyrosine-containing N-(2 hydroxypropyl) methacrylamide copolymers. Photochem Photobiol. 1999;70(2):130–7.
86. Silva E, Godoy J. Riboflavin sensitized photooxidation of tyrosine. Int J Vitam Nutr Res. 1994;64:253–6.
87. Bastian M, Sigel H. The self-association of flavin mononucleotide (FMN (2-)) as determined by (1) H NMR shift measurements. Biophys Chem. 1997;67(1–3):27–34.
88. Mazzotta C, Hafezi F, Kymionis G, Caragiuli S, Jacob S, Traversi C, Barabino S, Randleman JB. In vivo confocal microscopy after corneal collagen crosslinking. Ocul Surf. 2015;13(4):298–314.
89. Friedman MD, Kamaev P, Smirnov M, Mrochen M, Lytle G, Muller D. Can we safely cross-link thinner corneas? Pathways for optimized CXL treatment planning. Barcelona: ESCRS; 2015.
90. Yam JC, Chan CW, Cheng AC. Corneal collagen cross-linking demarcation line depth assessed by Visante OCT After CXL for keratoconus and corneal ectasia. J Refract Surg. 2012;28(7):475–81.
91. Kymionis GD, Tsoulnaras KI, Liakopoulos DA, Skatharoudi CA, Grentzelos MA, Tsakalis NG. Corneal stromal demarcation line depth following standard and a modified high intensity corneal cross-linking protocol. J Refract Surg. 2016;32(4):218–22.
92. Zygoura V, del Barrio JA, Gatzioufas Z, Saw V, Raiskup F. Evaluation of corneal stromal demarcation line depth following standard and a modified-accelerated collagen cross-linking protocol. Am J Ophthalmol. 2015;159(1):211–2.
93. Fontana L, Moramarco A. Esperienze personali con CXL accelerato. UOC Oculistica ASMN-IRCCS Reggio Emilia. CXL Course, Roma; 20 settembre 2014.
94. Mazzotta C. In vivo corneal micro-structural analysis in accelerated corneal collagen X-linking. CXL Course, Roma; 20 Sept 2014.
95. Mazzotta C, Paradiso AL, Baiocchi S, Caragiuli S, Caporossi A. Qualitative investigation of corneal changes after accelerated corneal collagen cross-linking (A-CXL) by in vivo confocal microscopy and corneal OCT. J Clin Exp Ophthalmol. 2013;4:6.
96. Ozgurhan EB, Sezgin Akcay BI, Yildirim Y, Karatas G, Kurt T, Demirok A. Evaluation of corneal stromal demarcation line after two different protocols of accelerated corneal collagen cross-linking procedures using anterior segment optical coherence tomography and confocal microscopy. J Ophthalmol. 2014;2014:981893.
97. Kymionis GD, Tsoulnaras KI, Liakopoulos DA, Grentzelos MA, Paraskevopoulos TA, Zacharioudaki ME, Zivkovic M, Kouroupaki AI, Tsilimbaris MK. Corneal stromal demarcation line determined with anterior segment optical coherence tomography following a very high intensity corneal collagen cross-linking protocol. Cornea. 2015;34(6):664–7.
98. Peyman A, Nouralishahi A, Hafezi F, Kling S, Peyman M. Stromal demarcation line in pulsed versus continuous light accelerated corneal cross-linking for keratoconus. J Refract Surg. 2016;32(3):206–8.
99. Mrochen M, Friedman MD, Kamaev P, Smirnov M, Lytle G, Muller D. Consistency, consistency, consistency: treatment standardization requirements for corneal cross-linking (CXL). Barcelona: ESCRS; 2015.
100. Wollensak G, Aurich H, Wirbelauer C, Sel S. Significance of the riboflavin film in corneal collagen crosslinking. J Cataract Refract Surg. 2010;36(1):114–20.
101. Ng AL, Kwok PS, Wu RT, Jhanji V, Woo VC, Chan TC. Comparison of the demarcation line on ASOCT after simultaneous LASIK and different protocols of accelerated collagen cross-linking: a bilateral eye randomized study. Cornea. 2017;36(1):74–7.
102. Rajpal RK, Wisecarver CB, Williams D, Rajpal SD, Kerzner R, Nianiaris N, Lytle G, Hoang K. Lasik Xtra® provides corneal stability and improved outcomes. Ophthalmol Ther. 2015;4(2):89–102.

103. Tan J, Lytle GE, Marshall J. Consecutive laser in situ keratomileusis and accelerated corneal crosslinking in highly myopic patients: preliminary results. Eur J Ophthalmol. 2014.
104. Mazzotta C, Balestrazzi A, Traversi C, Caragiuli S, Caporossi A. In vivo confocal microscopy report after Lasik with sequential accelerated corneal collagen cross-linking treatment. Case Rep Ophthalmol. 2014;5(1):125–31.
105. Lee H, Kang DS, Ha BJ, Choi JY, Kim EK, Seo KY, Kim TI. Changes in posterior corneal elevations after combined transepithelial photorefractive keratectomy and accelerated corneal collagen cross-linking: retrospective, comparative observational case series. BMC Ophthalmol. 2016;16:139.
106. Nguyen MK, Chuck RS. Corneal collagen cross-linking in the stabilization of PRK, LASIK, thermal keratoplasty, and orthokeratology. Curr Opin Ophthalmol. 2013;24(4):291–5.
107. Ng AL, Chan TC, Cheng GP, Jhanji V, Ye C, Woo VC, Lai JS. Comparison of the early clinical outcomes between combined small-incision lenticule extraction and collagen cross-linking versus SMILE for myopia. BMC Ophthalmol. 2016;16:139.
108. Seven I, Sinha Roy A, Dupps WJ. Patterned corneal collagen crosslinking for astigmatism: computational modeling study. J Cataract Refract Surg. 2014;40(6):943–53.
109. Mazzotta C, Moramarco A, Traversi C, Baiocchi S, Iovieno A, Fontana L. Accelerated corneal collagen cross-linking using topography-guided UV-A energy emission: preliminary clinical and morphological outcomes. J Ophthalmol. 2016;2016:2031031. https://doi.org/10.1155/2016/2031031.

2 Crosslinking Results and Literature Overview

2.1 Conventional Crosslinking

2.1.1 The Standard "Dresden Protocol"

Corneal crosslinking (CXL) is performed in an outpatient setting. Thirty minutes in advance, a systemic analgosedation can be administered. Some surgeons use Pilocarpin 2% eye drops in order to reduce potential thermal and photochemical effects of UVA-radiation on the retina and the lens.

The procedure is performed under sterile conditions in an operating room. After topical anesthesia, an eye lid retractor is inserted and the epithelium is removed with a diameter of 8 mm so that riboflavin can penetrate into the corneal stroma leading to a high UVA-absorption.

Riboflavin 0.1% is a photosensitizer which is installed every 2 min for 30 min, ensuring maximum penetration into the cornea. During this riboflavin application is the eyelid retractor removed. Before UV-irradiation, the surgeon checks the appearance of riboflavin in the anterior chamber via slit lamp with blue filter. Corneal thickness is measured (ultrasonic pachymetry) immediately after the epithelium removal (in order to decide which kind of riboflavin solution should be used: isoosmolar or hypoosmolar) and before irradiation in order to ensure that the corneal thickness is above 400 μm and endothelium remains protected from UV-light. A special UV-sensor is used in order to detect intensity of irradiation in advance of the procedure. An area of 8 mm of central cornea is irradiated with UV-light of a wave length of 370 nm and intensity of 3 mW/cm^2. The irradiation lasts 30 min and riboflavin is applied every 5 min.

Local antibiotics and lubricants are applied after the CXL and a soft contact lens is inserted till the epithelium is fully restored. The systemic use of painkillers is possible. After epithelial closure, topical steroids are prescribed for a duration of 3 weeks. Patients are followed-up every day till the re-epithelialization process is completed and after 1, 3, 6, 12 months and every year. Fitting of new rigid contact lenses is recommended about 6–8 months after the procedure [1, 2].

C. Mazzotta et al., *Management of Early Progressive Corneal Ectasia*,
DOI 10.1007/978-3-319-61137-2_2

2.1.2 Medical History

An exact medical history is crucial for differentiation of low and high risk keratoconus patients. High risk patients need a more frequent examination in order to early detect progression of the disease. For low risk patients an examination once a year seems to be sufficient. The following parameters are essential for division into the two groups: age, sex, regular medical intake, allergies, pregnancy, heavy exercising or body-building and smoking habits. In our experience, which is similar as the one of an Italian study group, in younger patients (up to 18 years) with keratoconus there is a clear dominance of male sex (M/F 4/1) [3].

In the group of children and adolescent patients, mostly male, keratoconus seems to be very aggressive with rapid progression compared to the older age groups. Also patients with a history of atopy are in a risk of more rapid keratoconus progression not only because of the atopy itself but also due to regular intake of steroids. Another study reported a change in biomechanical corneal properties in terms of decrease of corneal stiffness due to steroid exposure in vitro [4].

Regular systemic intake of steroids for example in patients with chronic systemic inflammatory diseases or estrogens (hormonal contraception) or anabolic steroids (body-building) seems to induce the progression of the ectasia in susceptible corneas [5]. There seems to be a negative influence of pregnancy due to changes in hormone levels on corneal biomechanical properties. Pregnant women with keratoconus should be examined more frequently and in case of keratoconus progression, CXL should be performed after the delivery [6].

We do not perform CXL in pregnant women, because of possible postoperative complications such as infections or corneal melting and consecutive necessity of systemic medical intake and surgery requiring general anesthesia. Female patients with keratoconus should be informed, that a pregnancy due to hormonal changes, especially estrogens, could lead to a progression of the disease [7].

There are several sports, hobbies and physical activities leading to a repeated long-standing elevation of intraocular pressure (IOP), for example during weight lifting, yoga, wind instrument playing, which might be a risk factor for progression in predisposed ectatic corneas [8, 9].

In contrast to previously described circumstances, there are systemic diseases such as diabetes or certain habits for example smoking, which induce a natural cross-linking in different human tissues. In these patients a mild or none progression is expected, thus frequent examinations are not necessary.

The protective effect of diabetes could be explained via the induction of crosslinks in the corneal stroma preventing from a weakening of the cornea [10, 11].

Smoking is also negatively associated with keratoconus progression. A strengthening effect for smokers was shown in skin and blood vessels [12, 13].

Smoke contains toxic substances inducing chemical cross-linking of the cornea. Nevertheless, due to its numerous negative effects on health, smoking should not be recommended as a prevention for keratoconus patients [14].

2.1.3 Evidence of Progression

Not every ectatic cornea needs to be crosslinked. A record of progression of the disease indicates CXL, which was the case in every of the above mentioned clinical trials, whereas the parameters for the definition of progression were slightly different. In Dresden, progression is defined according to an increase in Kmax at the apex of the cone of about 1 D within 1 year, decrease in BCVA, or frequent need for new contact lens fitting more than once within 2 years because of refraction changes [2]. Vinciguerra defined progression of keratoconus as changes in myopia and/or astigmatism of ≥3 D within the last 6 months, a mean change of central K-value of ≥1.5 D in three consecutive corneal topographic measurements within 6 months or a mean decrease in central corneal thickness ≥5% in three consecutive tomographic measurements within 6 months [15].

FDA study group in US performed CXL when one or more of the following changes within 24 months were reported: (a) increase of maximum K-value of ≥1 D, (b) increase of ≥1 D in astigmatism, (c) increase of ≥0.5 D in spherical equivalent (SE). Exclusion criteria were a history of corneal surgery and/or ocular surface pathology, pachymetric values less than 300 μm, pregnancy and current breastfeeding [16].

2.1.4 Clinical Studies

The last decade has seen a dramatic change in the management of corneal ectatic diseases. New treatment modalities such as corneal crosslinking (CXL) have moved the timing of intervention to much earlier in the disease process. No longer are we delaying invasive treatment until there is significant loss of vision. CXL is currently available and is performed by the majority of the panelists for the Global Delphi Panel of Keratoconus and Ectatic Diseases (83%) for keratoconus, using a variety of techniques. The panelists who do not have current access to CXL were willing to use this technique once it becomes available [17].

After years of experimental studies, it was the first clinical pilot study on CXL that was conducted in Dresden and published by Wollensak in 2003. This prospective, non-randomized study with follow-up time up to 4 years analyzed results of 23 eyes of 22 patients. The study found in all eyes cessation of the progression of keratoconus and in 70% of the eyes was recorded even decrease of keratometry readings with mild improvement of corrected visual acuity in 65% [1].

Meanwhile was the effectiveness and safety of the procedure for treatment of keratoconus demonstrated in various clinical trials in Europe, Australia and the US. In 2008, Dresden group reported results of a retrospective study of 241 eyes in 130 patients with a follow-up of 6 years after CXL. This analysis confirmed that CXL leads to a significant decrease in keratometric values at the apex of the cone, reduction of astigmatism and improvement of best corrected visual acuity [18].

Durability, stability and safety of this procedure could be demonstrated in a 10-year-follow-up as well, that was published by the same group in 2015 [2].

The first randomized controlled trial was initiated by Wittig-Silva et al. in Australia. This prospective study found similar results compared to those from Dresden [19].

The study was conducted in Melbourne in 2006 including refractive, topographic and clinical results of 46 eyes with progressive keratoconus after CXL. There was another control group of 48 eyes with a follow-up of 3 years. The standard protocol for CXL was used. The eyes in the control group showed both a statistically significant increase in Kmax and astigmatism and a decrease in BCVA. In contrast to this, the CXL-group revealed a statistically significant decrease of Kmax and an improvement of corrected and uncorrected visual acuity.

The 1-year results of a multicenter, prospective, randomized clinical trial revealed, according to FDA guidelines, an improvement of corrected and uncorrected visual acuity, Kmax, and mean K-values [16].

Another prospective study in the UK showed a significant and continuous improvement of topographic and wave front parameters with a follow-up of 5 years. Stability was achieved up to 7 years after CXL [20].

A prospective randomized trial in an Asian population with progressive keratoconus showed a statistical significant improvement of uncorrected VA and decrease in K-values in the treated group compared to control group [21].

A multicenter, prospective, randomized, double-blind clinical trial initiated in 2008 in Germany investigated efficacy and safety of CXL in patients with progressive keratoconus. Twenty-nine eyes were included in treatment and control group, respectively. Follow-up was 3 years. Results confirmed efficacy of CXL, but 4 out of 15 eyes in the treatment group showed an increase in K-values. Eleven eyes in the treatment and six eyes in a control group did not show any further progression. In the treatment group, a decrease in Kmax-value of 0.35 ± 0.58 D per year was recorded. The control group revealed a significant increase of 0.11 ± 0.61 D [22].

All these studies have been conducted according to the standard "Dresden protocol".

2.1.5 Complications

The clinical trials mentioned above could show, that CXL is effective in halting of keratectasia progression and stabilizes corneal architecture. None of these studies evaluated potential complications and failure rate of the procedure. CXL is technically easy to perform; but pain and reduced visual acuity after epithelial debridement within first postoperative days are common side effects, which are completely resolved after a few days when reepithelialization is completed. There are reports on corneal infections and melting with consecutive corneal perforation as sequelae of persistent epithelial defect and/or applying of therapeutic contact lenses [23–26].

Koller et al. investigated failure rate after CXL within the first postoperative year and analyzed 117 eyes of 99 patients with primary keratectasia [27].

Progression of keratectasia was recorded by Scheimpflug images over a period of 6 months (range: 6 months–2 years). Progression was assumed when Kmax value increased more than 1 D. The fellow eye was treated not earlier than 6 months after the first one.

Only eyes with mild to moderate keratoconus were included (Kmax <65 dpt, CCT >400 μm). Complication rate was defined as percentage of eyes losing two or more lines of BCVA in 1 year. Failure rate was defined as percentage of eyes with an increase of Kmax of more than 1 D. Ninety percent of patients completed follow-up of 1 year. Complication rate was 2.9% and failure rate 7.6%. Age above 35 years and preoperative BCVA better than 20/25 were identified as risk factors for complications.

If the age of 35 years had been defined as upper age limit for inclusion, complication rate would have been 1.04%. There was no clear cause sufficiently explaining the loss of visual acuity. A high preoperative Kmax-value was a negative predictor for failure. If Kmax of 58 D would have been the upper limit for inclusion instead of 65 D, failure rate would have decreased to 2.8%.

In 2.8% of eyes there were stromal scars and in 7.6% of eyes could be observed sterile infiltrates. The results of Koller's study suggested, that modification of inclusion criteria for CXL could minimize complication and failure rate respectively. Consequently, patients should be carefully counseled about individual risk factors, prognosis and potential postoperative complications of this procedure. Furthermore, they should be advised about postoperative behavior reducing the risk of microbial keratitis.

Kymionis et al. reported about a case where CXL induced herpes keratitis with iritis even if there was no history of herpes infection previously [23].

Typical changes after CXL is occurrence of corneal haze. It has been observed that the depth of the crosslinked stromal tissue can be estimated detected by visualizing of stromal demarcation line [28] or evaluating of haze via slit lamp finding [27].

Herrmann et al. reported a case with temporary subepithelial haze after CXL which completely resolved within a few months [29].

Mazzotta et al. investigated stromal haze using in vivo confocal microscopy, demonstrating that it occurred 2–3 months after CXL with no improvement after topical steroid treatment. Confocal microscopy revealed a tighter fibrillary matrix, which was even more intense in patients with advanced stages of keratoconus. These opacities completely disappeared after 30–40 days applying topical preservative free steroids. Preoperative confocal analysis of patients younger than 20 years revealed hyperactive keratocytes nuclei in the anterior stroma up to a depth of 80 μm. Patients above 20 years showed dark, reticular microstriae. This group also showed preoperative Vogt striae, which could be a risk factor for development of corneal haze after CXL [30, 31].

A multicenter, prospective randomized study investigated the natural development of CXL-associated haze using Scheimpflug-Imaging (densitometry) and slit-lamp evaluation of patients with keratoconus und iatrogenic induced ectasia. There was an objective quantification of the time course of haze formation. They found the maximum haze after 1 month after CXL with a consecutive plateau after 3 months and a significant decrease between the third and twelfth month. Changes of haze structure were not correlated to postoperative results [32].

Dresden group investigated retrospectively the development of stromal scaring after CXL [33].

The cohort comprised 163 eyes of 127 patients with keratoconus stage 1–3 according to Amsler-Krumeich scale. One year after CXL, 8.6% of eyes developed significant stromal scaring. Eyes with scaring revealed higher Kmax-value at the apex (mean 71.1 ± 13.2 D) and thinnest central corneal thickness (mean: 420.0 ± 33.9 μm). We therefore assume that the risk of scar formation is increased in patients with advanced keratoconus due to reduced CCT and a higher corneal curvature.

Another complication after CXL is loss of endothelial cells. Kymionis et al. treated 14 eyes of 12 patients with a mean CCT of 373.92 ± 22.92 μm after removal of epithelium. After 1 year there was a significant decrease in endothelial cell count from 2733 ± 180 cells/mm^2 to 2441 ± 400 cells/mm^2 [34].

They applied 0.1% riboflavin and 20% dextran solution. This combination could possibly cause intraoperative decrease of corneal thickness and increased thinning of the already thinned corneas. Reports of other investigators using similar procedure of CXL in patients with thin corneas did not record CCT after removal of epithelium [35, 36].

Corneal melting is another possible complication after CXL. There was a case described of a young patient, that within 1 day after CXL developed significant stromal haze, endothelial precipitates and cells in anterior chamber. Reepithelialization was very slow and progressive corneal thinning resulted in descemetocoele with spontaneous rupture 2 months after procedure [37].

Consequently, a careful and regular examination after CXL is essential. Patients with delayed reepithelialization could benefit from amnion membrane transplantation or the use of serum eye drops in order to support epithelialization preventing corneal perforation. Another keratoconus patient suffered from corneal melting 1 week after CXL because of uncontrolled use of diclofenac and proparacaine eye drops [38]. Faschinger et al. reported a case of patient with Down syndrome and keratoconus with thin corneas without signs of progression who underwent CXL on both eyes. This patient developed corneal melting and perforation in both eyes 1 and 4 weeks after procedure and had to undergo urgent penetrating keratoplasty [39].

Critically analyzing, these cases arise questions, whether patients without significant ectasia progression and potential postoperative risk factors such as eye rubbing, uncontrolled application of eye drops due to incompliance and thin corneas are good candidates for CXL? Eberwein et al. reported a case of a 45-year-old patient with a history of severe atopy and keratoconus, who developed corneal melting due to herpes simplex infection after CXL and deep anterior keratoplasty. In the course of this case a penetrating keratoplasty and intensive immunosuppressive and antiviral therapy were necessary to restore the ocular surface [40].

We are of the opinion, that patients with a history of atopy belong to a high risk group concerning postoperative complications after CXL, especially regarding postoperative corneal healing, delayed epithelialization and higher susceptibility to infections.

There was a one case described from Australia, reporting a poly-microbial keratitis occurring 1 day after CXL. This patient admitted to clean his therapeutic contact lens in his mouth before re-inserting it into the eye again [26].

All the mentioned complications and irreversible damage should force us to careful preoperative examination and thorough recording of patient's medical history. We should guarantee that patients are good candidates for CXL, fulfill all the inclusion criteria and that we shall be able to examine them regularly after the procedure.

2.1.6 Conclusion

Eighteen years ago, has been corneal crosslinking with riboflavin and UVA light proposed as a therapeutic procedure improving biomechanical properties in corneal ectatic diseases. Until that time, could the available conservative and surgical therapeutic options only improve refractive effect of keratoconus, whereas they had no impact on its progression. Corneal graft, an invasive surgical procedure, was the only definite therapeutic choice solving negative consequences of this corneal pathology—still, with possible intra- and postoperative complications limiting the outcomes in the long run.

There are many clinical trials proving that CXL can stop progression of corneal ectasia with a low complication rate. Apart from clinical aspects, there are several economic and psychosocial advantages of this procedure. CXL can be performed in an outpatient setting, it is minimal invasive, cost-efficient and with a manageable minimal stress for the patient [2, 16, 17, 19–21, 41–44].

2.2 Transepithelial Crosslinking

The clinical evidence, that epi-off CXL stabilizes progressive keratoconus and its effect lasts for at least 10 years was demonstrated by the results of a retrospective interventional case series study [2].

A systematic review and meta-analysis focusing on studies dealing with epi-off CXL procedure in progressing keratoconus expressed concerns about the quality of the available evidence [45]. Their analysis incorporated 49 studies that involved patients receiving epi-off CXL, of which 39 were graded as "very low quality evidence". A number of reasons were given, including study design, lack of a comparator arm, high loss to follow-up and incomplete reporting. The reviewers also stated uncertainty about duration of the benefit from this procedure. However, they recognized that the procedure delays or even avoids the need of corneal transplant and improves the fitting of contact lenses. They also recorded the most common side effects like pain, stromal edema, and corneal haze, which are associated with wound response, but usually resolve within a few days after procedure.

The Cochrane Database of Systematic Reviews analyzed three randomized controlled trials (RCTs) published till August 2014 where CXL with UVA light and riboflavin was used to treat patients with keratoconus and was compared to no treatment [46]. Its conclusion was that the evidence for the use of CXL in the management of keratoconus was limited due the lack of properly conducted RCTs.

Another evidence-based analysis reviewed 65 reports involving 1404 patients after CXL for corneal ectasia. This analysis found CXL stabilizing the underlying disease and in some cases even reverting disease progression. The quality of evidence for CXL of keratoconus was in this review graded as moderate [47].

The procedure itself and the postoperative period could be painful and epi-off CXL also carries a risk of delay of epithelial healing, sterile infiltrates, stromal haze, stromal melting, infectious ulceration, herpes simplex reactivation and the development of permanent stromal scars [48]. However, most of these adverse events are avoidable and manageable with topical antibiotics, steroids, lubricants and appropriate peri- and postoperative analgesia.

The reason why the standard protocol involves epithelial cell removal is the fact that riboflavin is a large hydrophilic molecule that cannot penetrate an intact epithelium [49] and besides that the epithelium blocks also about 20% of the administered UV light energy [50, 51]. Accordingly, a number of approaches have been taken to try and get the riboflavin into the corneal stroma, including pharmacological cleavage of epithelial tight junctions, intrastromal application of riboflavin through injections, perforators or femtosecond laser-created pockets and channels.

The transepithelial (TE) approach or "epi-on" CXL leaves the corneal epithelium intact and thus is supposed to eliminate or at least minimize wound-related complications and pain associated with epi-off CXL.

The current published data regarding the efficacy of TE-CXL showed generally inferiority comparing to standard epi-off procedure, although there is general consensus that it is a safe procedure without occurring any complications associated with healing process. An experimental study performed in rabbits has shown that pharmacological disruption of the epithelial tight junctions with the surfactant benzalkonium chloride (BAC) 0.005% (prior to the regular UV illumination and riboflavin application) increases corneal stiffness—but only by approximately one-fifth of what regular, epi-off CXL achieves [52]. Another experimental studies examining the biomechanical effect of the procedure leaving the epithelium intact and applying BAC on rabbits' corneas showed that treatment with BAC 0.02% induced sufficient epithelial permeability for the passage of riboflavin, which enabled its stromal diffusion and resulted in increase corneal stiffening [53]. Further experimental investigations revealed that hypoosmolar riboflavin solution without dextran but with 0.01% BAC and 0.44% NaCl promoted the permeability of riboflavin through the epithelium and resulted in a sufficient concentration of riboflavin in the corneal stroma [54]. Nevertheless, Brillouin microscopy of CXL-treated porcine eyes that had received either an epi-off or TE-CXL (with 0.02% benzalkonium chloride and 0.44% NaCl as the penetration enhancers) protocol showed that TE-CXL was 70% less effective in terms of biomechanically strengthening the cornea than standard CXL procedure [55].

When evaluated clinically, there is one study that used penetration enhancers both for a 30-min pretreatment soak and throughout the 30-min illumination period (riboflavin 0.1%, dextran T500, trometamol and EDTA) and appeared to halt keratoconus progression with a statistically significant improvement in visual acuity and topographic parameters—according to Placido topography [56]. Another studies analyzing results of TE-CXL performed by pharmacological cleavage of corneal epithelial sheet are rather more moderate with their conclusion statements and less enthusiastic. A study using benzalkonium chloride-assisted TE-CXL showed improved corrected distance visual acuity and stable corneal topography parameters measured on Placido disc (EyeSys), although the keratometry values recorded on Scheimpflug imaging (Oculus Pentacam) and I-S value on Placido topography deteriorated [48]. Treatment failure rate was 7% and no haze or other complications were noted in the 18-month follow-up period reported. A study comparing TE-CXL with epi-off CXL states that TE-CXL does not effectively halt the progression of keratoconus [57] and prospective case-series study showed that functional results after TE-CXL led to keratoconus instability, in particular in pediatric patients [58]. This study reported that "50% of pediatric patients were retreated with epi-off CXL due to significant deterioration of all parameters after 12 months of follow-up".

A recent randomized controlled trial using tetracaine 1% with BAC 0.02% without dextran compared to the standard procedure showed that epi-off was significantly more effective than TE-CXL [59]. Another randomized clinical study applying TE riboflavin solution with dextran and EDTA showed that TE-CXL was a safe procedure without epithelial healing problems, but 23% of these cases showed a continued keratoconus progression after 1 year [60]. A prospective, multicenter cohort study using a modified riboflavin solution with 0.01% BAC showed no sterile infiltrates, infection or corneal stromal haze after the procedure but in 46% of the eyes were found epithelial defects in the first postoperative day, 23% of the eyes had marked SPK's or loose epithelium also in this immediate postoperative period and in 46% of the eyes failed the procedure at 1-year follow-up time [61]. Another major reason driving clinicians to apply TE-CXL in their patients is to avoid early postoperative pain and temporary worsening of vision due to healing process [56]. A study focusing on these parameters: epithelial findings and pain score, comparing standard and TE-CXL revealed that the epithelial damage was observed in both procedures, the epithelial healing time was even longer in TE-CXL group and the group treated with standard procedure had less pain score than the TE-CXL group [62]. Riboflavin solution used in this study contained hydroxypropylmethylcellulose (HPMC), BAC, EDTA, TRIS and isotonic saline.

The studies focusing on morphological changes of the corneal stromal tissue after TE-CXL performed by pharmacological cleavage of epithelium showed also structural changes that were less pronounced comparing to the changes after epi-off CXL. Confocal analysis of these corneas showed a limited apoptotic effect of this treatment, about one-third of classic epi-off CXL procedure [63]; anterior segment OCT analysis revealed poorly evident corneal modifications in the TE-CXL group comparing to the traditional CXL [64]. Another confocal microscopy study showed that TE-CXL did not even appear to alter corneal morphology [65].

Among other methods concerning novel pharmacological modalities of transporting riboflavin into the cornea through an intact epithelium is a stromal penetration of a biocompatible riboflavin-based nanoemulsion system achieving in experimental set up in rabbit corneas greater stromal concentration when compared to debrided corneas with the standard protocol [66].

There are also surgical options how to introduce riboflavin solution into the corneal stroma, e.g. by injections into the corneal stroma or by a femtosecond laser creating a localized corneal channels or pockets for riboflavin infusion. Porcine eye studies have shown that though the biomechanical effect of CXL using the femtosecond laser pocket technique is about 50% less pronounced than that after standard CXL [67] but as the investigators state, it could be a feasible "epi-on" approach for CXL [68]. Investigators of this experiment are with their conclusions cautious demanding more experimental data before clinical testing. The surgical approach in creating of corneal pockets has been already tried in the clinical set up, taking eyes with early keratoconus, using the femtosecond laser to make an incision 100 μm in depth, and irradiating the eyes with UV-A illumination with a fluence of 7 mW/cm^2 for 15 min [69]. There was no ectasia progression (as determined by keratometry) noted during the mean 26 month follow-up period. The question that could arise observing these approaches of riboflavin application into the corneal stroma is, whether this modification truly fulfills the requirements for higher safety level regarding lower risk of infection, inflammation and haze formation and more comfort for patient comparing to the standard CXL treatment.

The positive, stabilizing effect of a standard, epi-off CXL in progressing keratoconus persists for at least a decade [2]. Removing the corneal epithelium might be uncomfortable for the patients, the healing process lasts several days longer and is more painful procedure than TE-CXL and it does carry a mild increase in risk of postoperative complications such as corneal infection, inflammation or other adverse events like development of corneal haze. These risks can easily be mitigated, and the pain and hazing can be with proper perioperative and postoperative local and systemic therapy managed. Transepithelial CXL would be a great option for patients with keratoconus, if it could work as effectively as epi-off CXL, but there is just not enough proof at the moment that either epi-off technique can.

There are two topics involving controversial aspects of transepithelial CXL treatment: one of them is the formulation of transepithelial solutions used in different studies and the second one is the dosage of total UVA energy [70]. It was also shown that the presence of dextran in transepithelial solution reduced the passage through the epithelium [52]. It is well documented that corneal epithelium and Bowman layer decreases the passage of UVA and it was determined that the amount of blockage was approximately 20–30% [51]. Considering this fact, the total dose of UVA energy in TE-CXL procedure should be increased. It seems to be plausible, that the combination of sufficient riboflavin uptake into the corneal stroma and sufficient duration or intensity of the UVA light could lead to optimizing of the effectiveness of transepithelial CXL procedure. These issues in different settings remain to be established [71].

2.3 Accelerated Crosslinking

2.3.1 Introduction

Recently, to shorten treatment time yet maintain the same efficiency of conventional CXL, accelerated crosslinking (ACXL) was proposed based on the physical concept of photochemical reactions indicated in Bunsen-Roscoe's law of reciprocity as described in Chap. 1. This theory demonstrated that the photochemical process behind crosslinking depends on the absorption of UVA energy, and its biological effect is proportional to the total dose of energy distributed to the tissue. In fact, based on the physical principal of the "equal dose", 9 mW/cm^2 for 10 min, 18 mW/cm^2 for 5 min, 30 mW/cm^2 for 3 min and 45 mW/cm^2 for 2 min (all at a constant Fluence of 5.4 J/cm^2) has the same photochemical impact as conventional 3 mW/cm^2 for 30 min. Most clinical trials highlighted the efficiency of this new accelerated procedures and will be briefly described.

2.3.2 The 9 mW/cm^2 Accelerated CXL

In 2013 Cinar et al. published a study in which they compared the accelerated procedure (9 mW/cm^2) and the conventional procedure (3 mW/cm^2) for the treatment of progressive keratoconus. They highlighted how the refractive and visual results of the two procedures were similar in the short term, but since the accelerated procedure was faster patients were more compliant [72]. The following year, the same authors published a clinical study evaluating the efficiency of accelerated crosslinking at 9 mW/cm^2 in the case of progressive keratoconus, and noted that with the patients treated early there was a significant change in the UDVA, although not in all. Only after 6 months did the CDVA show significant improvement [73]. The same result was observed by Hersh et al. at 6 months [16] while Vinciguerra et al. reported at a year [15]. The improvement in the CDVA could be attributed to changes in the keratometric indexes. Cinar further encountered that the flat keratometry, steep keratometry, average keratometry were significantly reduced 6-months after this procedure. It was noted that the reduction in the Kmax value could be due to an increase in the biomechanical stability of the cornea [73]. Instead, Legare reported a stabilization in the K values. Nonetheless, there are no significant Km and K changes after the 2-year follow-up [74]. In the study of Cinar there were no significant changes in thinnest corneal thickness (TCT) 6 months after 9 mW A-CXL [73]. Kymionis et al. carried out a prospective comparative study to evaluate the depth of the corneal demarcation lines in the two procedures increasing exposure time (9 mW/cm^2 in 14 min instead of 10 min) and standard Dresden Protocol (3 mW/cm^2). They highlighted that the difference in depth of the demarcation line was not statistically significant between the two groups [75]. One of the studies with the broadest follow-ups was carried out by Shetty et al. 18 patients were analysed over 2 years, with an average age of 12.7 years. Their evaluations showed an improvement in visual acuity in terms of average UDVA and average CDVA over 2 years.

Further, there was an improvement of the sphere, the cylinder and the spherical equivalent. As far as the keratometry was concerned, a statically significant flattening of average K 1 and average K 2 at the end of 2 years was observed [76].

Elbaz et al. in a retrospective study 1 year after the accelerated procedure (9 mW^2) concluded that the accelerated procedure is capable of stabilizing corneal parameters, but a larger and longer study with a more complete follow-up was required to validate it. They reported significant changes in CVDA, cylinder and spherical equivalent, but only a minimal change in the UDVA. All corneal parameters included: Ksteep, Kflat, Km, corneal astigmatism (Kcyl), and maximum curvature of the corneal apex, were stable from 6 to 12 months in all patients [77].

From December 2012 to September 2013 Jain et al. monitored corneal pachimetrical changes during accelerated treatment using isotonic riboflavin with HPMC. In 14 patients with a median age between 19 ± 8, they used pachimetry during the ACXL procedure. An isotonic solution was applied to the cornea after epithelium removal followed by the application of a riboflavin solution for 20 min, and lastly UV-A ray irradiation for 10 min with 9 mW/cm^2. No statistically significant changes of corneal thickness were noted before, during and after the procedure [78].

Pahuja N. et al. evaluated 33 eyes with a history of keratoconus, and looked at the correlation between the biomechanical results with the molecular operation of correlated ectasia genes. They evaluated visual acuity, keratometry, densitometry and results of corneal deformation after treatment, as well as the association with gene expression of proteins of the extracellular matrix (MMP 9, LOX, TGFβ, TNFα, IL10, IL6, COL A1 e COL IVA 1) using qPCR. They reported that the 9 mW ACXL procedure appears to be secure and provides biomechanical stability. Both keratometry and refraction remained stable after treatment, with a significant improvement of the cylindrical error. Pre-operative levels of the different proteins did not influence the clinical results described [79].

Cross-linking treatment is not only applied in the case of progressive keratoconus. Indeed, Marino et al., applied the 9 mW/cm^2 ACXL procedure to patients with post-LASIK ectasia. Analysing 40 eyes in 24 patients in terms of UDVA, CDVA, central corneal thickness, corneal topography, and endothelial cell density, they reported that the results are secure and efficient in the case of ectasia after a 2-year follow-up. Here, as well, they underlined that a larger group and longer follow-up is necessary to validate this new procedure [80].

In a recent study of Sadoughi et al. [81], the results of the conventional cross-linking (CXL) were compared to 9 mW ACXL in patients with bilateral progressive keratoconus (KC). Fifteen consecutive patients were enrolled with a 12-months follow-up. In each patient, the fellow eyes were randomly assigned to conventional CXL (3 mW/cm^2 for 30 min) or accelerated CXL (9 mW/cm^2 for 10 min) groups. Accelerated CXL with 9 mW/cm^2 for 10 min irradiation had a similar refractive, visual, keratometric and aberrometric result and less adverse effects on the corneal thickness and endothelial cells compared to the conventional method after 12 months of follow-up.

2.3.3 The 18 mW/cm^2 Accelerated CXL

As far as the 18 mW/cm^2/5 min procedure is concerned we can look to the trials of Cingu et al., who evaluated endothelial changes in the ACXL procedure comparing it with the standard procedure. No differences were stressed between the two groups that underwent different protocols, but nonetheless there is a reduction of 500 cell/mm^2 in the first post-operative period after ACXL. From the third to the sixth months the results were similar. Cingu advises that there could be a transient change in human endothelial cells in ACXL. The resolution of these changes during the follow-up indicate a secure recovery [82].

Hashemi et al. [83] evaluated the long and short term effects obtained with the 18 mW/cm^2/5 min ACXL compared to the standard CXL in two randomized studies made up of 31 patients. At 6-months follow-up, the two procedures had stopped the progression of keratoconus in a similar way. UDVA, CDVA, and the spherical equivalent do not show any significant changes between the two groups. In the standard procedure, the thickness of the central cornea results as higher compared to accelerated. The reduction of K max, K average, and average changes in corneal asphericity were not statistically different. Even changes in corneal hysteresis, factors of corneal resistance, and the area under apex were similar. Lastly, reduction in endothelial cells count (ECC) was not statistically significant in both groups [84].

The long-term comparison demonstrated that between the two groups, the results and security profile were similar, but the standard procedure produced higher corneal flattening. However, both methods have the ability to stop keratoconus progression in a similar way. This affirmation is confirmed evaluating 31 eyes with the accelerated procedure, compared to eyes treated with the standard procedure using the same energy dose of 5.4 J/cm^2. At 18 months from the procedure the group treated with the conventional method presented an improvement in the spherical equivalent, in K-readings, Q Value, improvement of the surface symmetry index and a temporary reduction in corneal thickness, but no significant changes in visual acuity, corneal hysteresis, corneal resistance factor, or endothelial cell density. As far as the group treated with the accelerated procedure was concerned, the corneal thickness was the only parameter that changed in any statically significant way. However, none of these parameters shows a significant difference between the standard and 18 mW/cm^2 ACXL procedures [84].

Chow et al. compared the results of the conventional procedure (3 mW/cm^2; 365-nm ultraviolet-A light, 30 min) with accelerated (18 mW/cm^2; 365-nm ultraviolet-A light, 5 min) in patients with progressive keratoconus. The effect of corneal flattening obtained with conventional CXL was statistically significant compared to that of the 18 mW accelerated procedure after a year follow-up. Except for the corneal thickness that results as thinner, the topographical and clinical parameters were stable in both groups, [85]. In this study, there was a significant improvement in the UCVA, BCVA and spherical equivalent in both groups. Previous studies have shown similar functional improvement after CXL [1, 16, 18, 19, 86–91]. This has been attributed to improvement in the regularity of the corneal shape after CXL. From the topographical point of view, there were no clinically significant changes, but a reduction in the keratometry was noted in both the accelerated and the conventional groups. Thus, like other studies demonstrated improvement of the topographical flattening obtainable in more curved corneas. Carrying out an association analysis, Chan et al. found a negative association among the baseline keratometry and the post-operative keratometric values found in the ACXL group. The higher values of maximum baseline keratometry were associated with a greater reduction in the maximum keratometry values. The same negative association was also found in standard procedure cases [92]. One recently published comparative study of four CXL protocols in homogeneous pre-operative keratoconic eyes (steep keratometry between 48.6 and 50.5 D), demonstrated that conventional CXL of 3 mW/cm^2 has a stronger effect on flattening compared to the ACXL protocol of 9, 18 and 30 mW/cm^2 over a year follow-up. This was found in another study with a different selection of patients: that 18 mW/cm^2 concluding that accelerated CXL treatment is not capable of inducing corneal flattening at 1 year in eyes with a base Kmax <58 D, and an average variation of 1.00 ± 1.63 D of Kmax at 1 year. The authors attributed this potential reduction to the biomechanical effect of the 18 mW/cm^2 ACXL treatment [93].

Wernli et al. observed that with 40–45 mW/cm^2 for 2 min an increase in the rigidity equivalent could be reached. For more elevated intensities that go from 50 to 90 mW/cm^2, no statistically significant increase in rigidity could be obtained citing the non-applicability of the Bunsen–Roscoe law of reciprocity for brief, high intensity illumination time [90].

Hammer et al. observed a tendency of the reduction in the Young model with increased irradiation, reaching some statistically significant differences between 18 mW/cm^2 and the controls group. The authors proposed the hypothesis that the intra-stromal capacity of diffusion and the increase in the consumption of oxygen associated with higher irradiation can be a limiting factor, with consequential reduction of the efficiency of the treatment [91].

A reduced depth of postoperative demarcation line was observed with 18 mW/cm^2 ACXL which suggests a reduced effect of treatment compared to conventional CXL treatment [94]. Kymionis et al. also discovered that a 40% increase in irradiation treatment was needed in the accelerated procedure to obtain a similar demarcation line depth like that obtained in the conventional procedure [95].

Kurt et al. evaluated the results of 18 mW/cm^2 for 5 min ACXL procedure in an 18-month follow-up in patients with progressive keratoconus. Forty-two eyes of forty-two patients with an age range from 24 to 36 years were studied. Finding a significant improvement in the UDVA and CDVA, a significant reduction of the Kflat, K steep and K apical curvature (AK), concluding that that the ACXL procedure was effective for the stabilization keratoconus progression during 18-month follow-up [96, 97].

2.3.4 The 30 mW/cm^2 Accelerated CXL

Mazzotta et al. performed a comparative study between 30 mW/cm^2 epithelium-off ACXL with pulsed light (pl-ACXL 8 min UVA exposure) and continuous light (cl-ACXL 4 min UVA exposure). Twenty eyes were treated, [98].

The dose of energy used was 7.2 J/cm^2 for both groups, according to Avedro 30 mW first protocol. Through comparative analysis efficiency in the stabilization of the progress of keratoconus was shown for both procedures at a 1-year follow-up. Further, the pulsed light procedure had slightly better results in terms of UCVA, even if a true significant difference was not found between the two treatment modalities. The slight improvement obtained in the UCVA could be attributed to an improvement in Kaverage values and a reduction of the KC apical curvature (AK). Further, the same study evaluated the effect of the two procedures regarding the degree of ACXL stromal penetration measured by corneal OCT and confocal documenting the demarcation line depth at 1 month. An apoptotic effect was discovered at 215 μm of depth on average in the pl ACXL with 8 min of UVA exposure and at 160 μm of depth on average in the cl ACXL with 4 min of UVA exposure [65, 98]. This was the first study documenting that 30 mW/cm^2 ACXL induced a more superficial cross-linking penetration especially if continuous light irradiation and shorter exposure time is used, opening a new way for the treatment of thin corneas. Moreover, the study demonstrated that pulsing the light intra-operatively the re-uptake of oxygen is induced and the increased exposure time at 8 min influenced a better penetration of the oxidative damage around 200 μm of corneal stroma. Both procedures reached the anterior part of the corneal stroma up to a depth of 200 microns [98–100]. The functional improvement of ACXL with pulsed light could be a way to optimize disposition of oxygen, thanks to the on/off cycle of oxygen delivery. In fact, treatments have observed a similar efficiency in keratoconus stabilization in all follow-up periods. Both modalities represent a safe procedure in the short-term evolution of keratoconus stabilization [65, 98, 100]. Even for Mazzotta et al., the efficiency of this technique must be evaluated with longer follow-ups and larger control groups. However, the inferior penetration of these ACXL protocols can be used for CXL customization in different ectatic pathways as showed in Chap. 6.

Another Italian study performed by Fontana et al. [101] compared the two methods of pulsed and continued light ACXL treatment. They evaluated the stromal demarcation line depth after ACXL with continued light (30 mW/cm^2 for 4 min), and pulsed light (30 mW/cm^2 for 8 min 1 s on - 1 s off) with a total energy dose of 7.2 J/cm.^{2} A month after the procedure, the stromal corneal demarcation line was measured by two different people using anterior segment optical coherence tomography (AS-OCT). After evaluating 60 patients they concluded that the average demarcation line depth was deeper in the pulsed light group (213 μm) compared to the continuous light group (149.32 μm) showing a statistically significant difference. This study substantially confirmed the findings of Mazzotta et al. concerning a more superficial penetration of 30 mW/cm^2 of ACXL treatment and advantages of pulsed-light treatment increasing depth of demarcation line and ACXL efficiency [98, 100].

Ozgurhan et al. carried out a retrospective study evaluating paediatric patients between 9 and 18 years of age (15.3 ± 2.1 years) treated with the accelerated procedure (30 mW/cm^2) for 24-months follow-up. In this trial as well they concluded that the procedure was capable of stopping the progression of keratoconus without side effects in paediatric patients. Visual acuity, keratometric values and corneal aberrations improved all [102].

Another fundamental aspect evaluated by Ozgurhan et al. in one of their precious works was the effect of 30 mW/cm^2 ACXL in the treatment of keratoconic thin corneas. They treated 34 eyes of 34 patients who had a corneal thickness inferior to 400 μm. UDVA and CDVA, manifested refraction and topography were evaluated at 1–6 and 12-month follow-up. The density of endothelial cells (cell/mm^2) was evaluated pre-and post-operatively at 12 months. Further, they measured the stromal demarcation line with anterior segment OCT 1 month after the procedure. The results show how UDVA, CDVA, average spherical and cylindrical refraction improve, but not in any significant way. They conclude that the accelerated procedure was able to stabilize the progression of keratoconus in thin corneas under 400 μm without a significant loss of endothelial cells (varying from 2.726.02 ± 230.21 to 2.714.58 ± 218.26 cells/mm^2) during the 12-month follow-up, [103].

A 6-month retrospective study by Mita et al. [104] evaluated the efficiency of the 30 mW/cm^2 ACXL procedure at 5.4 J/cm^2 and 3 min of UV-A exposure. They treated 39 eyes in 22 patients with progressive keratoconus by looking at changes in dioptric strength and corneal topography. Per the authors, the 30 mW/cm^2 ACXL procedure at 5.4 J/cm^2 and 3 min of UV-A exposure has the potential to be an effective and efficient way to arrest the progression of keratoconus, and it could also be an efficient therapy option for the treatment of other corneal ectasias. The check-ups were carried out pre-operatively at 1, 3 and 6 months. The changes after the procedure were similar to those of the standard CXL procedure. UDVA and Kmax values showed statistically significant improvement. Regarding the density of endothelial cells, however, there were no significant changes pre- and post-operatively. These results were encouraging and suggested that 30 mW/cm^2 ACXL could improve corneal steepening, and could prevent the progression of keratoconus and in many cases including the regression of keratoconus. The observed reduction in Kmax values could be the result in improved biomechanical stability of the cornea after accelerated CXL, a result found in numerous studies as well. Even the biomechanical parameters measured with the dynamic bidirectional applanation device (ocular response analyser) did not change after the procedure. Similar results were reported after having used the conventional protocol [105]. In Mita's study the degree of treatment penetration was checked by the Heidelberg Retinal Tomograph II in vivo confocal microscopy, reporting an average was depth approximately at 320 μm, however this data is in contrast will all the repeatable data reported in literature by various European research groups [30, 65, 98, 100, 106]. The typical initial damage of the procedure included the disappearance of stromal keratocytes associated with hyper-reflective extracellular matrix and lacunar stromal oedema, that are all changes similar to those demonstrated for the first time at international level by Mazzotta after the conventional procedure [30, 106].

Another study carried out by Tomita et al. [107] comparing the results obtained through the accelerated procedure (30 mW/cm^2 for 3 min) and the conventional one (3 mW/cm^2 in 30 min) with a 1-year follow-up considered 48 eyes of 39 patients (30 eyes underwent the 30 mW/cm^2 ACXL procedure and 18 the 3 mW/cm^2 conventional procedure). In both procedures, a similar dose of UVA rays

(5.4 J/cm^2) was used with the same riboflavin solution and soaking times. Accelerated CXL and conventional CXL both proved safe and efficient. The ACXL, being faster, seemed to be the most advantageous for both patients and surgeons. These authors, too, agreed that an 8–10-year follow-up is needed. There were no statistically significant differences regarding UDVA, CDVA or the spherical equivalent manifested in both procedures. Further, there were no significant changes in the keratinometric values measured with the Pentacam, or in the biomechanical response measured with the dynamic bidirectional applanation device ocular response analyser (ORA). There were no differences in pre-and post-operative endothelial cells count in the two procedures.

2.3.5 The 45 mW/cm^2 Accelerated CXL

Some studies also looked into a UVA ray intensity of 45 mW/cm^2 with a 2-min exposure time. The study carried out by Sherif et al. at the University of Cairo [108] compared two groups of eyes with mild to moderate keratoconus for 12 months, and evaluated the visual acuity, the keratometric parameters, corneal thickness, corneal hysteresis and the of corneal resistance factor (CRF). It was found that the progressive reduction of flat keratometry, steep keratometry and mean keratometry were highlighted in the whole follow-up period in the two groups. The improvement of the keratinometric values were not significant. Visual acuity expressed in BSCVA shows an improvement at both 6 and 12 months, up to obtaining a statistically significant improvement after a year compared to base levels. For the standard procedure, also, there is an improvement that at 6 months which seems insignificant, but at 12 months it is significant. The improvement of corneal hysteresis and factors of resistance, instead, resulted as non-significantly progressive in both groups. The corneal thickness was significant at 6 months in both groups and stable at 12 months. This way, like other authors, Sherif too concords on the fact that the two procedures can produce similar results, but to validate the procedure there must be more studies done with a longer follow-up and larger group of controls [108].

2.3.6 Conclusion

The introduction of accelerated cross-linking protocols represents something innovative and exciting. Favouring a reduction in procedure time compared to the standard CXL procedure is more comfortable for the patients. This reduction in time also allows for a higher turn-over of patients, leading to shorter waiting lists and thus more patients treated. There a lot of studies in progress concerning the accelerated cross-linking procedures. More studies, more patients, longer follow-ups and larger control groups are necessary to develop customized treatment protocols as a valid substitute to the standard procedure in treating progressive keratoconus.

2.4 Crosslinking for Paediatric Keratoconus: 10 Years-Follow-Up

2.4.1 Introduction

Keratoconus (KC) represents one of the most common causes of paediatric corneal transplantation causing about 15–20% of all corneal transplants in children [109]. Diagnosis of keratoconus before adulthood is a negative prognostic factor for KC progression, increasing the probability of the need for corneal transplant [110]. Young age was associated with more severe forms of KC and faster progression [111]. Indeed, an inverse correlation between age at onset and KC severity was reported in literature [112]. KC progression in paediatric patients 18 years and under was found to be with a sevenfold higher risk of requiring corneal grafting [113]. The 1-year progression rate of KC in children was seen in 88% of patients [114]. Moreover, paediatric patients were at higher risk of acute or post-acute corneal hydrops [115]. KC paediatric patients suffering from allergy and eye-rubbing KC could represent a particular population with faster deterioration of KC and visual acuity caused by chronic inflammatory events of the ocular surface as showed in Figs. 2.1 and 2.2 [116–119].

The age of the youngest child with KC diagnosis reported in the literature was 6 years [110]. Medium to long-term results up to 5-years of follow-up on corneal collagen crosslinking (CXL) for the treatment of progressive KC [58, 120, 121] have demonstrated the capacity of the procedure to slow-down or stop the

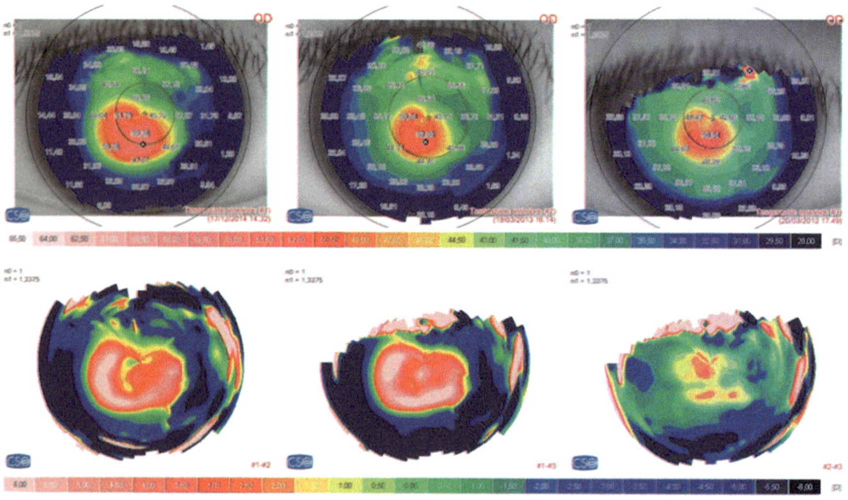

Fig. 2.1 Differential tomography map (Sirius™ C.S.O. Florence, Italy) shows a dramatic worsening of keratoconus in a 13 years-old patient suffering from uncontrolled oculo-rhinitis and eye-rubbing in a 12-months follow-up

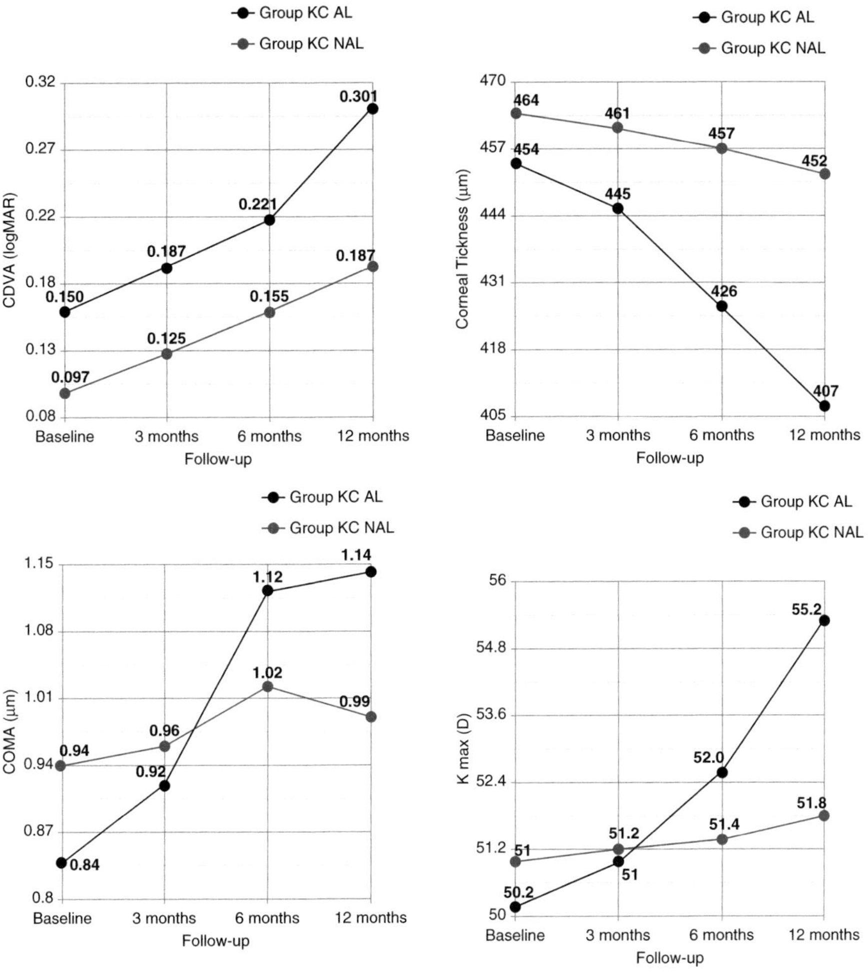

Fig. 2.2 Comparative functional and tomographic outcomes between a group of 52 keratoconic patients suffering from allergy (KC AL, *black lines*) and 48 keratoconic patients without allergic diseases (KC NAL, *gray lines*). Corrected distance visual acuity (CDVA), Minimum Corneal Thickness, K Max and Coma values worsened significantly at 1-year follow-up addressing a manifest correlation between keratoconus progression, allergy and eye-rubbing in paediatric population. Despite a tendency to Keratoconus progression (*gray lines*), no statistically significant worsening was recorded in the non allergic group

progression of KC through photo-polymerization of corneal collagen mediated by reactive oxygen species, increasing the biomechanical rigidity and biochemical resistance of the cornea [2, 86, 122, 123].

The effects of CXL against progression of the ectasia are not limited to the instantaneous formation of covalent bonds (cross-links) within and between collagen fibrils and/or to the inhibition of collagenase activity, but the long-term stabilizing effect is sustained by synthesis of new collagen, having different structure and resistance, capable of imparting variable lamellar compaction to the corneal stroma [30, 124, 125]. This compaction is responsible for functional changes recorded after treatment and improvement of functional results [106, 126].

2.4.2 Demographic Data

The study included all consecutive pediatric patients (<18 years and under) who underwent an epithelium-off CXL procedure for progressive KC from September 2004 through September 2007 at Department of Ophthalmology of Siena University, Italy. The diagnosis of KC was established in concordance with the global consensus on keratoconus and ectatic diseases report [127]. Following inclusion criteria were applied for CXL treatment: K max progression defined as a change of ≥1.0 diopter (D) within 1 year, a centrally clear cornea (no sub-apical scars, no Vogt's striae), and optical minimum corneal thickness (MCT) of 400 μm before ultraviolet-A (UV-A) irradiation. The "Siena CXL Long-Term Paediatrics" study was approved by the Ethical Committee of the University of Siena and was performed in accordance with the tenets established by the Declaration of Helsinki.

The prospective longitudinal cohort study comprised 48 eyes of 36 patients who completed the 10-years follow-up. Twenty-nine patients (82%) were male, and mean age at the time of treatment was 14.11 ± 2.43 years (range: 8–18 years). Average Uncorrected Distance Visual Acuity (UDVA) and Corrected Distance Visual Acuity (CDVA), Kmax (mean) 55.3 ± 3.23 diopters (D), Kavg (mean, D) 48.33 ± 3, Minimum Corneal Thickness (MCT) 453.33 ± 24.01 μm.

2.4.3 Surgical Procedure

Surgical procedure of Riboflavin-UVA CXL treatment was performed in all patients according to the Siena (Dresden modified) protocol [86] by using the Vega CBM (Caporossi-Baiocchi-Mazzotta) X-linker, Costruzione Strumenti Oftalmici (CSO), Florence, developed in Italy at the Department of Ophthalmology of Siena University by the same authors, under the intellectual property of the University of Siena, Italy. The treatment was conducted under topical anesthesia after premedication with 2% pilocarpine in the eye to be treated, instilled 30 min before the operation, topical anesthesia with 4% lidocaine 15 min before the treatment. After applying closed valves eyelid speculum, a 9 mm diameter Thornton marker was used to mark the corneal epithelium in a central circle, then epithelium was removed with a blunt metal spatula. After epithelial scraping, a disposable isotonic solution of Riboflavin 0.1% and Dextran 20% (Ricrolin Sooft, Montegiorgio, Italy) was instilled for 10 min [2, 58] of corneal soaking before starting UVA irradiation. The Riboflavin-Dextran solution was administered every 2.5 min for a total of 30 min of UVA exposure at 3 mW/cm^2, washing the eye surface with balanced saline solution and instillation of two to four drops of ofloxacin and cyclopentolate at the end of the procedure, and dressing the eye with a therapeutic soft corneal lens for 4 days. No adjunctive sedation was required before the procedure (except in one 8 years-old patient), and all children were able to tolerate the treatment. Sometimes, the presence of a parent (generally the mother) was needed in the operating room to effectively reduce the patient's anxiety [58]. After therapeutic corneal lens removal, fluoro-metholone 0.2% drops (tapered 3 times/day) and lacrimal substitutes were administered for 6–8 weeks.

Ophthalmic evaluations were performed before CXL and at all follow-up visits (1, 3, 6, 12, 24, 36, 48, 60, 72, 84, 96, 108 and 120 months) after undergoing CXL. The evaluation included uncorrected distance visual acuity (UDVA), corrected distance visual acuity (CDVA), Scheimpflug corneal tomography (Sirius, CSO, Florence, Italy). K max, K average, Coma variations, minimum corneal thickness (MCT) and a slit-lamp evaluation with particular focus on allergic eyes and sub-tarsal papillary hypertrophy. UDVA and CDVA were measured in LogMAR and used as main outcome measures together with Kmax and Kavg. Progression was defined as a change in Kmax and/or Kaverage ≥1.0 D. Contact lens wearers were instructed to remove their lenses 2 weeks before all evaluations. A two-tailed paired samples Student t test was used to compare each baseline measurement with the respective follow-up measurements. Differences with $P < 0.05$ were considered significant. Data were collected and analyzed with PRISM 6.0 GraphPad Software (California USA).

2.4.4 Clinical Results

The CDVA improved significantly after undergoing cross-linking at all follow-up visits, with the exception of the third month after treatment (P 0.3299) (Figs. 2.2 and 2.3).

The baseline and follow-up measurements documented that Kmax improved significantly 6 months after treatment, and this improvement remained significant throughout the entire follow-up period (P 0.292) (Fig. 2.4).

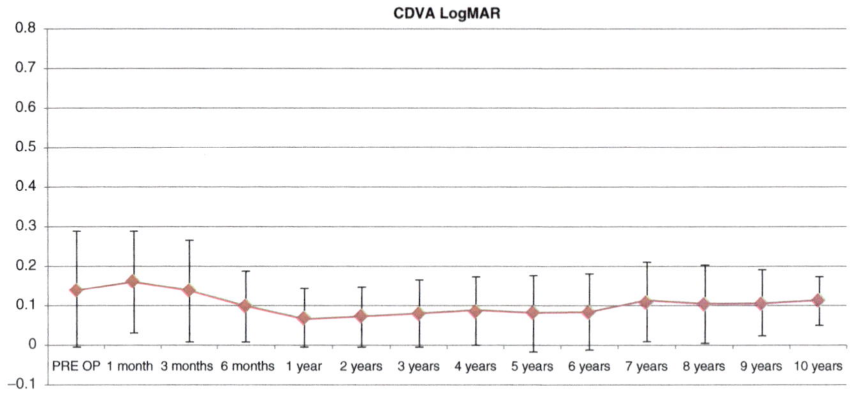

Fig. 2.3 CDVA improved significantly after standard epithelium-off CXL in pediatric population in a 10-years follow-up

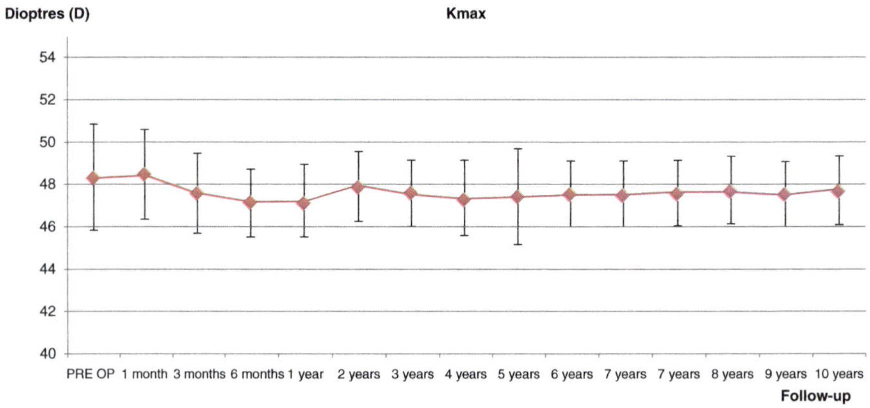

Fig. 2.4 Kmax improved significantly 6 months after treatment, and this improvement remained significant throughout the entire follow-up period

2.4.5 Complications

No postoperative infections, persistent haze or endothelial cell failure were encountered during the follow-up period in the study cohort.

In five eyes (10.4%) of three children (12%), K max increased by 1.2 D at the 36-month follow-up visit returning to baseline value despite an initial improvement of—1 D at the 12-month after CXL; two eyes (4.16%) of two children (5.55%) showed a KC instability at 36-month follow-up visit with Kavg progression up to 2 D and K max progression up to 3.2 D, requiring an additional epithelium-off CXL retreatment. Kmax values stabilized in both patients 12 months after retreatment. Both retreated children suffered from severe allergy and eye-rubbing.

2.4.6 Conclusion

According to these data, the overall Kmax progression >1 D occurred in seven eyes (14.58%) of five children (13.8%) at 36-month follow-up visit, stabilizing thereafter without retreatment in five eyes and after CXL retreatment in the other two eyes. One eye (2.03%) of one patient (2.77%) required a deep anterior lamellar keratoplasty 6 years after CXL respectively in the worst eye for hard gas permeable contact lenses intolerance and poor spectacle corrected visual acuity even if its KC was stable after CXL. Moderate stromal hyper-density (haze) was present in six eyes (12.5%) of four patients (11.11%) without negatively influencing visual acuity. No cases of persistent haze or infection was recorded in the follow-up. After the 48-months follow-up visit KC stability was observed throughout the remaining study period of 10-years in the whole study population.

The long-term results of the "*Siena CXL paediatrics study*" confirmed the Siena group previous study [58] and the long-term results reported by other research group in the Netherland [120] demonstrating that epithelium-off cross-linking can be considered both safe and effective, achieving stable long-term results up to 10 years in pediatric patients. Moreover, the *Siena long-term paediatric study* recorded significant functional improvement in 89.6% patients18 years and under after 10-years follow-up. Only a small number of eyes (10.4%), 24–36 months after CXL, showed a not statistically significant tendency of keratometry readings regression, returning at their baseline values, even this aspect not necessarily means instability or CXL inefficacy as only two eyes (4.16%) showed a KC instability at 36-month follow-up visit with a Kavg progression up to 2 D and K max progression up to 3.2 D requiring an additional epithelium-off CXL retreatment. This finding was similar to with the findings reported by Raiskup et al. [2]. Interestingly, none of these patients showed a decline of one or more lines in either UDVA or CDVA. Both patients suffered from atopy and allergic conjunctivitis with intense eye-rubbing that were considered as possible causes of unfortunate response after CXL beyond age less than 14 years in both patients.

Those findings are also similar with the findings reported by Chatzis and Hafezi [114] where the initial Kmax improvement was no longer significant at 2-year follow-up and revealing a not statistically significant trend toward deterioration at the 3-year follow-up visit. However, the improvement in CDVA did remain significant.

In the Siena long-term paediatric study cohort, the effect of cross-linking on Kmax did not decline over time except a return to baseline value in a small number of patients (10%); in fact, significant improvement was measured throughout the entire 10-year follow-up period.

No adverse events (no infections or permanent haze) were recorded in this paediatric series. Transient slight to moderate corneal haze (stromal hyperdensity) occurred within the first 6–12 months in four patients (11%) with a temporary (1–3 months) glare disability and without negatively influencing the final visual acuity. Haze was managed with topical preservative-free steroids fluorometholone drops, tapered 3 times a day for 4–6–8 weeks.

Topographic indices showed a statistically significant mean reduction of K max. The improvement in topographic K readings reflects improved corneal symmetry because of recentering of the corneal apex as demonstrated in the literature. Only one patient (2.7%) had a deep anterior lamellar keratoplasty (DALK) 6 years after CXL due to hard gas permeable contact lenses intolerance and poor spectacle corrected visual acuity since his enrolment in the treatment protocol, not for KC instability. The "*Siena long-term paediatric study*" demonstrates the effective capacity of CXL to stabilize and slow-down the progression of keratoconus in paediatric patients aged 18 years or younger, improving functional performance in 89.6% of patients 10 years after the operation. In a small percentage of cases (13.8%), a worsening of topographic data was initially observed during the follow-up between the 24 and 36-month follow-up visit, reasonably explained by the higher aggressiveness and progressiveness of keratoconus in paediatric patients suffering from allergy and atopy and other environmental factors such as eye-rubbing. On the other hand, the stability recorded in the long-term may be correlated not only to a good treatment response but also to natural age-related lisyl-oxidase (LOX) mediated corneal collagen crosslinking.

References

1. Wollensak G, Spoerl E, Seiler T. Riboflavin/ultraviolet-a-induced collagen crosslinking for the treatment of keratoconus. Am J Ophthalmol. 2003;135:620–7.
2. Raiskup F, Theuring A, Pillunat LE, et al. Corneal collagen crosslinking with riboflavin and ultraviolet-A light in progressive keratoconus: ten-year results. J Cataract Refract Surg. 2015;41:41–6.
3. Caporossi A, Mazzotta C, Baiocchi S, et al. Age-related long-term functional results after riboflavin UV A corneal cross-linking. J Ophthalmol. 2011;2011:608041.
4. Spoerl E, Zubaty V, Terai N, et al. Influence of high-dose cortisol on the biomechanics of incubated porcine corneal strips. J Refract Surg. 2009;25:S794–8.
5. Spoerl E, Zubaty V, Raiskup-Wolf F, et al. Oestrogen-induced changes in biomechanics in the cornea as a possible reason for keratectasia. Br J Ophthalmol. 2007;91:1547–50.
6. Bilgihan K, Hondur A, Sul S, et al. Pregnancy-induced progression of keratoconus. Cornea. 2011;30:991–4.
7. Hafezi F, Iseli HP. Pregnancy-related exacerbation of iatrogenic keratectasia despite corneal collagen crosslinking. J Cataract Refract Surg. 2008;34:1219–21.
8. Kappmeyer K, Lanzl IM. [Intra-ocular pressure during and after playing high and low resistance wind instruments]. Ophthalmologe. 2010;107:41–6.
9. McMonnies CW. The possible significance of the baropathic nature of keratectasias. Clin Exp Optom. 2013;96:197–200.
10. Kuo IC, Broman A, Pirouzmanesh A, et al. Is there an association between diabetes and keratoconus? Ophthalmology. 2006;113:184–90.
11. Seiler T, Huhle S, Spoerl E, et al. Manifest diabetes and keratoconus: a retrospective case-control study. Graefes Arch Clin Exp Ophthalmol. 2000;238:822–5.
12. Morita A. Tobacco smoke causes premature skin aging. J Dermatol Sci. 2007;48:169–75.
13. Mahmud A, Feely J. Effect of smoking on arterial stiffness and pulse pressure amplification. Hypertension. 2003;41:183–7.
14. Spoerl E, Raiskup-Wolf F, Kuhlisch E, et al. Cigarette smoking is negatively associated with keratoconus. J Refract Surg. 2008;24:S737–40.

15. Vinciguerra P, Albe E, Trazza S, et al. Refractive, topographic, tomographic, and aberrometric analysis of keratoconic eyes undergoing corneal cross-linking. Ophthalmology. 2009;116:369–78.
16. Hersh PS, Greenstein SA, Fry KL. Corneal collagen crosslinking for keratoconus and corneal ectasia: one-year results. J Cataract Refract Surg. 2011;37:149–60.
17. Gomes JA, Tan D, Rapuano CJ, et al. Global consensus on keratoconus and ectatic diseases. Cornea. 2015;34:359–69.
18. Raiskup-Wolf F, Hoyer A, Spoerl E, et al. Collagen crosslinking with riboflavin and ultraviolet-A light in keratoconus: long-term results. J Cataract Refract Surg. 2008;34:796–801.
19. Wittig-Silva C, Chan E, Islam FM, et al. A randomized, controlled trial of corneal collagen cross-linking in progressive keratoconus: three-year results. Ophthalmology. 2014;121:812–21.
20. O'Brart DP, Patel P, Lascaratos G, et al. Corneal cross-linking to halt the progression of keratoconus and corneal ectasia: seven-year follow-up. Am J Ophthalmol. 2015;160:1154–63.
21. Sharma N, Suri K, Sehra SV, et al. Collagen cross-linking in keratoconus in Asian eyes: visual, refractive and confocal microscopy outcomes in a prospective randomized controlled trial. Int Ophthalmol. 2015;35:827–32.
22. Lang SJ, Messmer EM, Geerling G, et al. Prospective, randomized, double-blind trial to investigate the efficacy and safety of corneal cross-linking to halt the progression of keratoconus. BMC Ophthalmol. 2015;15:78.
23. Kymionis GD, Portaliou DM, Bouzoukis DI, et al. Herpetic keratitis with iritis after corneal crosslinking with riboflavin and ultraviolet A for keratoconus. J Cataract Refract Surg. 2007;33:1982–4.
24. Pollhammer M, Cursiefen C. Bacterial keratitis early after corneal crosslinking with riboflavin and ultraviolet-A. J Cataract Refract Surg. 2009;35:588–9.
25. Rama P, Di Matteo F, Matuska S, et al. Acanthamoeba keratitis with perforation after corneal crosslinking and bandage contact lens use. J Cataract Refract Surg. 2009;35:788–91.
26. Zamora KV, Males JJ. Polymicrobial keratitis after a collagen cross-linking procedure with postoperative use of a contact lens: a case report. Cornea. 2009;28:474–6.
27. Koller T, Mrochen M, Seiler T. Complication and failure rates after corneal crosslinking. J Cataract Refract Surg. 2009;35:1358–62.
28. Seiler T, Hafezi F. Corneal cross-linking-induced stromal demarcation line. Cornea. 2006;25:1057–9.
29. Herrmann CI, Hammer T, Duncker GI. [Hazeformation (corneal scarring) after cross-linking therapy in keratoconus]. Ophthalmologe. 2008;105:485–7.
30. Mazzotta C, Traversi C, Baiocchi S, et al. Corneal healing after riboflavin ultraviolet-A collagen cross-linking determined by confocal laser scanning microscopy in vivo: early and late modifications. Am J Ophthalmol. 2008;146:527–33.
31. Mazzotta C, Balestrazzi A, Baiocchi S, et al. Stromal haze after combined riboflavin-UVA corneal collagen cross-linking in keratoconus: in vivo confocal microscopic evaluation. Clin Exp Ophthalmol. 2007;35:580–2.
32. Greenstein SA, Fry KL, Bhatt J, et al. Natural history of corneal haze after collagen crosslinking for keratoconus and corneal ectasia: Scheimpflug and biomicroscopic analysis. J Cataract Refract Surg. 2010;36:2105–14.
33. Raiskup F, Hoyer A, Spoerl E. Permanent corneal haze after riboflavin-UVA-induced cross-linking in keratoconus. J Refract Surg. 2009;25:S824–8.
34. Kymionis GD, Portaliou DM, Diakonis VF, et al. Corneal collagen cross-linking with riboflavin and ultraviolet-A irradiation in patients with thin corneas. Am J Ophthalmol. 2012;153:24–8.
35. Gokhale NS. Corneal endothelial damage after collagen cross-linking treatment. Cornea. 2011;30:1495–8.
36. Bagga B, Pahuja S, Murthy S, et al. Endothelial failure after collagen cross-linking with riboflavin and UV-A: case report with literature review. Cornea. 2012;31:1197–200.
37. Labiris G, Kaloghianni E, Koukoula S, et al. Corneal melting after collagen cross-linking for keratoconus: a case report. J Med Case Rep. 2011;5:152.

38. Gokhale NS, Vemuganti GK. Diclofenac-induced acute corneal melt after collagen crosslinking for keratoconus. Cornea. 2010;29:117–9.
39. Faschinger C, Kleinert R, Wedrich A. [Corneal melting in both eyes after simultaneous corneal cross-linking in a patient with keratoconus and Down syndrome]. Ophthalmologe. 2010;107:951–2, 954–5.
40. Eberwein P, Auw-Hadrich C, Birnbaum F, et al. [Corneal melting after cross-linking and deep lamellar keratoplasty in a keratoconus patient]. Klin Monbl Augenheilkd. 2008;225:96–8.
41. Sandvik GF, Thorsrud A, Raen M, et al. Does corneal collagen cross-linking reduce the need for keratoplasties in patients with keratoconus? Cornea. 2015;34:991–5.
42. Godefrooij DA, Gans R, Imhof SM, et al. Nationwide reduction in the number of corneal transplantations for keratoconus following the implementation of cross-linking. Acta Ophthalmol. 2016;94:675–8.
43. Rebenitsch RL, Kymes SM, Walline JJ, et al. The lifetime economic burden of keratoconus: a decision analysis using a Markov model. Am J Ophthalmol. 2011;151:768–73.e762.
44. Salmon HA, Chalk D, Stein K, et al. Cost effectiveness of collagen crosslinking for progressive keratoconus in the UK NHS. Eye (Lond). 2015;29:1504–11.
45. Craig JA, Mahon J, Yellowlees A, et al. Epithelium-off photochemical corneal collagen crosslinkage using riboflavin and ultraviolet a for keratoconus and keratectasia: a systematic review and meta-analysis. Ocul Surf. 2014;12(3):202–14.
46. Sykakis E, Karim R, Evans JR, et al. Corneal collagen cross-linking for treating keratoconus. Cochrane Database Syst Rev. 2015;(3):CD010621.
47. Pron G, Ieraci L, Kaulback K. Collagen cross-linking using riboflavin and ultraviolet-a for corneal thinning disorders: an evidence-based analysis. Ont Health Technol Assess Ser. 2011;11(5):1–89.
48. Koppen C, Wouters K, Mathysen D, et al. Refractive and topographic results of benzalkonium chloride-assisted transepithelial crosslinking. J Cataract Refract Surg. 2012;38(6):1000–5.
49. Baiocchi S, Mazzotta C, Cerretani D, et al. Corneal crosslinking: riboflavin concentration in corneal stroma exposed with and without epithelium. J Cataract Refract Surg. 2009;35(5):893–9.
50. Spoerl E. Chapter 20: corneal collagen cross-linking: epithelium-on versus epithelium-off treatments. In: Hafezi F, Randleman JB, editors. Corneal collagen cross linking. Thorofare: SLACK Incorporated; 2013. p. 139–42.
51. Podskochy A. Protective role of corneal epithelium against ultraviolet radiation damage. Acta Ophthalmol Scand. 2004;82(6):714–7.
52. Wollensak G, Iomdina E. Biomechanical and histological changes after corneal crosslinking with and without epithelial debridement. J Cataract Refract Surg. 2009;35(3):540–6.
53. Kissner A, Spoerl E, Jung R, et al. Pharmacological modification of the epithelial permeability by benzalkonium chloride in UVA/Riboflavin corneal collagen cross-linking. Curr Eye Res. 2010;35(8):715–21.
54. Raiskup F, Pinelli R, Spoerl E. Riboflavin osmolar modification for transepithelial corneal cross-linking. Curr Eye Res. 2012;37(3):234–8.
55. Scarcelli G, Kling S, Quijano E, et al. Brillouin microscopy of collagen crosslinking: noncontact depth-dependent analysis of corneal elastic modulus. Invest Ophthalmol Vis Sci. 2013;54(2):1418–25.
56. Filippello M, Stagni E, O'Brart D. Transepithelial corneal collagen crosslinking: bilateral study. J Cataract Refract Surg. 2012;38(2):283–91.
57. Kocak I, Aydin A, Kaya F, et al. Comparison of transepithelial corneal collagen crosslinking with epithelium-off crosslinking in progressive keratoconus. J Fr Ophtalmol. 2014;37(5):371–6.
58. Caporossi A, Mazzotta C, Baiocchi S, et al. Riboflavin-UVA-induced corneal collagen crosslinking in pediatric patients. Cornea. 2012;31(3):227–31.
59. Al Fayez MF, Alfayez S, Alfayez Y. Transepithelial versus epithelium-off corneal collagen cross-linking for progressive keratoconus: a prospective randomized controlled trial. Cornea. 2015;34(Suppl 10):S53–6.
60. Soeters N, Wisse RPL, Godefrooij DA, et al. Transepithelial versus epithelium-off corneal cross-linking for the treatment of progressive keratoconus: a randomized controlled trial. Am J Ophthalmol. 2015;159(5):821–8.e3.

61. Gatzioufas Z, Raiskup F, O'Brart D, et al. Transepithelial corneal cross-linking using an enhanced riboflavin solution. J Refract Surg (Thorofare, N.J.: 1995). 2016;32(6):372–7.
62. Yuksel E, Novruzlu S, Ozmen MC, et al. A study comparing standard and transepithelial collagen cross-linking riboflavin solutions: epithelial findings and pain scores. J Ocul Pharmacol Ther. 2015;31(5):296–302.
63. Caporossi A, Mazzotta C, Baiocchi S, et al. Transepithelial corneal collagen crosslinking for keratoconus: qualitative investigation by in vivo HRT II confocal analysis. Eur J Ophthalmol. 2012;22(Suppl 7):S81–8.
64. Mastropasqua L, Nubile M, Lanzini M, et al. Morphological modification of the cornea after standard and transepithelial corneal cross-linking as imaged by anterior segment optical coherence tomography and laser scanning in vivo confocal microscopy. Cornea. 2013;32(6):855–61.
65. Touboul D, Efron N, Smadja D, et al. Corneal confocal microscopy following conventional, transepithelial, and accelerated corneal collagen cross-linking procedures for keratoconus. J Refract Surg (Thorofare, N.J.: 1995). 2012;28(11):769–76.
66. Bottos KM, Oliveira AG, Bersanetti PA, et al. Corneal absorption of a new riboflavin-nanostructured system for transepithelial collagen cross-linking. PLoS One. 2013;8(6):e66408.
67. Wollensak G, Hammer CM, Sporl E, et al. Biomechanical efficacy of collagen crosslinking in porcine cornea using a femtosecond laser pocket. Cornea. 2014;33(3):300–5.
68. Seiler TG, Fischinger I, Senfft T, et al. Intrastromal application of riboflavin for corneal cross-linking. Invest Ophthalmol Vis Sci. 2014;55(7):4261–5.
69. Kanellopoulos AJ. Collagen cross-linking in early keratoconus with riboflavin in a femtosecond laser-created pocket: initial clinical results. J Refract Surg (Thorofare, N.J.: 1995). 2009;25(11):1034–7.
70. Yuksel E, Bektas C, Bilgihan K. Transepithelial versus epithelium-off corneal cross-linking for the treatment of progressive keratoconus: a randomized controlled trial. Am J Ophthalmol. 2015;160(2):399–400.
71. Lombardo M, Pucci G, Barberi R, et al. Interaction of ultraviolet light with the cornea: clinical implications for corneal crosslinking. J Cataract Refract Surg. 2015;41(2):446–59.
72. Cınar Y, Cingü AK, Türkcü FM, Çınar T, Yüksel H, Özkurt ZG, Çaça I. Comparison of accelerated and conventional corneal collagen cross-linking for progressive keratoconus. Cutan Ocul Toxicol. 2014;33(3):218–22.
73. Cınar Y, Cingü AK, Turkcu FM, Yüksel H, Sahin A, Yıldırım A, Caca I. Accelerated corneal collagen cross-linking for progressive keratoconus. Cutan Ocul Toxicol. 2014;33(2):168–71.
74. Legare ME, Iovieno A, Yeung SN, et al. Corneal collagen cross-linking using riboflavin and ultraviolet A for the treatment of mild to moderate keratoconus: 2-year follow-up. J Ophthalmol. 2013;48:63–8.
75. Kymionis GD, Tsoulnaras KI, Grentzelos MA, Liakopoulos DA, Tsakalis NG, Blazaki SV, Paraskevopoulos TA, Tsilimbaris MK. Evaluation of corneal stromal demarcation line depth following standard and a modified-accelerated collagen cross-linking protocol. Am J Ophthalmol. 2014;158(4):671–5.
76. Shetty R, Nagaraja H, Jayadev C, Pahuja NK, Kurian Kummelil M, Nuijts RM. Accelerated corneal collagen cross-linking in pediatric patients: two-year follow-up results. Biomed Res Int. 2014;2014:894095.
77. Elbaz U, Shen C, Lichtinger A, Zauberman NA, Goldich Y, Chan CC, Slomovic AR, Rootman DS. Accelerated (9-mW/cm2) corneal collagen crosslinking for keratoconus-A 1-year follow-up. Cornea. 2014;33(8):769–73.
78. Jain V, Gazali Z, Bidayi R. Isotonic riboflavin and HPMC with accelerated cross-linking protocol. Cornea. 2014;33(9):910–3.
79. Pahuja N, Kumar NR, Francis M, Shanbagh S, Shetty R, Ghosh A, Roy AS. Correlation of clinical biomechanical outcomes of accelerated crosslinking (9 mW/cm^2 in 10 minutes) in keratoconus with molecular expression of ectasia-related genes. Curr Eye Res. 2016;41(11):1419–23.
80. Marino GK, Torricelli AA, Giacomin N, Santhiago MR, Espindola R, Netto MV. Accelerated corneal collagen crosslinking for postoperative LASIK ectasia: two-year outcomes. J Refract Surg. 2015;31(6):380–4.

81. Sadoughi MM, Einollahi B, Baradaran-Rafii A, Roshandel D, Hasani H, Nazeri M. Accelerated versus conventional corneal collagen cross-linking in patients with keratoconus: an intrapatient comparative study. Int Ophthalmol. 2016. https://doi.org/10.1007/s10792-016-0423-0.
82. Cingü AK, Sogutlu-Sari E, Cınar Y, Sahin M, Türkçü FM, Yüksel H, Sahin A, Caça I. Transient corneal endothelial changes following accelerated collagen cross-linking for the treatment of progressive keratoconus. Cutan Ocul Toxicol. 2014;33(2):127–31.
83. Hashemi H, Fotouhi A, Miraftab M, Bahrmandy H, Seyedian MA, Amanzadeh K, Heidarian S, Nikbin H, Asgari S. Short-term comparison of accelerated and standard methods of corneal collagen crosslinking. J Cataract Refract Surg. 2015;41(3):533–40.
84. Hashemi H, Miraftab M, Seyedian MA, Hafezi F, Bahrmandy H, Heidarian S, Amanzadeh K, Nikbin H, Fotouhi A, Asgari S. Long-term results of an accelerated corneal cross-linking protocol (18 mW/cm2) for the treatment of progressive keratoconus. Am J Ophthalmol. 2015;160(6):1164–70.
85. Chow VW, Chan TC, Yu M, Wong VW, Jhanji V. One year outcomes of conventional and accelerated collagen crosslinking in progressive keratoconus. Sci Rep. 2015;5:14425. https://doi.org/10.1038/srep14425.
86. Caporossi A, Mazzotta C, Baiocchi S, Caporossi T. Long-term results of riboflavin ultraviolet a corneal collagen crosslinking for keratoconus in Italy: the Siena eye cross study. Am J Ophthalmol. 2010;149(4):585–93.
87. Asri D, Touboul D, Fournié P, Malet F, Garra C, Gallois A, Malecaze F, Colin J. Corneal collagen crosslinking in progressive keratoconus: multicenter results from the French National Reference Center for Keratoconus. J Cataract Refract Surg. 2011;37(12):2137–43.
88. Kanellopoulos AJ. Long term results of a prospective randomized bilateral eye comparison trial of higher fluence, shorter duration ultraviolet A radiation, and riboflavin collagen cross linking for progressive keratoconus. Clin Ophthalmol. 2012;6:97–101.
89. Gatzioufas Z, Richoz O, Brugnoli E, Hafezi F. Safety profile of high-fluence corneal collagen cross-linking for progressive keratoconus: preliminary results from a prospective cohort study. J Refract Surg. 2013;29(12):846–8.
90. Wernli J, Schumacher S, Spoerl E, Mrochen M. The efficacy of corneal cross-linking shows a sudden decrease with very high intensity UV light and short treatment time. Invest Ophthalmol Vis Sci. 2013;54(2):1176–80.
91. Hammer A, Richoz O, Arba Mosquera S, Tabibian D, Hoogewoud F, Hafezi F. Corneal biomechanical properties at different corneal cross-linking (CXL) irradiances. Invest Ophthalmol Vis Sci. 2014;55(5):2881–4.
92. Chan TC, Chow VW, Jhanji V, Wong VW. Different topographic response between mild to moderate and advanced keratoconus after accelerated collagen cross-linking. Cornea. 2015;34(8):922–7.
93. Shetty R, Pahuja NK, Nuijts RM, Ajani A, Jayadev C, Sharma C, Nagaraja H. Current protocols of corneal collagen crosslinking—visual, refractive and tomographic outcomes. Am J Ophthalmol. 2015;160(2):243–9.
94. Kymionis GD, Tsoulnaras KI, Grentzelos MA, Plaka AD, Mikropoulos DG, Liakopoulos DA, Tsakalis NG, Pallikaris IG. Corneal stroma demarcation line after standard and high-intensity collagen crosslinking determined with anterior segment optical coherence tomography. J Cataract Refract Surg. 2014;40(5):736–40.
95. Kymionis GD, Grentzelos MA, Plaka AD, Tsoulnaras KI, Diakonis VF, Liakopoulos DA, Kankariya VP, Pallikaris AI. Correlation of the corneal collagen cross-linking demarcation line using confocal microscopy and anterior segment optical coherence tomography in keratoconic patients. Am J Ophthalmol. 2014;157(1):110–5.
96. Kurt T, Ozgurhan EB, Yildirim Y, Akcay BI, Cosar MG, Bozkurt E, Taskapili M. Accelerated (18mW/cm^2) corneal cross-linking for progressive keratoconus: 18-month results. J Ocul Pharmacol Ther. 2016;32(4):186–91.
97. Razmjoo H, Peyman A, Rahimi A, Modrek HJ. Cornea collagen cross-linking for keratoconus: a comparison between accelerated and conventional methods. Adv Biomed Res. 2017;6:10.

98. Mazzotta C, Traversi C, Paradiso AL, Latronico ME, Rechichi M. Pulsed light accelerated crosslinking versus continuous light accelerated crosslinking: one-year results. J Ophthalmol. 2014;2014:604731.
99. Merwald H, Klosner G, Kokesch C, Der-Petrossian M, Hönigsmann H, Trautinger F. UVA-induced oxidative damage and cytotoxicity depend on the mode of exposure. J Photochem Photobiol B. 2005;79(3):197–207.
100. Mazzotta C, Traversi C, Caragiuli S, Rechichi M. Pulsed vs continuous light accelerated corneal collagen crosslinking: in vivo qualitative investigation by confocal microscopy and corneal OCT. Eye (Lond). 2014;28(10):1179–83.
101. Moramarco A, Iovieno A, Sartori A, Fontana L. Corneal stromal demarcation line after accelerated crosslinking using continuous and pulsed light. J Cataract Refract Surg. 2015;41(11):2546–51.
102. Ozgurhan EB, Kara N, Cankaya KI, Kurt T, Demirok A. Accelerated corneal cross-linking in pediatric patients with keratoconus: 24-month outcomes. J Refract Surg. 2014;30(12):843–9.
103. Ozgurhan EB, Akcay BI, Kurt T, Yildirim Y, Demirok A. Accelerated corneal collagen cross linking in thin keratoconic corneas. J Refract Surg. 2015;31(6):386–90.
104. Mita M, Waring GO 4th, Tomita M. High-irradiance accelerated collagen crosslinking for the treatment of keratoconus: six-month results. J Cataract Refract Surg. 2014;40(6):1032–40.
105. Spoerl E, Terai N, Scholz F, Raiskup F, Pillunat LE. Detection of biomechanical changes after corneal cross-linking using Ocular Response Analyzer software. J Refract Surg. 2011;27:452–7.
106. Mazzotta C, Caporossi T, Denaro R, Bovone C, Sparano C, Paradiso A, Baiocchi S, Caporossi A. Morphological and functional correlations in riboflavin UV A corneal collagen crosslinking for keratoconus. Acta Ophthalmol. 2012;90:259–65.
107. Tomita M, Mita M, Huseynova T. Accelerated versus conventional corneal collagen crosslinking. J Cataract Refract Surg. 2014;40(6):1013–20.
108. Sherif AM. Accelerated versus conventional corneal collagen cross-linking in the treatment of mild keratoconus: a comparative study. Clin Ophthalmol. 2014;8:1435–40.
109. Beltaief O, Farah H, Kamoun R, Ben Said A, Ouertani A. Penetrating keratoplasty in children. Tunis Med. 2003;81(7):477–81.
110. Reeves SW, Stinnett S, Adelman RA, et al. Risk factors for progression to penetrating keratoplasty in patients with keratoconus. Am J Ophthalmol. 2005;140:607–11.
111. Ertan A, Muftuoglu O. Keratoconus clinical findings according to different age and gender groups. Cornea. 2008;27(10):1109–13.
112. Al Suhaibani AH, Al-Rajhi AA, Al-Motowa S, Wagoner MD. Inverse relationship between age and severity and sequelae of acute corneal hydrops associated with keratoconus. Br J Ophthalmol. 2007;91(7):984–5.
113. Leoni-Mesplie S, Mortemosque B, Touboul D, et al. Scalability and severity of keratoconus in children. Am J Ophthalmol. 2012;154:156–62.
114. Chatzis N, Hafezi F, et al. Progression of keratoconus and efficacy of pediatric [corrected] corneal collagen cross-linking in children and adolescents. J Refract Surg. 2012;28(11):753–8.
115. Downie LE. The necessity for ocular assessment in atopic children: bilateral corneal hydrops in an 8 year-old. Pediatrics. 2014;134(2):e596–601.
116. Balasubramanian SA, Pye DC, Willcox MD. Effects of eye rubbing on the levels of protease, protease activity and cytokines in tears: relevance in keratoconus. Clin Exp Optom. 2013;96:214–8.
117. Weed KH, MacEwen CJ, Giles T, Low J, McGhee CN. The Dundee University Scottish Keratoconus study: demographics, corneal signs, associated diseases, and eye rubbing. Eye (Lond). 2008;22:534–41.
118. Wisse RP, Kuiper JJ, Gans R, Imhof S, Radstake TR, Van der Lelij A. Cytokine expression in keratoconus and its corneal microenvironment: a systematic review. Ocul Surf. 2015;13(4):272–83.
119. McMonnies CW. Inflammation and keratoconus. Optom Vis Sci. 2015;92(2):e35–41.

120. Godefrooij DA, Soeters N, Imhof SM, Wisse RP. Corneal cross-linking for pediatric keratoconus: long-term results. Cornea. 2016;35(7):954–8.
121. Vinciguerra P, Albé E, Frueh BE, Trazza S, Epstein D. Two-year corneal cross-linking results in patients younger than 18 years with documented progressive keratoconus. Am J Ophthalmol. 2012;154(3):520–6.
122. Raiskup F, Spoerl E. Corneal crosslinking with riboflavin and ultraviolet A. I. Principles. Ocul Surf. 2013;11(2):65–74.
123. Raiskup F, Spoerl E. Corneal crosslinking with riboflavin and ultraviolet A. Part II. Clinical indications and results. Ocul Surf. 2013;11(2):93–108.
124. Wollensak G, Spörl E, Mazzotta C, Kalinski T, Sel S. Interlamellar cohesion after corneal crosslinking using riboflavin and ultraviolet A light. Br J Ophthalmol. 2011;95(6):876–80.
125. Mazzotta C, Hafezi F, Kymionis G, Caragiuli S, Jacob S, Traversi C, Barabino S, Randleman JB. In vivo confocal microscopy after corneal collagen crosslinking. Ocul Surf. 2015;13(4):298–314.
126. Vinciguerra R, Romano MR, Camesasca FI, Azzolini C, Trazza S, Morenghi E, Vinciguerra P. Corneal cross-linking as a treatment for keratoconus: four-year morphologic and clinical outcomes with respect to patient age. Ophthalmology. 2013;120(5):908–16.
127. Magli A, Chiariello Vecchio E, Carelli R, et al. Pediatric keratoconus and iontophoretic corneal crosslinking: refractive and topographic evidence in patients underwent general and topical anesthesia, 18 months of follow-up. Int Ophthalmol. 2016;36(4):585–90.

Crosslinking Evidences In-Vitro and In-Vivo

3

3.1 Histology After Accelerated Cross-Linking (ACXL)

3.1.1 Introduction

Keratoconus is an ectatic disease of the cornea characterized by biochemical and biomechanical instability of stromal collagen leading to a reduction of corneal thickness [1], variation in posterior and anterior corneal curvatures and progressive deterioration of visual acuity due to irregular astigmatism [1, 2]. The recent advent of corneal collagen cross-linking in the panorama of ophthalmology of the last decade [3, 4] has transformed the conventional therapy of keratoconus, including in the best case scenario, rigid contact lens wearing for a lifetime or, at worst, corneal transplant. Conservative treatment has improved and thus reduced the necessity of a lamellar and penetrating corneal graft. Riboflavin UV-A induced corneal collagen cross-linking (CXL) demonstrated its efficacy in the conservative treatment of progressive keratoconus [3, 4] and secondary corneal ectasia [5] due to its ability to increase biomechanical corneal resistance [3, 4] and intrinsic anti-collagenase activity [6]. The physiochemical basis of cross-linking lies in the photo-dynamic type I-II reactions [7], induced by the interaction between 0.1% riboflavin molecules absorbed in the corneal tissue, and UV-A rays delivered at 3 mW/cm^2 for 30 min (5.4 J/cm^2 energy dose) releasing reactive oxygen species (ROS) that mediate cross-link formation between and within collagen fibers [8, 9]. The conventional epithelium-off cross-linking procedure (CXL) demonstrated its long-term efficacy stabilizing progressive keratoconus and secondary ectasia in different clinical trials [10–14]. Conventional CXL requires a long treatment time (1 h) [15]. A novel approach called Accelerated cross-linking (ACXL), based on the physical concept of photochemical reactions stated in the Bunsen–Roscoe's law of reciprocity [16–18], has been recently proposed to shorten treatment time while maintaining the same efficacy. This theory [16] demonstrated that the photochemical process behind cross-linking depends on the absorbed UV-A energy, and its biological effect is proportional to the total energy dose delivered in the

C. Mazzotta et al., *Management of Early Progressive Corneal Ectasia*,
DOI 10.1007/978-3-319-61137-2_3

tissue [16–19]. Indeed, according to the "*equal-dose*" [18, 19] physical principle, 9 mW/cm^2 for 10 min, 30 mW/cm^2 for 3 min, 18 mW/cm^2 for 5 min, 45 mW/cm^2 for 2 min, at a constant energy dose of 5.4 J/cm^2, have the same photochemical impact of conventional 3 mW/cm^2 for 30 min [18, 19]. Moreover, an energy dose of 7.2 J/cm^2 was demonstrated to be effective both in terms of corneal strengthening and anti-enzyme activity compared with the standard dose of 5.4 J/cm^2, respectively tested by biaxial corneal extensiometry and papain digestion [20]. Previous histological reports in literature on conventional and accelerated corneal cross-linking [20, 21] demonstrated keratocyte damage and repopulation of the corneal stroma by proliferating cells, and an increase in collagen fiber diameter. These modifications are the morphological correlate of the process leading to increased corneal biomechanical stability. These observations were confirmed by in vivo studies in humans provided by Mazzotta et al. with scanning laser confocal microscopy which demonstrated the reduction in anterior and intermediate stromal keratocytes followed by gradual repopulation [22]. Long term keratoconus stability after conventional cross-linking treatment was correlated *in vivo* to increased cross-links formation, synthesis of restructured collagen and new lamellar interconnections [23].

The technique of cross-linking is evolving. According to recent demonstrations [17, 20, 24] it is possible to deliver the same energy dose to corneal tissue while shortening treatment time by setting different UV-A powers from the conventional 3 mW/cm^2 up to 45 mW/cm^2 (ACXL), reducing conventional cross-linking treatment time and increasing patient's comfort. We evaluated the photochemical effects induced by conventional CXL and Accelerated CXL in ex vivo eye-bank human corneas unsuitable for corneal transplant by means of light microscopy (LM) and transmission electron microscopy (TEM).

3.1.2 Methods

3.1.2.1 Tissue Samples

Upon ethical approval from Siena University Hospital Institutional Review Board (IRB), 24 eye-bank human corneas unsuitable for transplant (provided by Tuscany Eye Bank of Lucca, Italy) were selected as samples and subdivided as follows:

- Group A (controls): Four corneas were used as control corneas and didn't undergo any riboflavin soaking and UV-A irradiation

Treatments with Epithelium Removal (EPI-OFF)

- Group B: Four corneas after epithelium removal were soaked for 20 min with Riboflavin 0.1%-dextran 20% solution and irradiated with UV-A at 3 mW/cm^2 for 30 min (5.4 J/cm^2 dose).

- Group C: Four corneas after epithelium removal were soaked for 20 min with Riboflavin 0.1%-dextran 20% solution and irradiated with UV-A at 12 mW/cm^2 for 10 min (7.2 J/cm^2 dose).
- Group D: Four corneas after epithelium removal were soaked for 15 min with Riboflavin 0.1%-dextran 20% solution and irradiated with continuous UV-A 30 mW/cm^2 for 4 min (7.2 J/cm^2 dose).

Treatments without Epithelium Removal (EPI-ON)

- Group E: Four corneas with epithelium on, were soaked for 30 min with Riboflavin 0.1% plus BAC, EDTA, TRIS solution and irradiated with UV-A at 10 mW/cm^2 for 9 min (5.4 J/cm^2 dose).
- Group F: Four corneas were soaked with epithelium on for 10 min with Riboflavin 0.25% plus BAC, EDTA, TRIS, HPMC solution and irradiated with UV-A 45 mW/cm^2 for 2.4 min (7.2 J/cm^2 dose).

Riboflavin solutions used in the study comprised the standard Riboflavin 0.1%-Dextran 20% solution (VibeX™ Avedro Inc., Waltham, Massachusetts, USA) for the EPI-OFF treatments (Groups B, C, D), which was recently granted orphan designation by the FDA (Food and Drug Administration) for the treatment of keratoconus and corneal ectasia following refractive surgeries [25].

For the EPI-ON treatments the solutions used were: Riboflavin 0.1%, Dextran 15% plus EDTA, BAC, TRIS solution (Ricrolin TE™ Sooft, Montegiorgio, Italy) at 10 mW UV-A power (Group E) and the 0.25% Riboflavin plus BAC, EDTA, TRIS, HPMC solution (ParaCel™ Avedro Inc., Waltham, Massachusetts, USA) at 45 mW UV-A power (Group F) respectively.

Group B corneas underwent the conventional EPI-OFF CXL treatment at 3 mW/cm^2 by C.B.M. (Caporossi, Baiocchi, Mazzotta) Vega X-Linker UV-A emitter (C.S.O. Florence, Italy); Group C and Group D corneas underwent the accelerated EPI-OFF A-CXL treatment by the KXL I UV-A emitter (Avedro Inc. Waltham MS, USA).

Group E corneas underwent the trans-epithelial (TE) CXL treatment by the C.B.M. Vega X-Linker UV-A emitter (C.S.O. Florence, Italy).

Group F corneas underwent the EPI-ON A-CXL treatment by the KXL I UV-A emitter (Avedro Inc. Waltham MS, USA).

Treatment Groups and protocols are summarized in Table 3.1.

3.1.2.2 Light Microscopy and Transmission Electron Microscopy

After UV-A irradiation, samples were immediately fixed in 2.5% cacodylate-buffered glutaraldehyde pH 7.3 for 6 h at 4 °C. The specimens were washed overnight in the same buffer, post-fixed in buffered 1% osmium tetroxide for 2 h, washed, dehydrated through a graded series of ethanol, cleared in propylene-oxide and embedded in Epoxy resin (Araldite). For each sample, semi-thin sections of

Table 3.1 Overall study treatment protocols

	Treatment modality	Solution	Power (mW/cm^2)	Dose (J)	Soaking time (min)	Irradiation time (min)	Total time (min)
Group A (Control)	None	None	0	0	0	0	0
Group B (CXL)	EPI-OFF	Riboflavin 0.1%, Dextran 20%	3	5.4	20	30	50
Group C (A-CXL)	EPI-OFF	Riboflavin 0.1%, Dextran 20%	12	7.2	20	10	30
Group D (A-CXL)	EPI-OFF	Riboflavin 0.1%, Dextran 20%	30	7.2	15	4	19
Group E (TE-CXL)	EPI-ON	Riboflavin 0.1%, Dextran 15%, EDTA, BAC, TRIS	10	5.4	30	9	39
Group F (A-CXL)	EPI-ON	Riboflavin 0.25%, EDTA, BAC, TRIS, HPMC	45	7.2	10	2.40	12.40

full-thickness corneas were cut with glass knives on an LKB V Ultratome (Leica, Wetzlar, Germany), stained with toluidine blue and evaluated by light microscopy to select the appropriate areas. The blocks were trimmed around areas of interest, and ultra-thin sections were cut with a diamond knife using the same ultra-microtome, retrieved onto copper grids, double-stained with uranyl-acetate and lead citrate and examined at 100 kV with a Philips 208 S Transmission Electron Microscope (FEI Company, Eindhoven, The Netherlands) at 100 kV, at magnification ranging from ×5600 to ×89,000. Digital electron micrographs were acquired with a Mega-View III CCD (Olympus, Tokyo, Japan) and image analysis and measurements were performed using the Soft Imaging System (SIS) software, which is embedded in the TEM computer. For each Group, semithin-section evaluation included the full-thickness cornea measurement (409–561 μm); the Bowman's layer thickness measurement (8–15 μm) and the cross-linking depth estimation (38–290 μm) related to different UV-A power and protocol. The number of the keratocytes nuclei was determined by counting the cell nuclei in six fields at 250× magnification. For each specimen, ultra-structural characteristics, including qualitative findings and quantitative measurements, were examined at specific depths (50, 100, 150, 200, 300, 400 μm and pre-Descemetic stroma) on a field column through the entire thickness of the cornea. The measurements were calculated by fitting the ultrathin corneal sections on micrometric close-mesh net reticulum at ×94,000 magnification measuring fibrils number in each mesh.

3.1.3 Results

3.1.3.1 Treatment Penetration

Group B corneas (conventional CXL, 3 mW/cm^2 for 30 min) showed the maximum treatment penetration among the EPI-OFF treatments at 287 μm of corneal stroma on average; a depth of 158 μm and 87 μm on average was measured in Group C (A-CXL, 12 mW/cm^2 for 10 min) and Group D (A-CXL, 30 mW/cm^2 for 4 min) respectively, Fig. 3.1 **(top left, blue bars)** (Table 3.2).

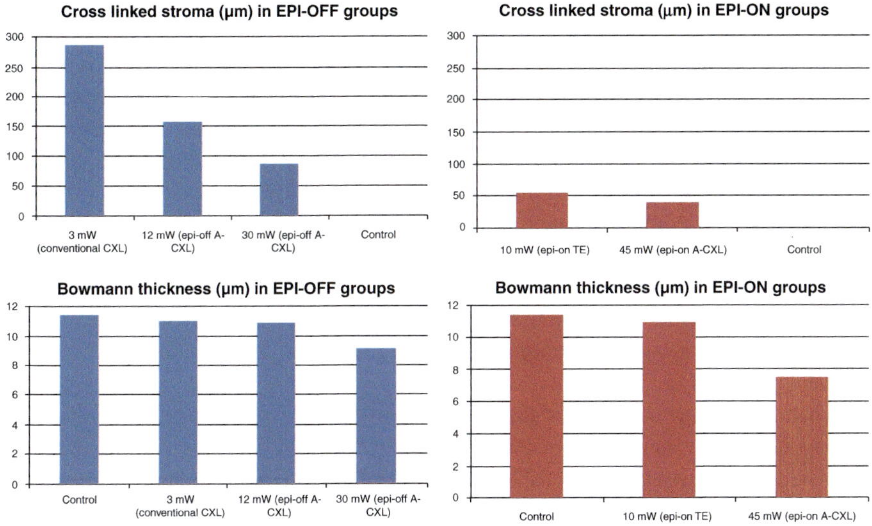

Fig. 3.1 (**a**) Cross linked stroma (μm), *top left* and *right*; (**b**) Bowmann thickness (μm), *bottom left* and *right*

Table 3.2 Overall study results

EPI-OFF	Treatment modality	Cross-linked stroma (μm)	Bowmann thickness (μm)	n° fibrils at 50 μm depth	n° fibrils at 100 μm depth	n° fibrils at 200 μm depth
Group A (Control)	None	0	11.40	44.10	42.20	30.80
Group B (CXL 3 mW/cm^2)	EPI-OFF	287	10.94	55.80	52.40	39.30
Group C (A-CXL 12 mW/cm^2)	EPI-OFF	158	10.90	56.40	51.60	30.80
Group D (A-CXL 30 mW/cm^2)	EPI-OFF	90	9.10	62.20	43.60	31.40
Group E (TE-CXL 10 mW/cm^2)	EPI-ON	56	10.96	45.20	42.30	30.70
Group F (A-CXL 45 mW/cm^2)	EPI-ON	40	7.50	72.50	43.20	31.10

EPI-ON treatments showed a depth of 56 μm on average in Group E (TE-CXL, 10 mW/cm^2 for 9 min) and 38 μm on average in Group F (A-CXL, 45 mW/cm^2 for 2 min and 40 s of irradiation time) respectively, Fig. 3.1 **(top right red bars)**.

3.1.3.2 Bowman's Layer Thickness

The Bowman's layer thickness measured demonstrated a slight decrease after EPI-OFF A-CXL at 30 mW/cm^2 for 4 min (Group D), and the most relevant thickness reduction after EPI-ON A-CXL at 45 mW/cm^2 for 2 min and 40 s of UV-A irradiation time (Group F), Fig. 3.1 (bottom left and right bars).

3.1.3.3 Semi-thin Sections

Semi-thin sections of control corneas showed the transition between the stiff cornea and the deeper corneal layers. The stiff cornea in control samples was estimated at 160 μm ± 149–171 μm depth on average, and showed a dense and compacted collagen lamellae compared to less packaged deeper layers (Fig. 3.2a).

Group B corneas (conventional CXL treatment, 3 mW/cm^2 for 30 min) showed deeper collagen compaction and keratocytes apoptosis approximately at 287 μm (274–300 μm) duplicating the appearance of the stiff cornea as clearly showed in Fig. 3.2b.

Group C Corneas (Accelerated CXL, 12 mW/cm^2 for 10 min) showed collagen compaction and keratocytes apoptosis approximately at 158 μm (145–171 μm) of corneal stroma, Fig. 3.2d.

Group D Corneas (Accelerated CXL, 30 mW/cm^2 for 4 min) showed stromal collagen compaction and keratocytes apoptosis at 90 μm (76–98 μm), Fig. 3.2c.

Group E Corneas (TE-CXL, 10 mW/cm^2 for 9 min) showed collagen compaction and keratocytes apoptosis approximately at 56 μm (32–44 μm), Fig. 3.2f.

Group F Corneas (EPI-ON Accelerated CXL, 45 mW/cm^2 for 2 min and 40 s) showed collagen compaction and keratocytes apoptosis approximately at 40 μm (53–59 μm), Fig. 3.2e.

3.1.3.4 Number of Collagen Fibrils Estimated at TEM Ultrathin Sections

The average number of collagen fibrils estimated at TEM ultrathin sections was assumed an indicative parameter of CXL-induced corneal collagen compaction at different stromal depths (50–100–200 μm) compared to control corneas, as shown in Fig. 3.3.

At a depth of 50 μm the number of collagen fibrils was, on average, 55.8 for conventional CXL, 45.2 for TE-CXL, 56.4 for A-CXL at 12 mW/cm^2, 62.2 for A-CXL at 30 mW/cm^2, 72.5 for epi-on A-CXL at 45 mW/cm^2 and 44.1 in the control group, as shown in Figs. 3.3 and 3.4.

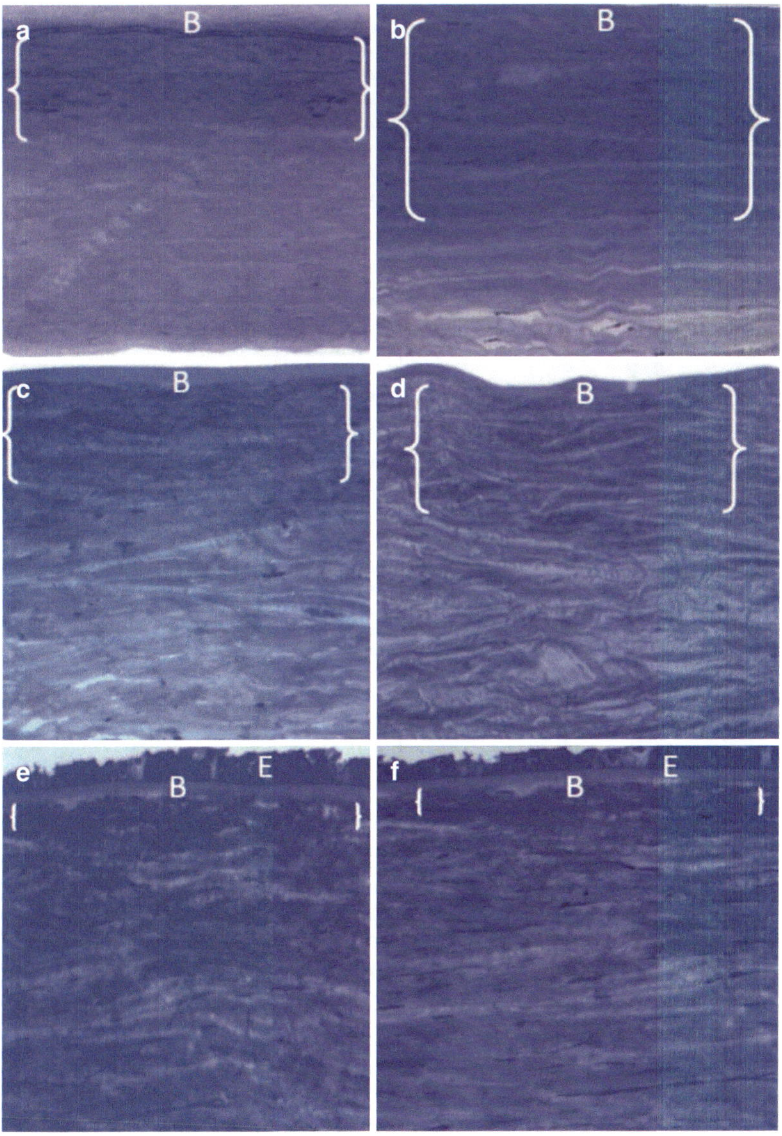

Fig. 3.2 Semi-thin sections. Group A (control) is placed at the *top left* (**a**) showing high lamellar compaction in the first 150 μm (stiff cornea). Group B (conventional CXL at 3 mW/cm^2) placed at the *top right* (**b**) showing the deeper keratocytes apoptosis associated with lamellar compaction approximately at 300 μm depth duplicating the stiff cornea; Group D (epi-off A-CXL at 30 mW/cm^2) placed at the *mid left* (**c**) showing apoptosis and collagen compaction approximately at 100 μm; Group C (epi-off A-CXL at 12 mW/cm^2) placed at the *mid right* (**d**) showing keratocytes apoptosis and collagen compaction approximately at 180 μm; Group F (CXL at 45 mW/cm^2) is placed at the *bottom left* (**e**) showing a collagen compaction and keratocytes apoptosis approximately at 50 μm; Group E (epi-on TE at 10 mW/cm^2) is placed at the *bottom right* (**f**) showing a collagen compaction and keratocytes apoptosis approximately at 50 μm. *E* Epithelium, *B* Bowman's layer; *Curly brackets* define the stromal area and depth where the tissue is denser

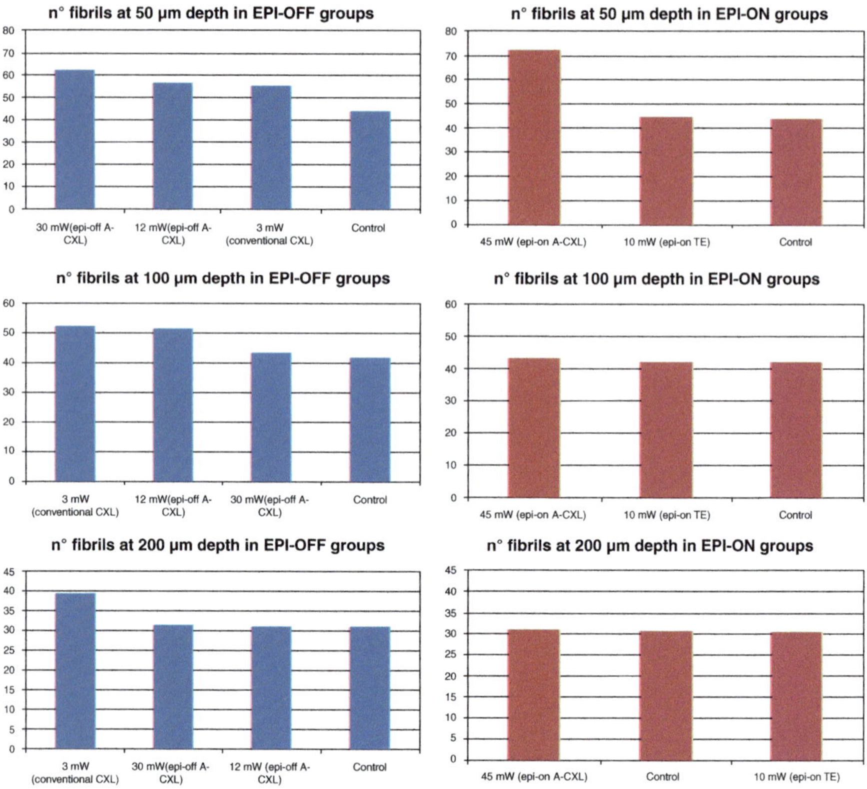

Fig. 3.3 (**a**) Number of fibers per area at 50 μm depth; (**b**) Number of fibers per area at 100 μm depth; (**c**) Number of fibers per area at 200 μm depth

At a depth of 100 μm the number of collagen fibrils was, on average, 52.4 for conventional CXL, 42.3 for epi-on TE, 51.6 for A-CXL at 12 mW/cm^2, 43.6 for A-CXL at 30 mW/cm^2, 43.2 for epi-on A-CXL at 45 mW/cm^2 and 42.2 in the control group, as shown in Figs. 3.3 and 3.5.

At a depth of 200 μm the number of fibrils was, on average, 39.3 per mesh-area for conventional CXL, 30.7 for epi-on TE, 30.8 for A-CXL at 12 mW/cm^2, 31.4 for A-CXL at 30 mW/cm^2, 31.1 for epi-on A-CXL at 45 mW/cm^2 and 30.8 per area in the control group, as shown in Figs. 3.3 and 3.6. ACXL induced a diffuse keratocytes apoptosis in the anterior corneal stroma reached by the treatment which is well evident at TEM, as shown in Fig. 3.7.

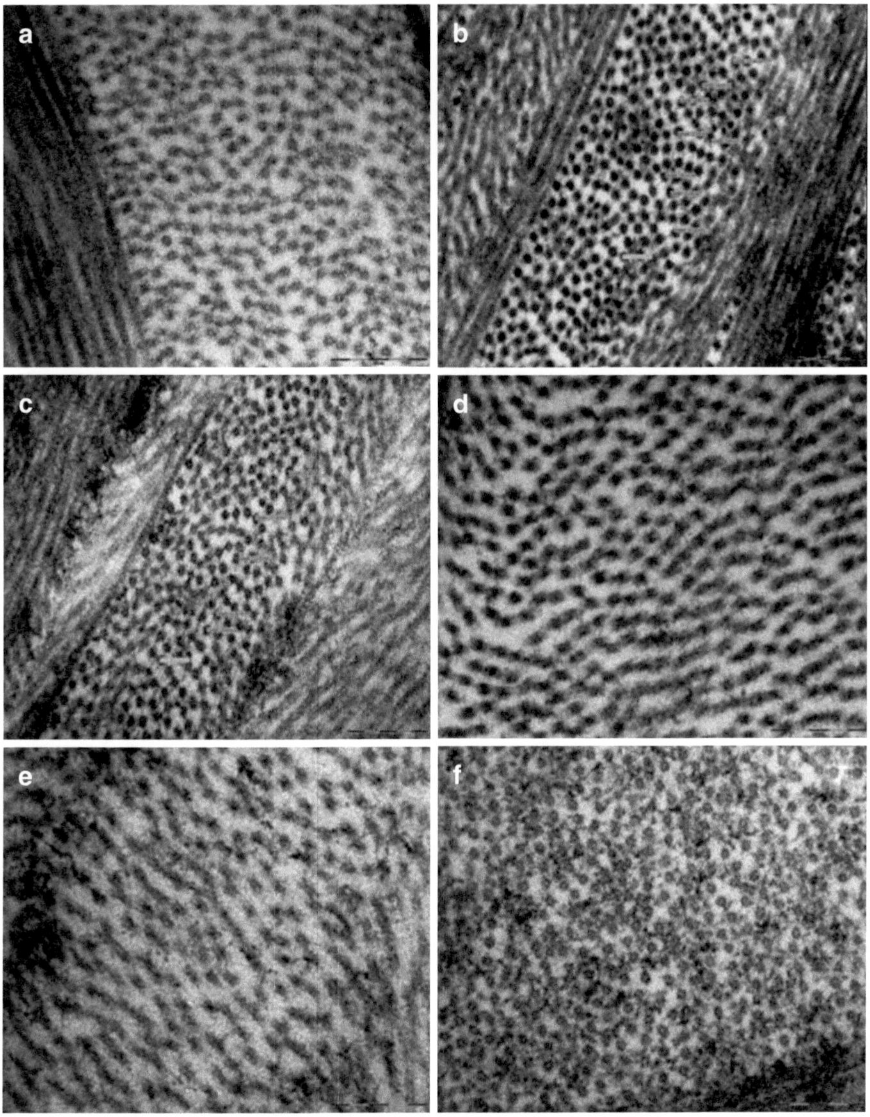

Fig. 3.4 Photomicrograph of collagen fibrils density at 50 μm depth for (**a**) Group A (control); (**b**) Group B (conventional CXL at 3 mW/cm^2); (**c**) Group E (epi-on TE at 10 mW/cm^2); (**d**) Group C (epi-off A-CXL at 12 mW/cm^2); (**e**) Group D (epi-off A-CXL at 30 mW/cm^2); (**f**) Group F (CXL at 45 mW/cm^2) (Uranyl acetate-lead citrate ×89,000)

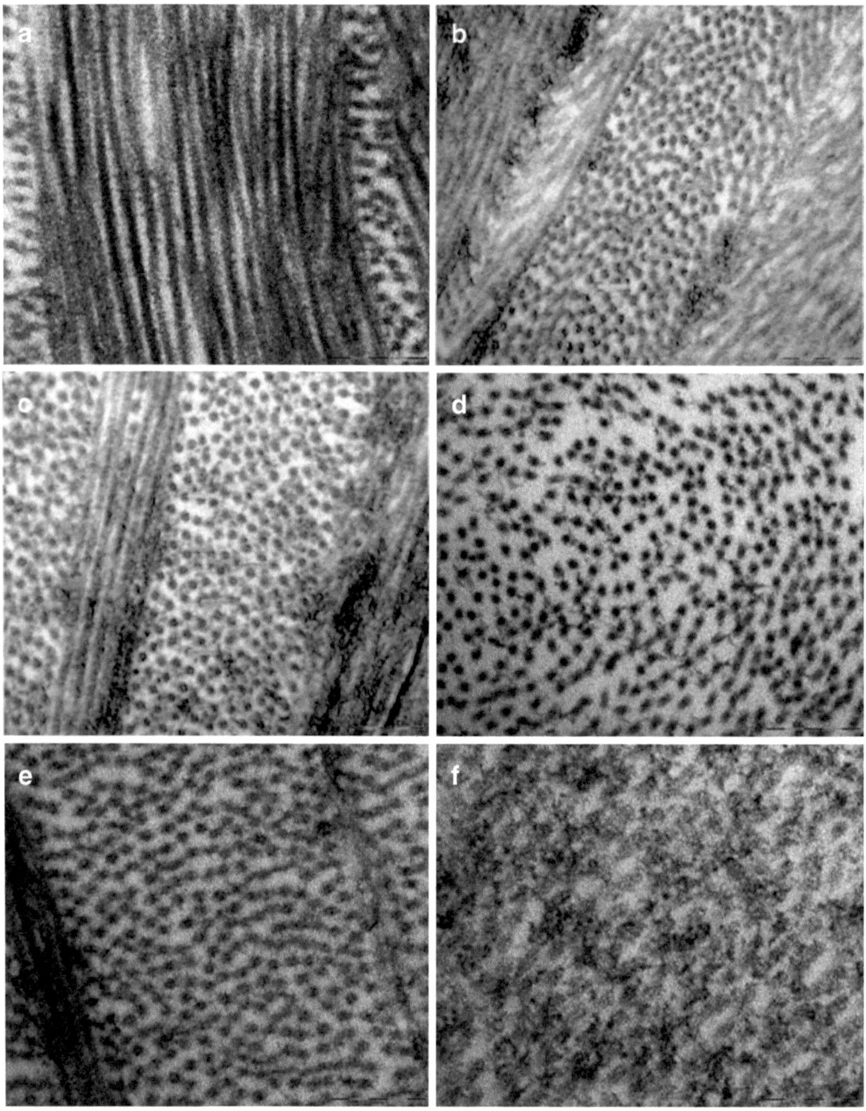

Fig. 3.5 Photomicrograph of collagen fibrils density at 100 μm depth for (**a**) Group A (control); (**b**) Group B (conventional CXL at 3 mW/cm^2); (**c**) Group E (epi-on TE at 10 mW/cm^2); (**d**) Group C (epi-off A-CXL at 12 mW/cm^2); (**e**) Group D (epi-off A-CXL at 30 mW); (**f**) Group F (CXL at 45 mW/cm^2) (Uranyl acetate-lead citrate ×89,000)

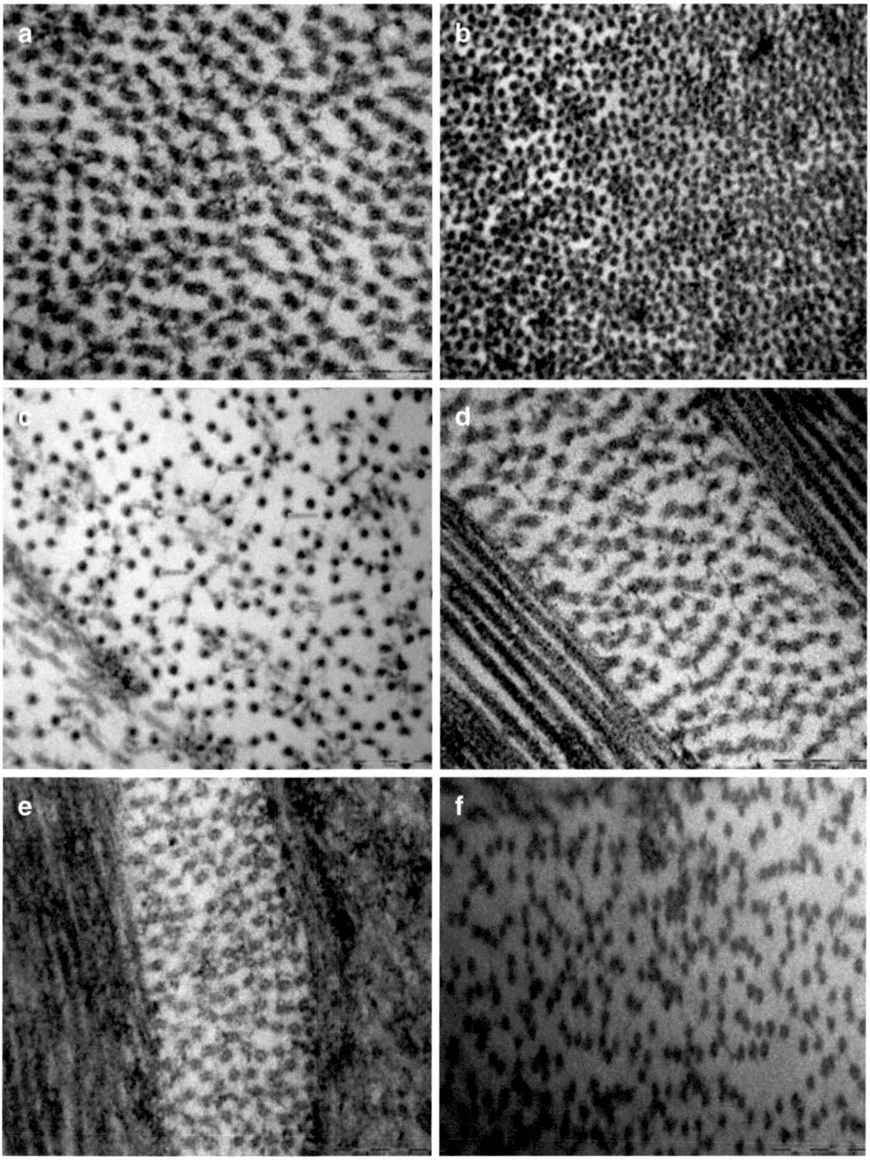

Fig. 3.6 Photomicrograph of collagen fibrils density at 200 μm depth for (**a**) Group A (control); (**b**) Group B (conventional CXL at 3 mW/cm^2); (**c**) Group E (epi-on TE at 10 mW/cm^2); (**d**) Group C (epi-off A-CXL at 12 mW/cm^2); (**e**) Group D (epi-off A-CXL at 30 mW/cm^2); (**f**) Group F (CXL at 45 mW/cm^2) (Uranyl acetate-lead citrate ×89,000)

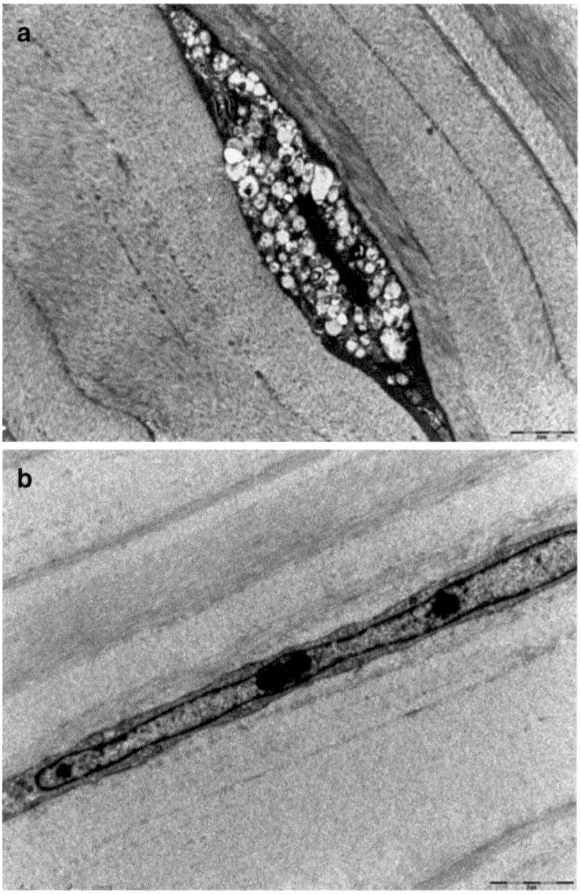

Fig. 3.7 (**a**) Apoptotic stromal keratocyte; (**b**) Normal stromal keratocyte (Uranyl acetate-lead citrate ×5600)

3.1.4 Discussion

The study provided in vitro descriptive evidences concerning 7.2 J dose Accelerated CXL compared to conventional 5.4 J dose CXL in a representative series of 24 ex vivo human corneas, identifying the differences between treatment depths based on different UV-A power settings, exposure times and delivered doses [4, 11, 21].

Accelerated CXL treatment depth, estimated in terms of CXL keratocytes induced apoptosis and collagen fibers density, resulted as inversely proportional to UV-A power (higher UV-A power induced lower treatment depth) and directly proportional to exposure time (longer exposure induced deeper cells apoptosis) in all epithelium-off corneas (Groups B, C and D). Conversely, the higher UV-A power seemed to increase the number of fibrils × analyzed area, but this outcome only resulted clearly at a depth of 50 μm. At this depth, the density of collagen fibrils was higher (higher UV-A fluency induced higher fibrils density). Superior to 50 μm, the increased density of collagen fibrils became less evident, and at 100 μm there was no difference among the various groups. The study demonstrated that by increasing exposure time while maintaining equal UV-A energy doses, treatment depth was increased favouring deeper compacted corneal tissue.

No substantial differences were found in term of fibrils density between control corneas and groups D and F (with 30 and 45 mW of UV-A power, respectively) with shorter exposure times (30 mW for 4 min and 45 mW for 2.40 min). These findings suggested that A-CXL with high UV-A irradiance and shorter exposure time induced the cross-linking of the corneal stroma under a depth of 150 μm, on average, covering the so called "stiff-cornea". Beyond a depth of 150 μm (200 μm with epithelium) there were no substantial differences between treated and untreated corneas (controls).

According to this data Accelerated cross-linking may penetrate deeper in the corneal stroma if UV-A fluency is kept at 15 mW, and under with exposure time of at least 10 min with continuous or pulsed light [26].

3.1.5 Conclusions

According to biomechanical studies [17], CXL treatment should cover at least 200 μm of corneal stroma (exceeding the stiff cornea) and UV-A power and exposure time should be calibrated to achieve this depth. *This is possible after epithelium removal ACXL, calibrating the UV-A power between 9 and 15 mW/cm^2 at constant Fluence (E dose) of 5.4 J/cm^2*. This data emerged from the laboratory study performed by Krueger, Herekar and Spoerl [26], demonstrating that high-irradiance CXL with UV-A exposures of 9 and 15 mW/cm^2 was equally efficacious, indicating a comparable efficacy in stiffening corneal collagen with standard irradiance of 3 mW/cm^2 but with the advantage of considerably less exposure time.

In conclusion, the rapidity of high-irradiance cross-linking offers great advantages in clinical applications as a practical consideration, where 30 min is too long for most clinicians and their patients. TEM analysis demonstrated that the depth of keratocytes apoptosis depends on UV-A power and exposure time. The laboratory study performed by S. Baiocchi, C. Mazzotta and M. de Santi at the Ophthalmic Operative Unit and Anatomy and Pathology Unit of the University of Siena, suggested that keratocytes apoptosis well complies with the treatment depth, as previously demonstrated in histological studies performed by Mencucci et al. [21] and in vivo confocal analysis performed by Mazzotta et al., after conventional and accelerated CXL [22, 23, 27].

Conventional cross-linking treatment determined the higher penetration depth with an appreciable fibrils compaction up to 250–300 μm of corneal stroma, allowing deeper crosslinking impact (the stiff cornea at semi-thin sections seemed duplicated as shown in Fig. 3.2b). On the other hand, accelerated corneal collagen cross-linking at 30 mW for 4 min reduced treatment time to under 20 min, inducing a detectable cross-linking impact (keratocytes apoptosis and fibrils compaction) under a depth of 160 μm, demonstrating that higher UV-A power induced lower treatment penetration reaching the stiff cornea, not beyond. The higher fibre density was limited to the anterior 50 μm, and further experimental investigations should be attempted in order to differentiate if this is linked to higher UV-A irradiance or to higher energy dose (7.2 J/J/cm^2).

In vivo measurements of corneal elastic modulus are necessary to determine the biomechanical resistance induced by the different treatment protocols, and the overall biomechanical effect in terms of ectasia stabilization should also be determined in different clinical settings according to patients age and ectasia staging. A recently published laboratory study in porcine corneas reported a decreased biomechanical effect of accelerated CXL using high UV-A irradiance with short irradiation time settings, concluding that intra-stromal oxygen diffusion capacity and increased oxygen consumption associated with higher irradiances may be a possible limiting factor, leading to reduced treatment efficiency [28].

On the other hand, the data which emerged from the laboratory study performed by Krueger, et al. [26] demonstrated that high-irradiance CXL with continuous or fractionated UV-A light exposure of 9 and 15 mW/cm^2 was equally efficacious, indicating a comparable efficacy in stiffening corneal collagen with standard irradiance of 3 mW/cm,^{2} but with the advantage of considerably less exposure time. This is the scientific point of reference of the new ACXL Siena Protocol performed by Mazzotta [29] at the Siena Crosslinking Center® (See Chap. 4).

In the Siena experimental study, the structure of Bowman's lamina was also modified in high-irradiance accelerated cross-linking performed with epithelium in situ. The effect (keratocytes apoptosis, fibrils compaction) of both trans-epithelial accelerated CXL treatment at 100 μm depth was superimposable.

This preliminary histological data may contribute to a better understanding of accelerated CXL impact using high UV-A power and exposure times. Brillouin microscopy allowed imaging and quantifying CXL-induced mechanical changes without contact in a depth-dependent manner at high spatial resolution (See this chapter). This technique may be useful to evaluate the mechanical outcomes of CXL procedures, to compare different crosslinking agents, and for real-time monitoring of CXL in clinical and experimental settings [30, 31].

3.2 In Vivo Confocal Microscopy

3.2.1 Introduction

First described by Marvin Minsky [32] in the last century, in vivo confocal microscopy (IVCM) provides a powerful, high resolution, minimally invasive, steady-state and dynamic assessment of the ocular surface at the cellular level (Fig. 3.8).

The basic principle of IVCM involves the optical sectioning of the cornea. Light is passed through an aperture and focused by an objective lens onto a small area of the examined specimen. The light reflected from the specimen then passes through a second objective lens, and focuses on a second aperture that is arranged so that out-of-focus light is eliminated. Because the illumination and detection paths share

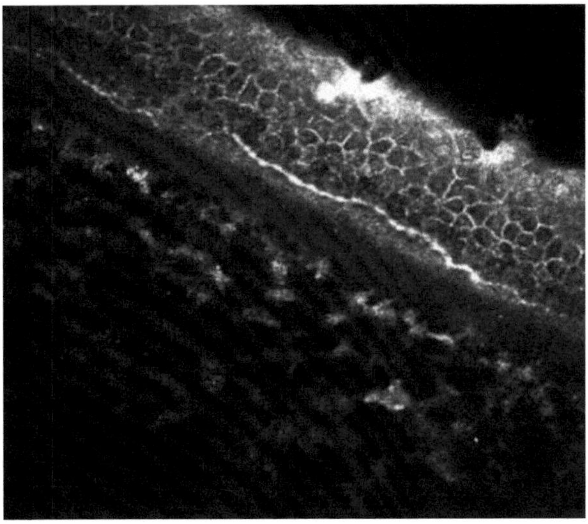

Fig. 3.8 IVCM scan provides a similar level of structural detail as light microscopy. Epithelium with cellular stratification, sub-basal nerve plexus, upon the Bowman's lamina, stroma and keratocytes

the same focal plane, the term "*confocal*" is used. The ability of the system to discriminate between light that is not on the confocal plane yields images of higher lateral and axial resolution (1 μm) and variable depth *z*-axis with a range of 4–25 μm, despite the limitation of a small field of view. Although the first IVCM analysis were essentially qualitative, the HRT III-Rostock Cornea Module (RCM) confocal microscope has been improved for manual and automated quantitative analysis of keratocytes, epithelial, endothelial cells and nerves densities measurement [33] (Table 3.3).

Quantitative analysis of keratocytes density varies with cornea depth, [34]. Due to high image contrast of the stromal cell nuclei, keratocytes density is reliable both in manual and automated measurements 39,392 + 652 cells/mm^3 vs. 40,781 + 1526 cells/mm^3. Nerve structure and quantification still needs standardizing, in point of fact measurements of normal nerve fiber density can vary widely across the cornea, with ranges from 62.5 fibers/mm^2 to 706.3 fibers/mm. Haze quantitative analysis can be assessed by measuring stromal light back-scattering in μm × pixel intensity expressed by Confocal Backscatter Units (CBU); however, measurement incorporates all factors that might contribute to interface backscatter, such as keratocyte activation, edema, and fibrosis. As consequence of small fields of view, reproducible investigation and quantification of the same areas over time is virtually impossible, [35]. The safety of riboflavin and UVA-induced corneal collagen cross-linking (CXL) was demonstrated in vivo in humans for the first time at international level with direct laser scanning IVCM by Mazzotta [22, 23, 34, 36–42] both in conventional and accelerated CXL protocols with and without epithelium removal. After Mazzotta first international reports, other important Authors performed the In Vivo confocal microscopy after standard and accelerated CXL protocol, substantially confirming the previous findings [43–50], as showed in Tables 3.4 and 3.5.

Table 3.3 In vivo confocal microscopy findings after conventional CXL

Author	Country	Treatment	N. eyes	F-up (months)	Epithelial healing (days)	Nerves regeneration (months)	Keratocytes repopulation (months)	Endothelium
Mazzotta et al. 2006	Italy	CXL	10	6	5	6	n.a.	Unaltered
Mazzotta et al. 2007	Italy	CXL	10	6	4	6	6	Unaltered
Mazzotta et al. 2008	Italy	CXL	44	36	4	12	6	Unaltered
Kymionis et al. 2009	Greece	CXL	10	6	4	6	6	Unaltered
Croxatto et al. 2010	Argentina	CXL	18	36	4	6	6	Unaltered
Knappe et al. 2011	Germany	CXL	8	12	14	12	6	Unaltered
Mazzotta et al. 2012	Italy	TE-CXL	10	6	4	No nerve loss	Unchanged	Unaltered
Toboul et al. 2012	France	TE-CXL	8	6	3	No nerve loss	Unchanged	Unaltered
Jordan et al. 2014	N. Zealand	CXL	38	12	n.a.	12 (to baseline values)	12 (to baseline values)	Unaltered
Sharma et al. 2015	India	CXL	23	6	7	6	6	Unaltered
Mazzotta et al. Review 2015	Italy	CXL	44	10 y	4	12	12	Unaltered

Table 3.4 In vivo confocal microscopy findings after ACXL

Author	Country	Treatment	N. eyes	F-up (months)	Epithelial healing (days)	Nerves regeneration (months)	Keratocytes repopulation (months)	Endothelium
Toboul et al. 2012	France	ACXL	8	6	3	n.a.	6	Unaltered
Mazzotta et al. 2014	Italy	ACXL	20	6	4	6	6	Unaltered
Bouheraoua et al. 2014	France	ACXL	15	6	n.a.	6 (partial)	6 (partial)	Unaltered
Mazzotta et al. Review 2015	Italy	ACXL	30	5 y	4	12	12	Unaltered

Table 3.5 HRT quantitative analysis of keratocyte density after CXL, ACXL, TE CXL, and ACXL

Keratocyte/mm^2 100 μm depth	Pre op	1 m	6 m	12 m	24 m
CXL	588 ± 39	No	444 ± 38	589 ± 34	622 ± 44
ACXL	464 ± 72	No	359 ± 34	450 ± 40	446 ± 39
TE CXL	502 ± 42	489 ± 30	511 ± 42	601 ± 35	599 ± 41
TE ACXL	699 ± 35	594 ± 32	690 ± 65	804 ± 69	769 ± 52

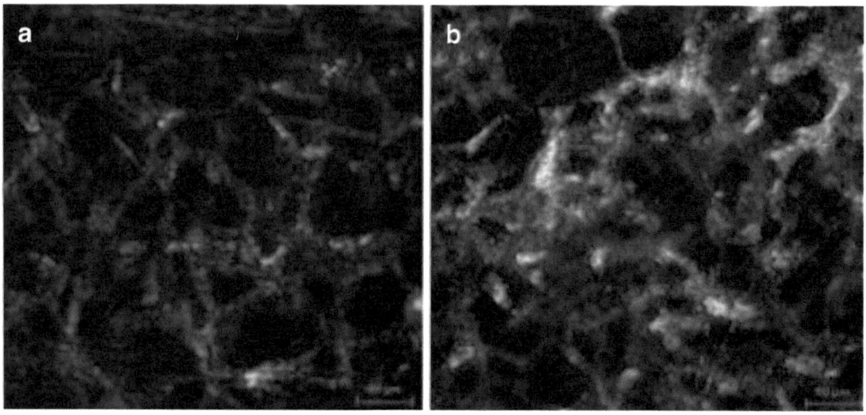

Fig. 3.9 IVCM scan of lacunar edema and keratocyes apoptosis of the anterior-mid stroma 1-month after epithelium-off standard (**a**) and accelerated CXL (**b**)

3.2.2 Stromal Healing After CXL

Review IVCM studies [34] after epithelium-off CXL and ACXL protocols invariably revealed the disappearance of keratocytes from the anterior and intermediate stroma due to cells apoptosis and photo-necrosis. This condition was associated with uneven stromal edema, which assume a lacunar appearance, Fig. 3.9.

Early postoperative keratocyte apoptosis was found in conventional CXL, TE-CXL, ACXL with continuous light, and ACXL with pulsed light, representing different depths and intensities based on the absence or presence of the epithelium and on different UV-A power settings.

Associated postoperative stromal edema tends to persist after the operation (it is detectable in epithelium-off treatment for at least 3 months and clinically for 1–2 months), progressively reducing after topical steroid therapy. A dense network of *trabecular patterned* fibrils, in which hyper-reflecting clustered *phantom cells* were visible (presumably keratocytes apoptotic bodies) and other elongated residues of degenerating keratocytes. The intensity of corneal edema increased linearly with intensifying UV-A power simultaneously with the reflectivity of extracellular *trabecular patterned* tissue surrounding the edematous lacunae.

IVCM demonstrated a progressive stromal repopulation by keratocytes from deeper (not-irradiated) layers, and in a centripetal direction from the non-irradiated periphery surrounding epithelial removal (beyond a diameter of 9 mm). It starts between the second and third month after treatment, with the reappearance of activated cell nuclei in the anterior and intermediate stroma. Six months after the treatment, cell re-colonization was still incomplete. Quantitative analysis showed complete cells repopulation 1 year after treatment as shown in Table 3.5, Fig. 3.10.

The demarcation lines detected after epithelium-off CXL and ACXL represent an expression of light-scattering through different tissue densities. This underlies the transition from an edematous area devoid of cells (stromal edema and apoptosis spreading ±20–50 microns) to an area unreached by irradiation and commonly populated by cells. The deep corneal stroma (beyond 300 μm in conventional CXL, 200 μm in A-CXL, 100 μm in TE CXL and TE ACXL) and lateral stroma (beyond 9 mm diameter) did not undergo tissue changes beyond vertical and lateral demarcation lines. In addition, no changes in density or morphology of the endothelium could be detected by the standard and accelerated cross-linking methods (Table 3.6).

The depth of demarcation lines represents an indirect expression of CXL penetration, and correlates well with its biomechanical and functional impact [34]. The results

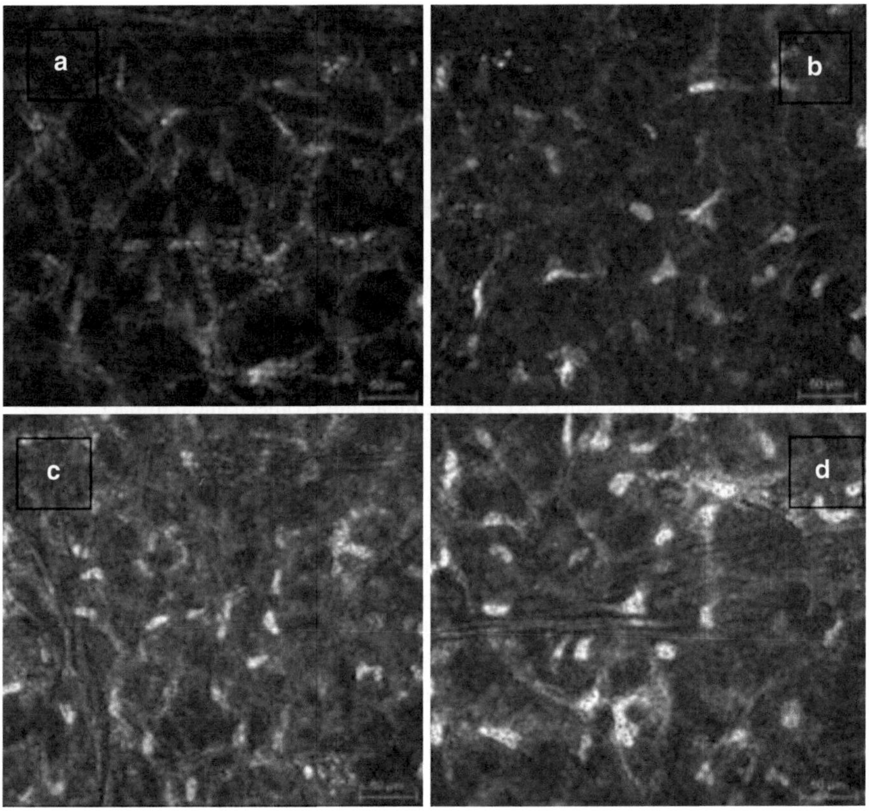

Fig. 3.10 Progressive stromal repopulation after CXL. Scan (**a**) first postoperative month with absence of keratocytes and lacunar edema; Scan (**b**) initial repopulation at third postoperative month with gradual disappearing of postoperative edema; Scan (**c**) increased cell repopulation of the anterior-mid stroma by activated keratocytes nuclei and increased extracellular matrix density. Scan (**d**) complete keratocytes repopulation 1 year after CXL treatment

Table 3.6 Demarcation line depth

IVCM in CXL	Conventional CXL 3 mW	C-light ACXL 30 mW	P-light ACXL 30 mW	TE CXL 3 mW	TE ACXL 45 mW
Average demarcation line depth	350 ± 20 μm	200 ± 20 μm	250 ± 20 μm	100 ± 20 μm	100 ± 20 μm

[a]Average epithelial thickness: 50 ± 5 μm

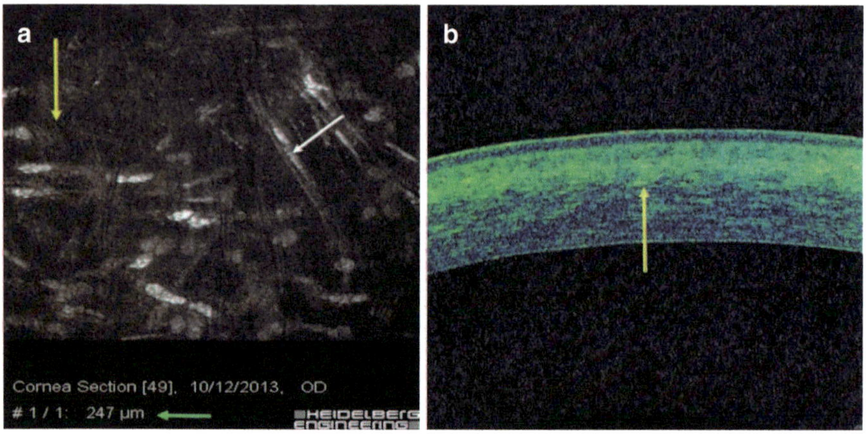

Fig. 3.11 *Yellow arrows* indicate the IVCM Demarcation line (**a**) and Spectral Domain Corneal OCT (**b**) after high-irradiance fractionated or pulsed light (1 s on/1 s off) 30 mW Accelerated-CXL

of the first confocal pilot studies in humans showed that treatment penetration varies to some extent and connects with CXL biochemical and biomechanical impact.

IVCM after continuous-UV-A light exposure A-CXL, after continuous-UV-A light exposure A-CXL, IVCM resulted in the anterior stromal tissue presenting high reflectivity in the anterior stroma with keratocytes loss (apoptosis hence photo-necrosis) up to 150 μm of depth with classical spongy or lacunar edema, as previously demonstrated in conventional epithelium-off CXL. These aspects were evident until the third postoperative month, gradually disappearing thereafter.

IVCM data of increased stromal reflectivity (corneal edema associated with cells apoptosis, nerve disappearance with hyper-dense extracellular matrix), and demarcation lines were comparatively verified and confirmed by corneal OCT at a mean depth of 150 μm (range 140–200 μm) after continuous light ACXL and 240 μm (range 200–250 μm) after pulsed light ACXL, Fig. 3.11.

Transepithelial (TE) CXL and A-CXL showed a more diffuse than lacunar edema associated with limited and uneven cell apoptosis confined in the anterior stroma under the Bowman lamina at a mean depth of 80 μm (range 50–100 μm), no

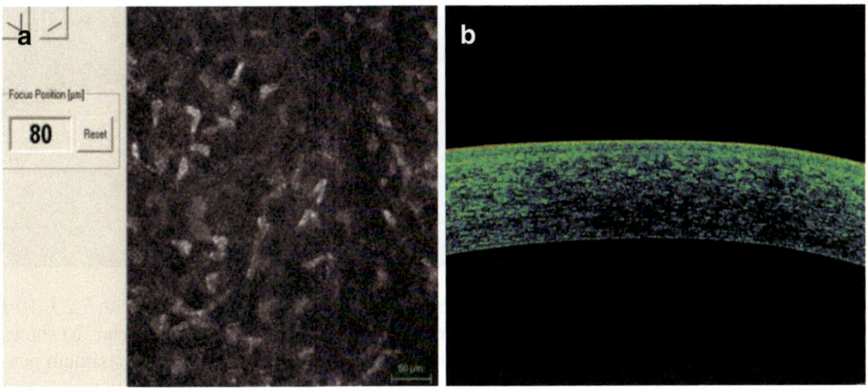

Fig. 3.12 IVCM and corneal OCT after TE CXL and ACXL. No Demarcation line was evident at IVCM (**a**) and Spectral Domain Corneal OCT (**b**) after transepithelial UV-A exposure with conventional (3 mW) and high-irradiance (10 and 45 mW) CXL. A limited and uneven apoptotic affect is detectable in the anterior stroma at a mean depth of 80 μm. OCT corneal scans confirmed a slightly increased reflectivity under the Bowman lamina without an evident demarcation line

demarcation lines were detected both at IVCM and spectral domain OCT corneal postoperative investigation as showed in Fig. 3.12.

IVCM analysis documented that by increasing the UV-A power while reducing treatment exposure times, limited penetration is achieved. As well demonstrated after continuous light ACXL with 30 mW/cm.^{2} On the other hand, fractionating UV-A exposure IVCM evidenced better penetration. In any case, deeper cell viability is achieved by prolonging exposure time while maintaining the Energy dose delivered in the corneal tissue, [42].

In our experience, by using Energy doses of 10 and 15 J/cm^2 like in the photorefractive intra-stromal crosslinking protocol (PiXL), keratocytes apoptosis was found between 250 and 300 μm. IVCM and corneal OCT scans revealed a type of multiple demarcation lines underlying the different energy doses used according to topography-guided zonal CXL protocol [42], Figs. 3.13 and 3.14.

IVCM permits a novel introduction in understanding CXL induced biodynamic interactions: treatment volume is not only related to exposure time and UV A power, but also to Energy dose. Conforming to our IVCM analysis, by using the conventional energy dose of 5.4 J/cm^2 the CXL stromal penetration (cell apoptosis) appeared to be inversely proportional to UV-A power (the lower UV power, the deeper penetration, the higher UV power, the lower penetration), directly proportional to Exposure time (the shorter time, the lower penetration, the longer time the deeper penetration). The same basic concepts are applicable to 7.2 J/cm^2 E dose. After high irradiance, fractionated ACXL with 7.2 J/cm^2, our published IVCM data showed a bit more hyper-reflective stromal tissue that could be correlated with higher collagen compaction compared to 5.4 J E dose. Nevertheless, no dose-depending substantial differences were found. IVCM showed that by using an

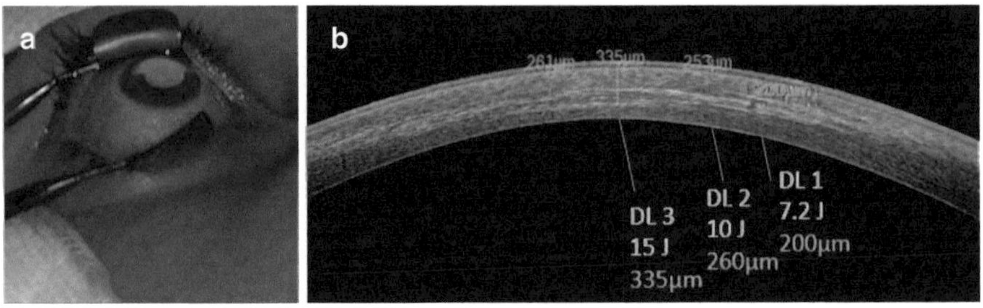

Fig. 3.13 Photorefractive intra-stromal high irradiance fractionated crosslinking with 7.2 J, 10 J and 15 J/cm^2 according to different corneal curvatures (PiXL protocol (**a**). OCT scan (**b**) shows multiple demarcation lines according to different Energy and Exposure time. The maximum penetration was recorded with 10 and 15 J/cm^2, at 260 and 340 µm respectively.

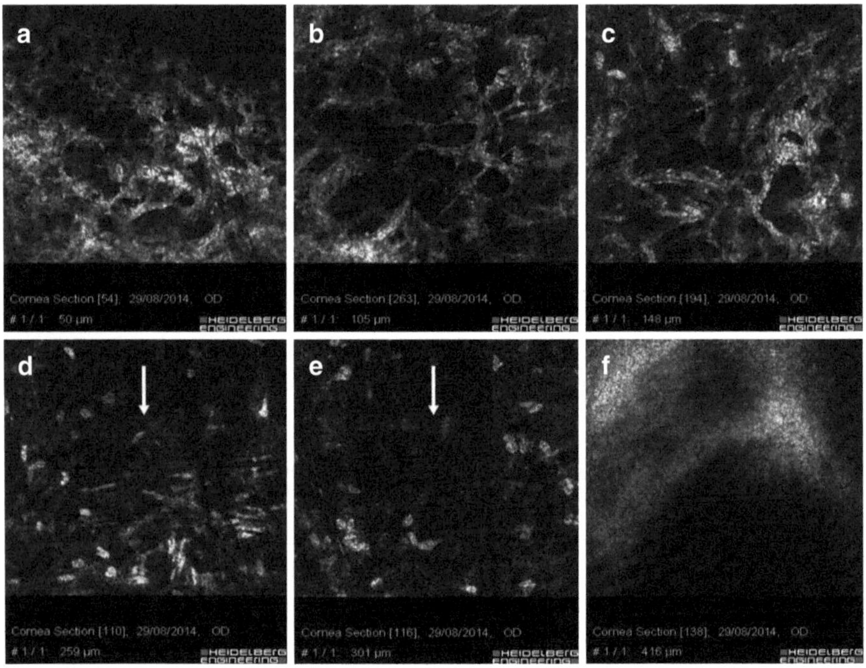

Fig. 3.14 IVCM scans in the first month after high-irradiance topography-guided CXL. Different apoptosis-based demarcation or vertical transition lines were documented at 200 µm depth in the flattest areas 48 D and under) irradiated at 7.2 J/cm^2 (scans **a**–**c**); at 260 µm depth in the area (>48 D and ≤52 D) irradiated at 10 J/cm^2 E dose (scan **d**); at 335 µm depth in the steepest cone area (>52 D) irradiated at 15 J/cm^2 E dose (scan **e**). Regular endothelium mosaic (Scan **f**)

energy dose over 7.2 J/cm^2 we achieve higher penetration as well as if with reduced exposure time and increased UV power [42]. This aspect should be further investigated and could change CXL technique application or customization.

Other important variables influencing postoperative cell apoptosis is riboflavin concentration (higher concentration lower penetration) and soaking time (shorter time, lower penetration).

3.2.3 Epithelium

Basal corneal epithelium regenerates quickly (within 3–4 days) under a therapeutic soft contact lens bandage after epi-off CXL and ACXL. One month after CXL, it was very thin (10–20 μm), and after 3 months the thickness increased to 30–40 μm on average, slightly under the normal value (50 μm). IVCM showed a full return to baseline pachymetry data between the third and sixth month after procedure (50–55 μm). IVCM revealed time-dependent postoperative regeneration and successive stratification of the corneal epithelium, smoothing corneal surface irregularities and improving corneal optical properties without limbal damage, Fig. 3.15.

3.2.4 Nerves

Micro-morphological analysis of the sub-epithelial nerve plexus by confocal microscopy showed the disappearance of sub-epithelial nerve fibres from the central treated area for up to a month after treatment. Riboflavin concentrates 95% of the UVA energy in the sub-epithelial and anterior-mid stroma, causing necrosis of nerve fibres in the 9 mm diameter irradiated area. Sub-epithelial nerve regeneration was microscopically detected between the first and second months after treatment, with the return of corneal sensitivity. One year after treatment, the anatomy of these

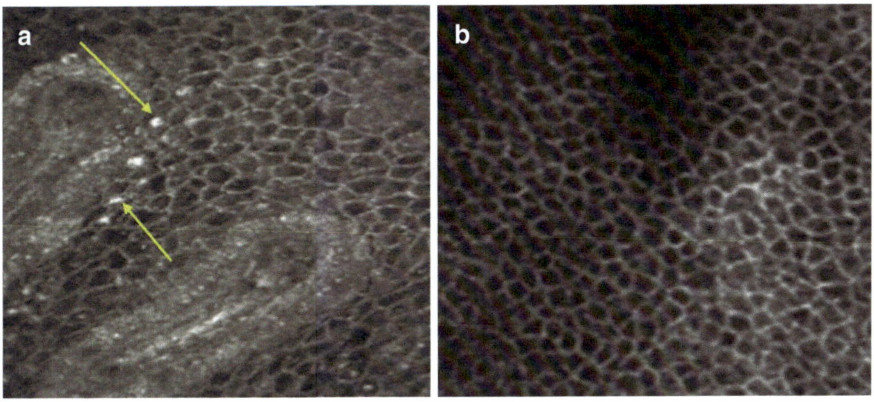

Fig. 3.15 Limbus and corneal epithelium after CXL. *Yellow arrows* indicate basal regenerating cells from Vogt's palisades in the first month after CXL (**a**); regular basal cells are shown by IVCM between the third and sixth postoperative month

sub-epithelial and stromal nerve plexus reached baseline values with the presence of interconnected fibres. Changes in corneal transparency and trophism related to kerato-neuro-dystrophic denervation mechanisms were not found after standard and ACXL, Fig. 3.16.

IVCM after transepithelial ACXL with high-irradiance UV-A power at 45 mW/cm^2 and 7.2 J/cm^2 energy revealed the same pattern of nerve loss as conventional CXL and epithelium-off ACXL, while IVCM analysis performed after transepithelial-CXL at 3 mW/cm^2 showed that SEP and anterior-mid stromal nerves did not disappear, Fig. 3.17.

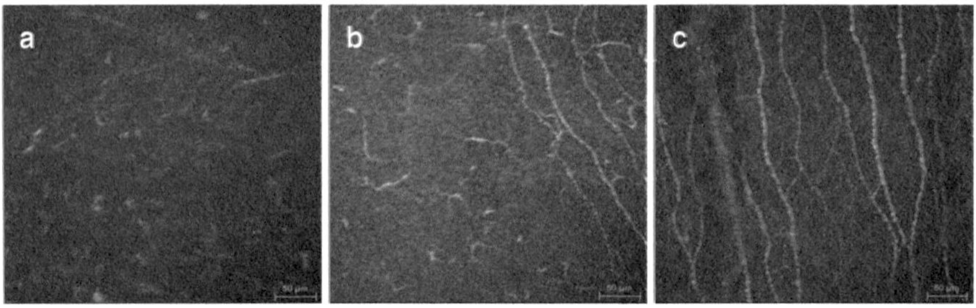

Fig. 3.16 Sub-Epithelial Plexus (SEP) nerves after epithelium-off Conventional and Accelerated CXL. IVCM Scan (**a**) shows the immediate postoperative after CXL, ACXL with epithelium removal with disappeared nerve fibres. Scan (**b**) shows reinnervation in progress between the third and sixth postoperative month. Scan (**c**) reveals complete nerve regeneration after 12 months. Corneal sensitivity showed normal limits within 6 months in both conventional and accelerated CXL

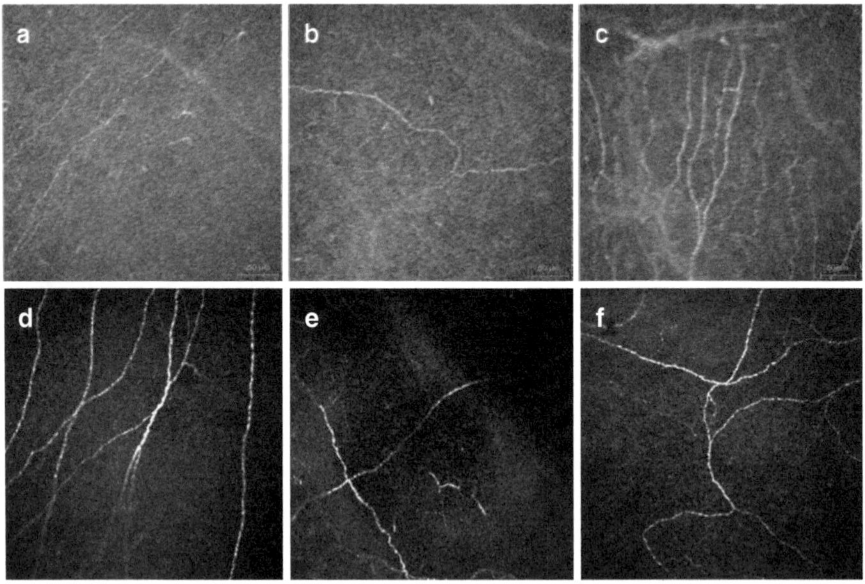

Fig. 3.17 IVCM after high irradiance 45 mW transepithelial ACXL shows the disappearance of SEP fibres analogous to epithelium off CXL and ACXL, due to high intensity UV-A power delivered. Nerve loss is often associated with diffuse actinic-like epitheliopathy. Scans (**b**) and (**c**) showed the regeneration of SEP nerves after 3 and 6 months, respectively. IVCM Scans (**d**), (**e**), (**f**) show an unaltered SEP after TE CXL with 3 mW

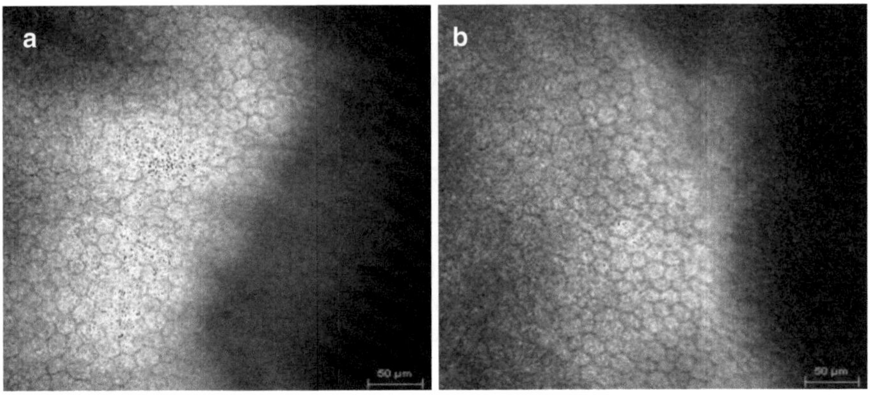

Fig. 3.18 IVCM Endothelial scans after conventional (**a**) and accelerated CXL (**b**). Long-term IVCM qualitative and quantitative analysis confirms the absence of alterations with a physiological reduction in cell count around 2% per year

3.2.5 Endothelium

The IVCM micro-morphological analysis at current state of the art after conventional and high irradiance accelerated CXL (both with 5.4 J/cm^2 7.2 J/cm^2) confirm long term (10 years) endothelial safety treatment, with no morphological or functional alterations of the corneal endothelium, Fig. 3.18.

3.2.6 Conclusion

We therefore conclude that IVCM is a powerful diagnostic tool for in vivo, in depth analysis, and for the validation of CXL protocols identifying cornea tissue modifications at a cellular level. It further represents a prognostic tool for the evolution of the development of the CXL technique, managing complications and monitoring post-operative outcomes. IVCM has not only proven important for assessing the safety and efficacy of CXL procedures, but also in revealing some of the basic mechanisms through which CXL works, showing strong correlations between IVCM micro-morphological findings and CXL biomechanical and functional power.

3.3 Biomechanical Measurement: Brillouin Microscopy

3.3.1 Introduction

Corneal collagen crosslinking (CXL) is a clear example of the importance of understanding corneal biomechanics. CXL is used to stop the progression of corneal ectasia by increasing the elasticity of the corneal tissue. The technique employs the resulting photoactivation of a photosensitizer (e.g. riboflavin) by means of ultraviolet light exposure to promote covalent bonding between adjacent collagen fibers in the stroma. Increasing the crosslinks between fibers increases the overall corneal strength. Due to the widespread development of CXL, great effort is currently underway to develop methods to assess corneal mechanical properties.

3.3.2 Measuring Corneal Biomechanics

Mechanical properties of a material are generally assessed via stress/strain tests, in which the material endures a stress and the resulting strain is measured to find the material's elastic modulus. While effective ex vivo, the destructive nature and low spatial resolution of these tests [3] make them unsuitable for in vivo studies. Therefore, a novel approach to assess the mechanical properties of the cornea in vivo is needed.

In recent years, a number of advances have been centered around measuring the biomechanics of the eye. The Ocular Response Analyzer (ORA), the first clinically approved method of its kind, utilizes the noncontact tonometry process by observing the cornea's dynamic response after it is exposed to a systematic air-pulse [10]. Doing so, ORA measures cornea hysteresis, the pressure difference during the inward and outward bending of the cornea, which has been shown to correlate to advanced keratoconus [11]. However, hysteresis is not considered a true corneal mechanical property, and due to the variance with measurement technique its clinical usefulness has been questioned [12, 13].

Building on the Ocular Response Analyzer principle, several methods have been developed that combine physical deformation of the cornea and dynamic imaging modalities. For example, a commercially available instrument (Corvis, Oculus) combines an air-puff with anterior-segment Schleimpfug's imaging in order to allow dynamic measurements of corneal deformation. Along the same direction, further advancement has focused on rapid imaging modalities, such as anterior-segment Optical Coherence Tomography (OCT), which allows for an extremely accurate reconstruction of the corneal deformation. Combining the air-puff and rapid imaging methods creates a more feasible clinical application, however, extracting pristine cornea mechanical properties remains a challenge due to the geometric and intraocular pressure variations between samples [14, 15]. To attack this problem, numerous OCT adaptations have been implored. In one case, micro-air-puffs are applied to the cornea and their propagation through the corneal tissue is recorded; in another technology, sound waves are sent to the cornea to induce very small mechanical perturbation, which are captured by rapid OCT.

3.3.3 Brillouin Microscopy

Brillouin microscopy is based on radically different principles from the previous techniques. The technology stems from spontaneous Brillouin light scattering, in which a frequency shift is induced from the interaction between applied light and acoustic phonons present in the material due to spontaneous thermal fluctuations. The frequency of the phonons, which is the frequency shift measured between incident and scattering light is given by

$$\nu_B = \pm \frac{2n}{\lambda_P} \sqrt{\frac{M'}{\rho}} \cos\left(\frac{\theta}{2}\right) \quad (3.1)$$

where n is the refractive index of the sampled material, M' is the real part of the longitudinal elastic modulus of the material on which we will focus the next section, ρ is the density of the material and θ is the angle between incident and scattered optical radiation.

Since the acoustic vibrations are a function of the collective motion of molecules present in a respective material, Brillouin microscopy allows the extraction of true tissue mechanical and material properties. Because of the all-optical operation, Brillouin microscopy can provide biomechanical characterization of the cornea without contact and with high three-dimensional (3D) resolution.

More generally, the Brillouin scattering spectrum is related to the complex longitudinal modulus ($M = M' + iM''$) of the sample, where the real part expresses the elastic response and the imaginary part expresses the viscous response. The real and imaginary parts of the complex longitudinal modulus are linked to Brillouin spectral signatures using the following equation [16]:

$$M' = \frac{\rho}{n^2} \left(\frac{\lambda_P}{2\cos(\theta/2)} \right)^2 \nu_B^{\,2}; M'' = \frac{\rho}{n^2} \left(\frac{\lambda_P}{2\cos(\theta/2)} \right)^2 \nu_B^{\,2} \Delta\nu_B^{\,2} \quad (3.2)$$

While the factor ρ/n^2 is not constant or uniform across samples, it can be approximated to a constant while dealing with a specific tissue. For example, for corneal tissue, from literature values of the refractive index and density, which are spatially varying [51, 52], the ratio of ρ/n^2 is found to be approximately constant with a value of 0.57 g/cm^3 and a variation of less than 0.3% throughout the cornea [53, 54].

While Brillouin spectroscopy can extract the local longitudinal modulus directly, the longitudinal modulus is not the quantity that traditional gold-standard tests provide, i.e. the Young's or shear moduli. In crystalline materials, the relationship between longitudinal modulus and Young's Modulus is well known. However, for soft material (i.e. corneas), no correlation formula has been shown yet. Therefore, we set out to investigate experimentally if a correlation existed between Brillouin-derived longitudinal modulus and traditional Young's or shear moduli. To do so, we took advantage of the depth-dependent variation of corneal modulus by acquiring Brillouin depth profiles, or maps, of porcine corneas. The longitudinal modulus values were computed using fixed index/density data taken from the literature. After Brillouin imaging, cornea tissue samples were cut with a biopsy punch in order to retrieve thin flaps from anterior, central and posterior portion of the cornea. The shear modulus of the thin flaps was measured at 0.5 Hz frequency with 0.1% strain amplitude with a stress-controlled rheometer (AR-G2, TA Instruments). For each flap, thickness was accurately measured in order to calculate the corresponding average longitudinal modulus from the Brillouin depth profile. Figure 3.19 shows a logarithmic plot of Brillouin-related longitudinal modulus vs. quasi-static shear modulus, showing a strong correlation between the two quantities and a log-log linear trend:

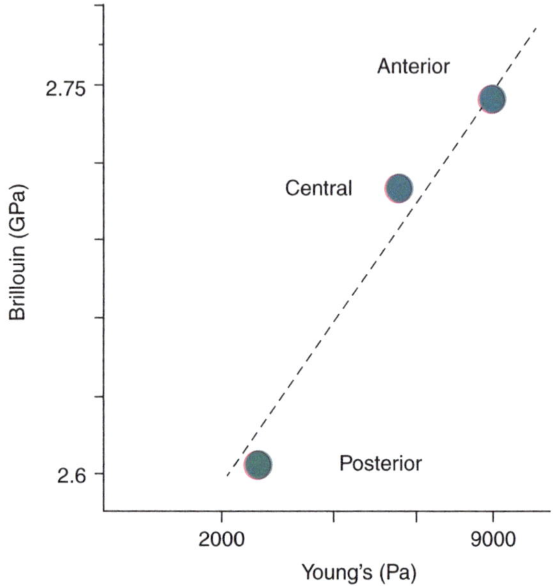

Fig. 3.19 Comparison of Brillouin-related longitudinal modulus and quasi-static shear modulus of thin flaps (100–300 microns) cut from anterior (N = 4), central (N = 6) and posterior (N = 12) corneal tissue. *Circles*, experimental data; error bars, s.e.m.; *solid line*, log-log linear fit

$$\log(M') = a \log(E') + b \tag{3.3}$$

where coefficients a and b represent intrinsic properties of the measured material ($R > 0.99$).

The logarithmic relationship demonstrated between mechanically-measured and Brillouin-measured moduli, which is consistent with what we previously found for crystalline lens and other polymeric materials [55], provides a quantitative characterization of tissue mechanical properties via Brillouin microscopy.

3.3.4 Brillouin Microscopy to Assess CXL Mechanical Outcome

Brillouin microscopy provides a unique way of measuring the mechanical properties of a material with 3D resolution. For this reason, Brillouin is promising to measure the efficacy of corneal cross-linking. We can use Eq. 3.3 to relate the changes of elastic modulus induced by CXL when comparing two different procedures via the following equation:

$$\frac{\Delta M_1^{'}}{\Delta M_2^{'}} = \frac{\Delta E_1^{'}}{\Delta E_2^{'}} \tag{3.4}$$

The traditional CXL protocol, the Dresden protocol, is the gold-standard of CXL procedures and therefore can be used as a term of comparison for different procedures. Thus far, we have been able to use demonstrate Brillouin's ability to assess the efficacy of several cross-linking protocols while varying parameters of the CXL procedure [34].

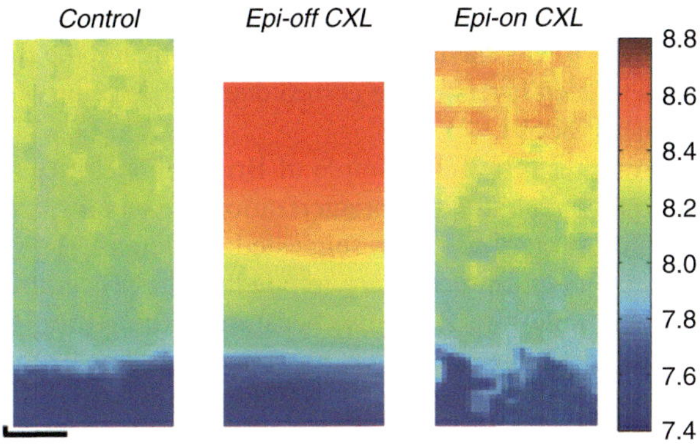

Fig. 3.20 Representative depth-sectional images of corneas treated with epi-off vs. epi-on crosslinking procedures. Biomechanical efficacy of transepithelial CXL results approximately 20% of standard CXL

For example, corneal cross-linking currently requires an epithelium debridement prior to exposure to Vitamin-B and UV-A. However, recent efforts have been given towards assessing the efficacy of the procedure without removing the epithelium and, thereby, decreasing patient discomfort. Figure 3.20 shows typical depth-sectional Brillouin maps of animal corneas. Using these measurements, we were able to compare the stiffness at varying depths of the cornea prior and post CXL procedure. Namely, we compared the images of a standard procedure in which the epithelium is removed (Fig. 3.20a, b) to a novel approach in which the epithelium was remained intact (Fig. 3.20c, d). For the standard CXL samples (Fig. 3.20b), porcine corneas debrided of their respective epitheliums, followed by a 30-min soak in riboflavin solution and 30-min UV-A light exposure. The CXL protocol in Fig. 3.20d mimicked that of the standard without initially removing the cornea's epithelium layer. Both CXL samples, both epi-on and -off, were compared to respective controls in which no procedure was performed.

For both samples, corneal cross-linking shows a depth depending variation in Brillouin shift, and, therefore, elastic modulus, in both of samples. However, it is evident that the magnitude and strengthened area of the CXL was limited in the epi-on sample, and the stiffened parts of the cornea are confined to the anterior portion. To further estimate CXL efficacy between the two CXL procedures, the ratio as in Eq. 3.4 was employed by averaging the modulus over the entire corneal depth. The epi-on CXL procedure was estimated to induce about 33% of the stiffening done by the epi-off mimicking procedure. For comparison, the mechanical stiffening of the epi-on procedure was tested with gold-standard quasi-static rheology and was found to induce approximately 39% of the stiffening of epi-off CXL. Prior studies [56] found the mechanical efficacy of transepithelial CXL to be approximately 20% of standard CXL. The increased mechanical efficacy found by our methods could be due to the improved protocol used for photosensitizer diffusion developed by Raiskup et al. [57].

The results obtained with Brillouin microscopy are consistent with what is known from the literature [29]. The epi-off CXL stiffness increase is remarkable in the anterior third of the cornea, less pronounced in the mid-stromal region, and minimal in the posterior stromal region. This can be understood by considering the gradient of riboflavin diffusion along depth and the diminished light energy delivered to deep layers of the cornea due to absorption of the riboflavin in the anterior cornea [58, 59].

Another relevant example of Brillouin's ability to assess corneal mechanics is in the mechanical characterization of changes involved with LASIK surgery. LASIK surgery has been suggested to decrease the stiffness of the cornea due to the flap creation necessary to conduct the procedure and due to the subsequent corneal ablation. Recently, because of the stiffening effects CXL has on corneas, an accelerated CXL procedure has been proposed in combination with LASIK surgery to combat the weakening of the cornea. We used Brillouin microscopy to observe the properties of the cornea at different intervals of the LASIK/CXL combined procedure. To do so, Brillouin depth-sections were measured of porcine eyes before any procedure (virgin eyes: Fig. 3.21a), after a LASIK flap was created (Fig. 3.21b), and following post-flap CXL (Fig. 3.21c). By extracting the information from the maps, we were able to show the Brillouin shift (correlating to stiffness) of each sample as a function of depth (Fig. 3.21d). The images of the virgin corneas are consistent with previous measurements, and show a gradient in stiffness from the anterior to the posterior of the cornea. After the LASIK flap was created, the cornea lost a significant amount of stiffness primarily closer to the anterior and central portions. Finally, while we observed a slight increase in stiffness, no significant difference was found after the flap-induced cornea was exposed to accelerated CXL. Using Brillouin microscopy, we were able to conclude that LASIK flaps decreased the overall stiffness of the cornea. Following the decrease, the commonly paired accelerated CXL procedure demonstrated no significant benefits towards increasing the

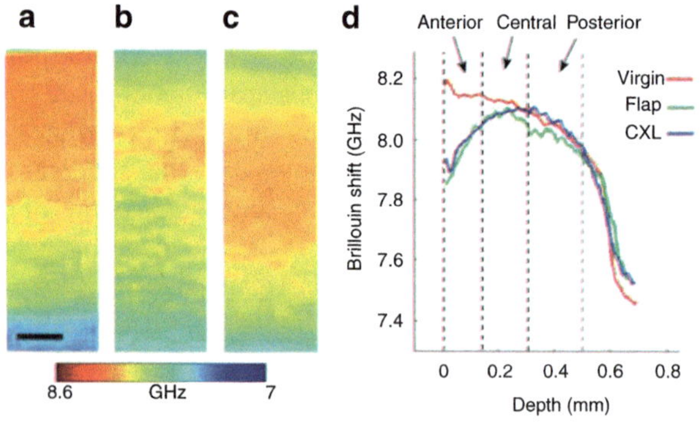

Fig. 3.21 Brillouin shift characterization of the standard Flap-CXL procedure. (**a**) Representative cross-sectional Brillouin image of virgin porcine cornea. (**b**) Brillouin image of cornea after flapping by micro keratotomy. (**c**) Brillouin image of cornea after standard CXL. (**d**) Brillouin depth profiles of the virgin cornea, after LASIK flap creation, and after rapid CXL. Scale bars are 100 μm

compromised stiffness. The maps also made it possible to see the most dramatic shift was confined to the anterior portion of the cornea, an observation not possible without the Brillouin technology.

3.3.5 The Future of Brillouin Technology

Recent years have shown a rapid development of Brillouin instrumentation [60, 61]. Specifically, the development of a clinically applicable and in vivo method was reported in 2012. The instrument employs low-power laser light at 780 nm which is scanned across each location of the eye for about 100 ms and a Brillouin spectrometer optimized for the infrared wavelength [62] (Fig. 3.22).

Using this first instrument prototype, a first clinical trials was started and focused on measuring the difference in mechanical properties of keratoconus corneas [37, 38]. Brillouin imaging was performed on tissue samples from normal donor corneas used in Descemet's stripping endothelial keratoplasty (DSEK) and advanced keratoconic corneas from patients undergoing deep anterior lamellar keratoplasty (DALK). Brillouin microscopy showed evident differences between the normal and kertoconic corneas. As expected, the Brillouin shift, and therefore, elastic modulus, was significantly lower in a coned-cornea with advanced keratoconus. However, outside the cone, Brillouin mechanical signatures appeared comparable to that of normal corneas. These findings prove that spatial asymmetry in the distribution of elastic modulus exists solely in keratoconic corneas, and

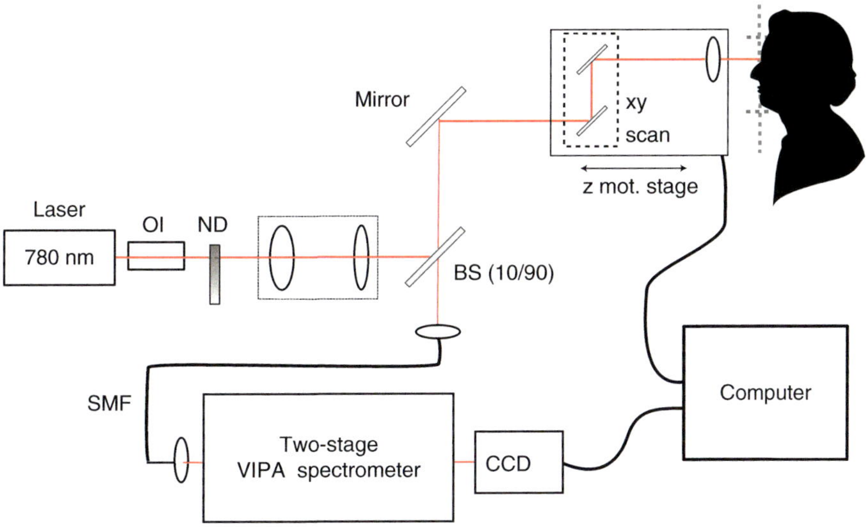

Fig. 3.22 Schematic representation of a Brillouin microscope composed by a laser-scanning confocal microscope connected to a Brillouin spectrometer via a single-mode optical fiber

confirm that corneal biomechanics provide a large diagnostic tool for the diagnostic and progression of keratoconus [41].

Due to its non-invasive and non-contact nature, Brillouin microscopy promises to become a widespread technology to assess corneal mechanical properties. The future challenges still lie in the instrument development portion of the research. Future technological improvements are aimed at enhancing the sensitivity of the mechanical measurements and the speed of the mechanical tests. Engineering efforts will need to make Brillouin microscopy portable, easy to operate by non-experts. Such technological development is crucial for the widespread use of the technology.

3.3.6 Conclusion

Measuring biomechanical properties of the cornea may provide information not currently available with traditional imaging techniques. This could lead to progress in several areas, including the early diagnosis of ocular mechanical conditions (keratoconus) and investigating the efficiency of cornea strengthening procedures (CXL). While a variety of mechanical tests can sufficiently measure a sample's material properties, they are often destructive and thus are not feasible in the clinic. Brillouin microscopy provides a novel approach in measuring the material properties of a sample with no contact or harm to the patient. Using this approach, we have been able to characterize several corneal procedures, including corneal collagen cross-linking as a function of depth, irradiation dose and epithelium debridement. Technology development is still crucial for the widespread use of Brillouin microscopy in the clinic.

References

1. Krachmer JH, Feder RS, Belin MW. Keratoconus and related noninflammatory corneal thinning disorders. Surv Ophthalmol. 1984;28(4):293–322.
2. Rabinowitz Y. Major review: keratoconus. Surv Ophthalmol. 1998;42(4):297–319.
3. Wollensak G, Spoerl E, Seiler T. Riboflavin/ultraviolet-a-induced collagen crosslinking for the treatment of keratoconus. Am J Ophthalmol. 2003;135(5):620–7.
4. Caporossi A, Baiocchi S, Mazzotta C, Traversi C, Caporossi T. Parasurgical therapy for keratoconus by riboflavin-ultraviolet type A rays induced cross-linking of corneal collagen: preliminary refractive results in an Italian study. J Cataract Refract Surg. 2006;32(5):837–45.
5. Hafezi F, Kanellopoulos J, Wiltfang R, Seiler T. Corneal collagen crosslinking with riboflavin and ultraviolet A to treat induced keratectasia after laser in situ keratomileusis. J Cataract Refract Surg. 2007;33(12):2035–40.
6. Spoerl E, Wollensak G, Seiler T. Increased resistance of crosslinked cornea against enzymatic digestion. Curr Eye Res. 2004;29(1):35–40.
7. Kamaev P, Friedman MD, Sherr E, Muller D. Photochemical kinetics of corneal cross-linking with riboflavin. Invest Ophthalmol Vis Sci. 2012;53(4):2360–7.
8. Spoerl E, Huhle M, Seiler T. The induction of cross links in corneal tissue. Exp Eye Res. 1998;66:97–103.
9. Spoerl E, Seiler T. Techniques for stiffening the cornea. J Refract Surg. 1999;15(6):711–3.

10. Raiskup-Wolf F, Hoyer A, Spoerl E, Pillunat LE. Collagen crosslinking with riboflavin and ultraviolet-A light in keratoconus: long-term results. J Cataract Refract Surg. 2008;34(5):796–801.
11. Caporossi A, Mazzotta C, Baiocchi S, Caporossi T. Long-term results of riboflavin ultraviolet a corneal collagen cross-linking for keratoconus in Italy: the Siena eye cross study. Am J Ophthalmol. 2010;149(4):585–93.
12. Wittig-Silva C, Whiting M, Lamoureux E, Lindsay RG, Sullivan LJ, Snibson GR. A randomized controlled trial of corneal collagen cross-linking in progressive keratoconus: preliminary results. J Refract Surg. 2008;24(7):S720–5.
13. Caporossi A, Mazzotta C, Baiocchi S, Caporossi T, Denaro R. Age-related long-term functional results after riboflavin UV A corneal cross-linking. J Ophthalmol. 2011;2011:608041.
14. Caporossi A, Mazzotta C, Baiocchi S, Caporossi T, Denaro R, Balestrazzi A. Riboflavin-UVA-induced corneal collagen cross-linking in pediatric patients. Cornea. 2012;31(3):227–31.
15. Spoerl E, Mrochen M, Sliney D, Trokel S, Seiler T. Safety of UVA-riboflavin cross-linking of the cornea. Cornea. 2007;26(4):385–9.
16. Brindley GS. The Bunsen-Roscoe law for the human eye at very short durations. J Physiol. 1952;118(1):135–9.
17. Schumacher S, Oeftiger L, Mrochen M. Equivalence of biomechanical changes induced by rapid and standard corneal cross-linking, using riboflavin and ultraviolet radiation. Invest Ophthalmol Vis Sci. 2011;52(12):9048–52.
18. Wernli J, Schumacher S, Spoerl E, Mrochen M. The efficacy of corneal cross-linking shows a sudden decrease with very high intensity UV light and short treatment time. Invest Ophthalmol Vis Sci. 2013;54(2):1176–80.
19. Celik HU, Alagöz N, Yildirim Y, Agca A, Marshall J, Demirok A, Yilmaz OF. Accelerated corneal crosslinking concurrent with laser in situ keratomileusis. J Cataract Refract Surg. 2012;38(8):1424–31.
20. Mazzotta C, Paradiso AL, Baiocchi S, Caragiuli S, Caporossi A. Qualitative investigation of corneal changes after accelerated corneal collagen cross-linking (A-CXL) by in vivo confocal microscopy and corneal OCT. J Clin Exp Ophthalmol. 2013;4:313.
21. Mencucci R, Marini M, Paladini I, Sarchielli E, Sgambati E, Menchini U, Vannelli GB. Effects of riboflavin/UVA corneal cross-linking on keratocytes and collagen fibres in human cornea. Clin Exp Ophthalmol. 2010;38(1):49–56.
22. Mazzotta C, Balestrazzi A, Traversi C, Baiocchi S, Caporossi T, Tommasi C, Caporossi A. Treatment of progressive keratoconus by riboflavin-UVA-induced cross-linking of corneal collagen: ultrastructural analysis by Heidelberg Retinal Tomograph II in vivo confocal microscopy in humans. Cornea. 2007;26(4):390–7.
23. Mazzotta C, Traversi C, Caragiuli S, Rechichi M. Pulsed vs continuous light accelerated corneal collagen crosslinking: in vivo qualitative investigation by confocal microscopy and corneal OCT. Eye (Lond). 2014;28(10):1179–83. https://doi.org/10.1038/eye.2014.163. Epub 25 Jul 2014.
24. Schumacher S, Mrochen M, Spoerl E. Absorption of UV-light by riboflavin solutions with different concentration. J Refract Surg. 2012;28(2):91–2.
25. Mazzotta C, Traversi C, Baiocchi S, Caporossi O, Bovone C, Sparano MC, Balestrazzi A, Caporossi A. Corneal healing after riboflavin ultraviolet-A collagen cross-linking determined by confocal laser scanning microscopy in vivo: early and late modifications. Am J Ophthalmol. 2008;146(4):527–33.
26. Krueger RR, Herekar S, Spoerl E. First proposed efficacy study of high versus standard irradiance and fractionated riboflavin/ultraviolet A cross-linking with equivalent energy exposure. Eye Contact Lens Sci Clin Pract. 2014;40(6):353–7.
27. Mazzotta C, Traversi C, Paradiso AL, Latronico ME, Rechichi M. Pulsed light accelerated crosslinking versus continuous light accelerated crosslinking: one-year results. J Ophthalmol. 2014;2014:604731. https://doi.org/10.1155/2014/604731. Epub 3 Aug 2014.
28. Hammer A, Richoz O, Arba Mosquera S, Tabibian D, Hoogewoud F, Hafezi F. Corneal biomechanical properties at different corneal cross-linking (CXL) irradiances. Invest Ophthalmol Vis Sci. 2014;55(5):2881–4.

29. Mazzotta C, Baiocchi, Bagaglia SA, Fruschelli M, Meduri A, Rechichi M. Accelerated 15 mW pulsed-light crosslinking in treatment of progressive keratoconus: Two-year clinical results. Accepted. 2017, in Press.
30. Scarcelli G, Besner S, Pineda R, Yun SH. Biomechanical characterization of keratoconus corneas ex vivo with Brillouin microscopy. Invest Ophthalmol Vis Sci. 2014;55(7):4490–5. https://doi.org/10.1167/iovs.14-14450.
31. Scarcelli G, Kling S, Quijano E, Pineda R, Marcos S, Yun SH. Brillouin microscopy of collagen crosslinking: noncontact depth-dependent analysis of corneal elastic modulus. Invest Ophthalmol Vis Sci. 2013;54(2):1418–25. https://doi.org/10.1167/iovs.12-11387.
32. Minsky M. Memoir on inventing the confocal scanning microscope. Scanning. 1988;10:128–38.
33. Efron N, Hollingsworth JG. New perspectives on keratoconus as revealed by corneal confocal microscopy. Clin Exp Optom. 2008;91(1):34–55. https://doi.org/10.1111/j.1444-0938.2007.00195.x.
34. Mazzotta C, Hafezi F, Kymionis G, Caragiuli S, Jacob S, Traversi C, Barabino S, Randleman JB. In vivo confocal microscopy after corneal collagen cross-linking. Ocul Surf. 2015;13(4):298–314.
35. Petroll WM, Robertson DM. In vivo confocal microscopy of the cornea: new developments in image acquisition, reconstruction, and analysis using the HRT-Rostock corneal module. Ocul Surf. 2015;13(3):187–203.
36. Mazzotta C, Traversi C, Baiocchi S, et al. Conservative treatment of keratoconus by riboflavin-UVA-induced cross-linking of corneal collagen: qualitative investigation. Eur J Ophthalmol. 2006;16(4):530–5.
37. Mazzotta C, Traversi C, Baiocchi S, et al. Corneal healing after riboflavin ultraviolet-A collagen cross-linking determined by confocal laser scanning microscopy in vivo: early and late modifications. Am J Ophthalmol. 2008;146:527–33; Mazzotta C, Paradiso AL, Baiocchi S, et al. Qualitative investigation of corneal changes after accelerated corneal collagen cross-linking (A-CXL) by in vivo confocal microscopy and corneal OCT. J Clin Exp Ophthalmol. 4:313. https://doi.org/10.4172/2155-9570.1000313.
38. Mazzotta C, Balestrazzi A, Baiocchi S, et al. Stromal haze after combined riboflavin-UVA corneal collagen cross-linking in keratoconus: in vivo confocal microscopic evaluation. Clin Exp Ophthalmol. 2007;35:580–2.
39. Caporossi A, Mazzotta C, Baiocchi S, et al. Transepithelial corneal collagen crosslinking for keratoconus: qualitative investigation by in vivo HRT II confocal analysis. Eur J Ophthalmol. 2012;22(Suppl 7):S81–8.
40. Mazzotta C, Balestrazzi A, Traversi C, et al. In vivo confocal microscopy report after Lasik with sequential accelerated corneal collagen cross-linking treatment. Case Rep Ophthalmol. 2014;5:125–31.
41. Mazzotta C, Caporossi T, Denaro R, et al. Morphological and functional correlations in riboflavin UV A corneal collagen cross-linking for keratoconus. Acta Ophthalmol (Copenh). 2012;90:259–65.
42. Mazzotta C, Baiocchi S, Denaro R, et al. Corneal collagen cross-linking to stop corneal ectasia exacerbated by radial keratotomy. Cornea. 2011;30:225–8.
43. Mazzotta C, Moramarco A, Traversi C, Baiocchi S, Iovieno A, Fontana L. Accelerated corneal collagen cross-linking using topography-guided UV-A energy emission: preliminary clinical and morphological outcomes. J Ophthalmol. 2016;2016:2031031. https://doi.org/10.1155/2016/2031031.
44. Kymionis GD, Diakonis VF, Kalyvianaki M, et al. One-year follow-up of corneal confocal microscopy after corneal cross-linking in patients with post laser in situ keratosmileusis ectasia and keratoconus. Am J Ophthalmol. 2009;147(5):774–8.e1. https://doi.org/10.1016/j.ajo.2008.11.017.
45. Croxatto JO, Tytiun AE, Argento CJ. Sequential in vivo confocal microscopy study of corneal wound healing after cross-linking in patients with keratoconus. J Refract Surg (Thorofare NJ 1995). 2010;26(9):638–45. https://doi.org/10.3928/1081597X-20091111-01.
46. Touboul D, Efron N, Smadja D, Praud D, Malet F, Colin J. Corneal confocal microscopy following conventional, transepithelial, and accelerated corneal collagen cross-linking procedures for keratoconus. J Refract Surg (Thorofare NJ 1995). 2012;28(11):769–76. https://doi.org/10.3928/1081597X-20121016-01.

47. Kymionis GD, Grentzelos MA, Plaka AD, et al. Correlation of the corneal collagen cross-linking demarcation line using confocal microscopy and anterior segment optical coherence tomography in keratoconic patients. Am J Ophthalmol. 2014;157(1):110–5.e1. https://doi.org/10.1016/j.ajo.2013.09.010.
48. Bouheraoua N, Jouve L, El Sanharawi M, et al. Optical coherence tomography and confocal microscopy following 3 different protocols of corneal collagen-crosslinking in keratoconus. Invest Ophthalmol Vis Sci. 2014;55(11):7601–9. https://doi.org/10.1167/iovs.14-15662.
49. Jordan C, Patel DV, Abeysekera N, McGhee CN. In vivo confocal microscopy analyses of corneal microstructural changes in a prospective study of collagen cross-linking in keratoconus. Ophthalmology. 2014;121(2):469–74.
50. Sharma N, Suri K, Sehra SV, Titiyal JS, Sinha R, Tandon R, Vajpayee RB. Collagen cross-linking in keratoconus in Asian eyes: visual, refractive and confocal microscopy outcomes in a prospective randomized controlled trial. Int Ophthalmol. 2015;35(6):827–32.
51. Kikkawa Y, Hirayama K. Uneven swelling of corneal stroma. Invest Ophthalmol. 1970;9(10):735–41.
52. Wilson G, Oleary DJ, Vaughan W. Differential swelling in compartments of the corneal stroma. Invest Ophthalmol Vis Sci. 1984;25(9):1105–8.
53. He X, Liu J. A quantitative ultrasonic spectroscopy method for noninvasive determination of corneal biomechanical properties. Invest Ophthalmol Vis Sci. 2009;50(11):5148–54.
54. Ortiz S, et al. Optical distortion correction in Optical Coherence Tomography for quantitative ocular anterior segment by three-dimensional imaging. Opt Express. 2010;18(3):2782–96.
55. Scarcelli G, Kim P, Yun S. In vivo measurement of age-related stiffening in the crystalline lens by Brillouin optical microscopy. Biophys J. 2011;101(6):1539–84.
56. Wollensak G, Iomdina E. Biomechanical and histological changes after corneal crosslinking with and without epithelial debridement. J Cataract Refract Surg. 2009;35(3):540–6.
57. Raiskup F, Pinelli R, Spoerl E. Riboflavin osmolar modification for transepithelial corneal cross-linking. Curr Eye Res. 2012;37(3):234–8.
58. Bueno JM, Gualda EJ, Giakoumaki A, Perez-Merino P, Marcos S, Artal P. Multiphoton microscopy of ex vivo corneas after collagen cross-linking. Invest Ophthalmol Vis Sci. 2011;52(8):5325–31.
59. Sondergaard AP, Hjortdal J, Breitenbach T, Ivarsen A. Corneal distribution of riboflavin prior to collagen cross-linking. Curr Eye Res. 2010;35(2):116–21.
60. Scarcelli G, Kim P, Yun SH. Cross-axis cascading of spectral dispersion. Opt Lett. 2008;33(24):2979–81.
61. Scarcelli G, Yun SH. Multistage VIPA etalons for high-extinction parallel Brillouin spectroscopy. Opt Express. 2011;19(11):10913–22.
62. Scarcelli G, Yun SH. In vivo Brillouin optical microscopy of the human eye. Opt Express. 2012;20:9197.

Accelerated Crosslinking Protocols

4

4.1 Dresden Accelerated CXL Protocol

Corneal cross-linking was in experimental setting introduced by Seiler and Spoerl in 1997 in Dresden and the first clinical pilot study was conducted and published by Wollensak et al. in 2003 also in Dresden [1, 2]. A standardized protocol that we refer to as a "Dresden protocol" involves abrasion of the corneal epithelium, followed by riboflavin application for 30 min as a photosensitizer and subsequent UVA illumination of 3 mW/cm^2 of its intensity applied to a 9-mm zone in the cornea for another 30 min. This corresponds to a total energy dose of 3.4 J or a radiant exposure of 5.4 J/cm^2 [3].

One major disadvantage of the standard CXL procedure so far is the long total treatment time of 1 h, therefore, in order to increase patient's comfort and the surgeon's work-flow in a clinical practice, a shorter CXL procedure would be desirable.

According to the photochemical law of reciprocity (Bunsen-Roscoe law), the same photochemical effect can be achieved with reduced illumination time and correspondingly increased irradiation intensity, meaning that 3-min irradiation at 30 mW/cm^2, 5-min irradiation at 18.0 mW/cm^2, and 10-min irradiation at 9.0 mW/cm^2 should provide the same effect obtained with a 30-min irradiation at 3.0 mW/cm^2, all delivering 5.4 J/cm^2 of energy [4].

In 2011, Schumacher et al. published an experimental study that used higher intensity and a shorter treatment time and showed an equivalent result in the biomechanical stability of the corneal stroma with standard CXL (3 mW/cm^2 and 30 min) and accelerated CXL (10 mW/cm^2 and 9 min). Using stress–strain measurements in porcine corneas, they found a similar increase in stiffness in both groups [4]. In an in vitro study using different irradiances (2, 3, 9, 15 mW/cm^2 continuously and 15 mW/cm^2 fractionated with alternate cycles of 30 s "on" and 30 s "off"), Krueger et al. found comparable efficacy in stiffening corneal collagen with the standard method and methods that achieved equivalent exposure of 5.4 J/cm^2. They used extensiometry to determine the stiffness and strength of treated porcine corneas [5].

C. Mazzotta et al., *Management of Early Progressive Corneal Ectasia*,
DOI 10.1007/978-3-319-61137-2_4

A large ex vivo study investigated the efficacy of CXL at higher intensities and corneal stiffness changes to irradiances between 3 mW/cm^2 and 90 mW/cm^2 with illumination times between 30 min and 1 min, respectively. Their results showed that the Bunsen-Roscoe reciprocity law is valid only for illumination intensities up to 40–50 mW/cm^2 with illumination longer than 2 min. At higher intensities and shorter duration, the stiffness could rapidly decrease [6].

Hafezi et al. observed even more pronounced decreased stiffening effect with increasing UV-A intensity. Young's modulus at 10% strain showed significant differences between 3 mW/cm^2 and used higher UV-A intensities (9 mW/cm^2 and 18 mW/cm^2). The biomechanical effect of CXL decreased significantly when using high irradiance and short irradiation time settings. These results confirmed authors' hypothesis that intrastromal oxygen diffusion capacity and increased oxygen consumption associated with higher irradiances may be a limiting factor leading to reduced treatment efficiency [7].

According to our results in experimental studies, we decided to use for the clinical setting an accelerated protocol UV-intensity of **9 mW/cm^2 for 10 min**. As a riboflavin solution we use **0.1% riboflavin** in 1.1% **hydroxypropyl methylcellulose (HPMC)**. The recent animal experiments with porcine corneas measuring riboflavin concentration gradient in the anterior corneal stroma showed, that riboflavin concentration decreased with increasing depth and increased with longer application times. In the deep layers of corneal stroma yielded HPMC-assisted riboflavin imbibition high concentrations [8].

The HPMC-assisted imbibition of corneal stroma leads to a mild tissue swelling and that's why it is suitable as a first choice riboflavin solution option also for a treatment of corneas with thickness after epithelial removal is slightly under 400 μm (up to 380 μm). If the corneal thickness is after epithelial removal under 380 μm, we use hypoosmolar riboflavin solution [9].

The crosslinking procedure is performed in our outpatient service of the Department as a day-surgery procedure. Thirty minutes before the procedure, pain medication is administered and if necessary also tranquilizers. The procedure is conducted under sterile conditions in operating room. After topical anesthesia of proxymetacaine hydrochloride 0.5% eyedrops is administered, lid speculum is applied, corneal thickness measured and the corneal epithelium is removed in a central 9-mm–diameter area with a hockey-knife. After measuring the corneal thickness again, is 0.1% riboflavin solution in HPMC instilled every minute for 15 min. After this period of time is the riboflavin solution layer removed from the corneal surface with Merocel sponge and the corneal thickness is measured again to prove, that corneal thickness before irradiation is above 400 μm. When required, a hypoosmolar riboflavin solution is instilled to promote corneal swelling. A **7.5-mm diameter** of the central cornea then is **irradiated with an irradiance of 9 mW/cm^2** (UV-X System, AVEDRO, Massachusetts, USA, former Innocross) for 10 min. During irradiation time, the riboflavin solution is not applied on the ocular surface anymore. A calibrated ultraviolet A meter (LaserMate-Q; Laser 2000, Wessling, Germany) is used before treatment to check the irradiance at a 1.0-cm distance. Topical anesthesia is added as needed during the procedure. A soft therapeutic contact lens is applied until re-epithelialization of cornea is complete. After surgery, analgesics systemically are prescribed and drops ofloxacin three times a day and artificial tears six times a day are applied. After the corneal reepithelialization is the contact lens removed and drops of dexamethasone three times a day for 3 weeks after discontinuation of the antibiotics are together with artificial tears further on applied. Postoperative follow-up examinations are performed daily until complete reepithelialization. Subsequent examinations are at 1, 3, 6, and 12 months and then annually. At each examination, refraction, best corrected visual acuity with glasses or with contact lenses, corneal topography, tomography, ocular response analyzer and intraocular pressure are recorded. At 6-month follow-up is a fitting of a new contact lens recommended.

There were two irradiation sources of ultraviolet light with the high intensity used in our patients with progressive keratoconus: UV-X device with energy of 9 mW/cm^2 and an irradiation time of 10 min ($\lambda = 370$ nm) (AVEDRO, Massachusetts, USA, former Innocross) which offered a top-hat beam profile (group 1) and UV-X 2000 (AVEDRO, Massachusetts, USA, former Innocross) that treated the ectatic corneas with a modified beam optimized profile (group 2), Fig. 4.1. Laboratory measurements of both profiles confirm that the beam optimized profile (BO) has a

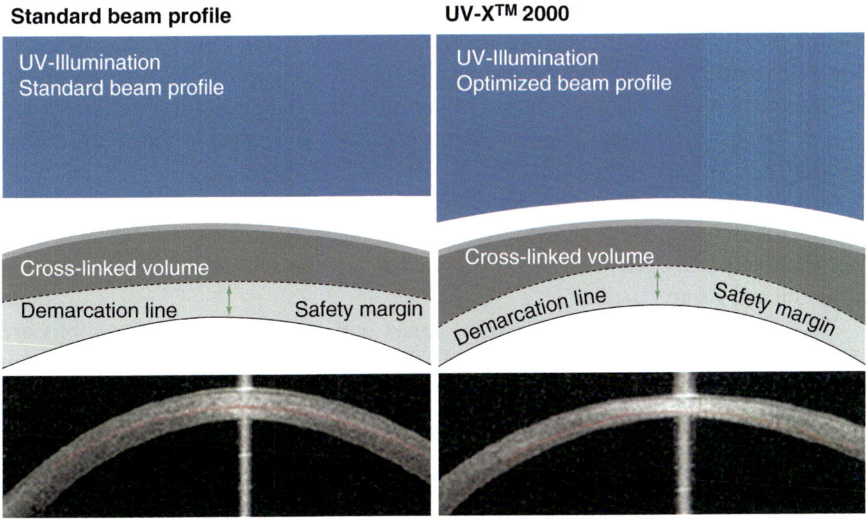

Fig. 4.1 Comparison of both illumination sources with provably deeper cross-links on OCT (source: UV-X 2000 Brochure, IROC Innocross AG [offline])

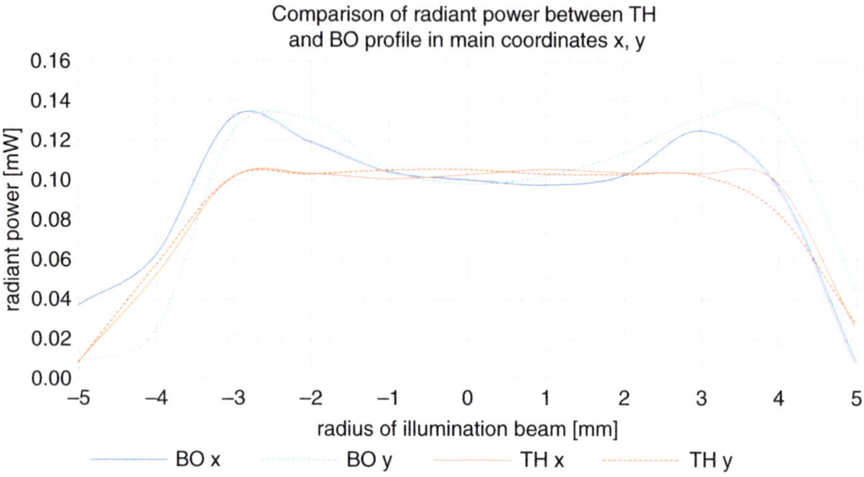

Fig. 4.2 Laboratory measurements of radiant power for both profiles, peripheral radiant power of BO at 3 mm has a factor of 1,3 in comparison to the central of both devices, "laser-mate Q" with a range of 1 mW, pinhole 0.05 mm

higher intensity in the peripheral area than in the center. As opposed to this the top-hat profile (TH) has a constant intensity, Fig. 4.2.

In these two groups we could compare the top-hat beam profile with the optimized beam profile at high intensity CXL protocol. The UV-X 2000 offers such a modified beam profile which has a higher peripheral intensity (12 mW/cm^2, center: 9 mW/cm^2) to get deeper outside the corneal center, Fig. 4.1. Accordingly, the demarcation line fits better the peripheral corneal thickness distribution and increases the cross-linking volume. In contrast, the standard illumination source has a flat profile concerning the light intensity with the previous described properties.

There was recorded a significant flattening in Kapex for both devices after 1 year follow up. Seiler et al. demonstrated a similar significant decrease of Kapex after high intensity BO-CXL [10]. In addition to that, we observed a significant reduction of Kmin and Kmax ($p < 0.05$).

The significant flattening of Kmin, Kmax and Kapex in our observations are comparable with well-known studies [11–13]. However, our differences between pre- and postoperative are less pronounced than previously described outcomes. The reason for this may be the different follow up time and the stage of keratoconus, Fig. 4.3.

Our results show a significant reduction of lowest corneal thickness (LCT) after 11 months which are partially comparable with other described results [11, 14] (Fig. 4.4). In some cases, the LCT reached the preoperative thickness after a longer follow up [15]. Some of these studies detected a significant decrease of the minimal

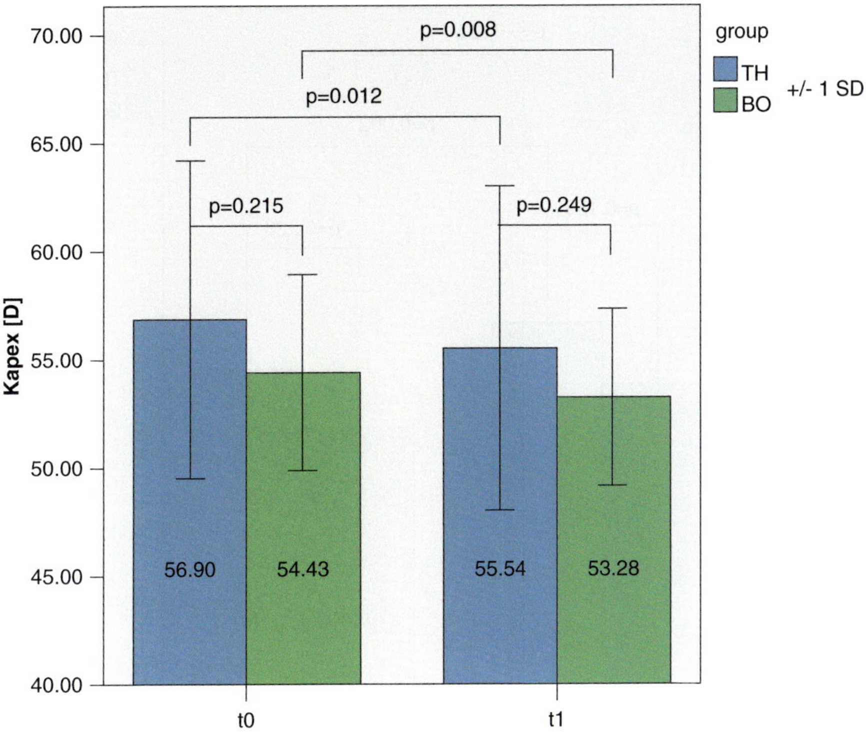

Fig. 4.3 Comparative analysis of Kapex, pre- (t0) and postoperative (t1) measurements, TH-profile (*left*) and BO-profile (*right*)

corneal thickness 1 up to 3 months after CXL followed by an increase of LCT with Pentacam or Orbscan. Other studies showed a constant LCT after CXL measured by ultrasound pachymetry or optical coherence tomography (OCT). The attempts to explain these findings reach from anatomical structural changes up to measurement errors of optical detection of corneal thickness [13, 16].

The "top hat" profile seems to have a higher influence on Keratoconus indices than the beam optimized profile. According to Greenstein et al. we detected a significant decrease in ISV, IVA and IHD for group 1, which results in apparently stronger regularization of corneal surface [17, 18]. Previous studies are not compliant concerning the effects of CXL on the several indices [17, 18]. However CXL ensures an improvement of indices in comparison to untreated keratoconic eyes [18]. The beam optimized profile shows also a decrease in all parameters, except KI, but is only significant in CKI and IHA. A reason for that could be the lower preoperative values than in group 1, associated with a lower stage of keratoconus in group 2.

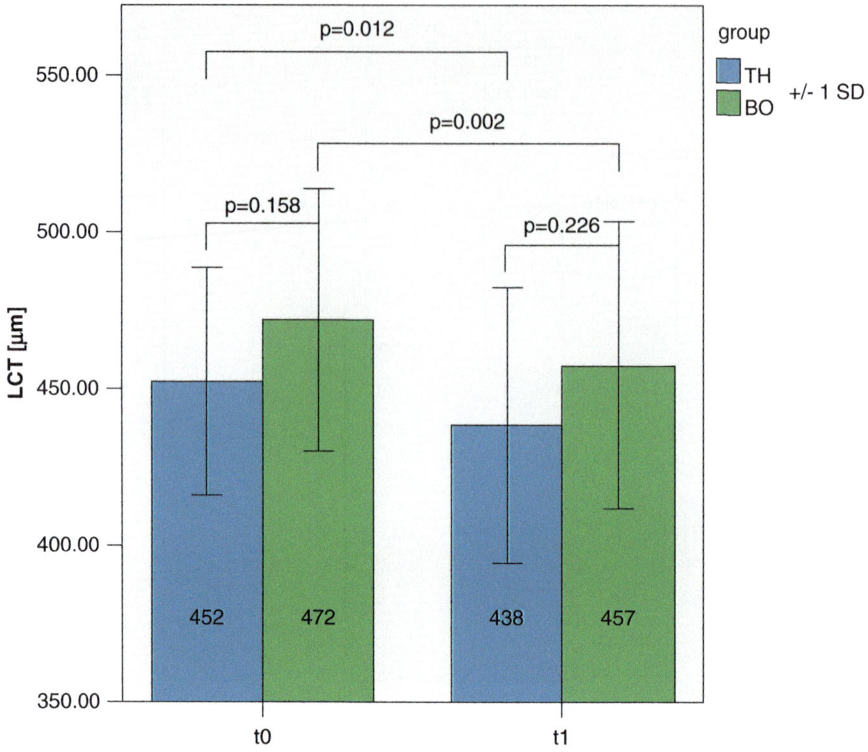

Fig. 4.4 Comparative analysis of lowest corneal thickness, pre (t0) and postoperative (t1) measurements, TH-profile (*left*) and BO-profile (*right*)

4.2 Siena Crosslinking Center® Accelerated CXL Protocol

4.2.1 Introduction

Conventional Riboflavin UV-A induced corneal collagen Crosslinking (CXL) with epithelium removal (Epithelium-Off) represents an evidence-based and scientifically well-supported treatment with documented long-term efficacy in stabilizing progressive keratoconus and secondary ectasia in a series of non-randomized and randomized clinical trials [11, 13, 19, 20], reducing the need of corneal transplants in patients affected by progressive keratoconus or secondary ectasia [21]. The standard irradiance of 3 mW/cm^2 for 30 min was effective in stiffening the cornea in primary and iatrogenic keratoectasia [22] cases but also demonstrated its potential in sterilizing antibiotic-resistant infectious keratitis due to the cytotoxic effect of the reactive oxygen species (ROS) generated during the CXL process [23], otherwise known as photoactivated chromophore CXL (PACK-CXL) [24, 25]. Since the conventional CXL procedure requires long treatment time (1 h approximately) [22], high-irradiance or accelerated crosslinking (A-CXL) protocols have been proposed to shorten CXL treatment time [26–30], improving patient's comfort and reducing hospital waiting lists. According to equal dose principles stated in the Bunsen Roscoe Law [31], by setting UV-A power at 9 mW/cm^2 × 10 min, 30 mW/cm^2 × 3 min, 18 mW/cm^2 × 5 min, 45 mW/cm^2 × 2 min while maintaining a constant energy (Fluence) of 5.4 J/cm^2 we can achieve the same effect as the conventional Dresden protocol at 3 mW/cm^2 for 30 min [4, 6]. Recent studies [32] have shed light on the chain of chemical events occurring during the photochemical activation of riboflavin with UV light, highlighting the importance of corneal oxygenation during treatment. With pulsed or fractionated ultraviolet-A (UV-A) radiation, CXL efficiency may be improved by allowing re-diffusion of oxygen during UV-A light exposure pauses [5, 32].

A preclinical laboratory study conducted by Krueger, Herekar and Spoerl [5] demonstrated that riboflavin 0.1% with 15 mW/cm^2 UV-A exposure, using an equivalent total energy exposure of 5.4 J/cm^2, was as effective as conventional 3 mW/cm^2 CXL and 9 mW/cm^2 ACXL in biomechanical strengthening of the cornea. Moreover, when fractionating the UV-A exposure with multiple cycles of pulsing light, the corneal extensiometry was equally as effective as without pulsing the light [32]. The study [5] established that, in theory, pulsed UV-A delivery should improve the degree of cross-linking, especially with the faster higher-irradiance exposures where oxygen is consumed more quickly. Fractionating UV-A exposure by pulsing the light, IVCM analysis proved better penetration treatment as demonstrated in vivo by Mazzotta et al. [33–35] and recently confirmed by Peyman et al. [36]. Deeper cell viability is reachable, prolonging exposure time while maintaining the same energy dose delivered into the corneal tissue [37, 38].

The present study evaluated the induced corneal micro-structural changes [35] (biomicroscopic, corneal SD-OCT, IVCM) and the 2-years functional results (UCVA, CDVA, Tomographic) after 15 mW/cm^2 high-irradiance pulsed-light cross-linking at the standard 5.4 J/cm^2 Fluence performed for the first time at international level by Cosimo Mazzotta at the Siena Crosslinking Center® in a cohort of patients with progressive stage-II keratoconus, based on the data reported in the aforementioned laboratory study [5].

4.2.2 Methods

The Siena ACXL protocol was based on a prospective interventional study following the tenets of the Declaration of Helsinki, and included 132 eyes of 96 patients, 76 males and 20 females (M/F ratio 3.8) with progressive stage II keratoconus collected at the Siena Crosslinking Center, Italy. Mean age was 23.7 ± 4.3 years. Informed consent was obtained from all the subjects after explanation of the nature and objective of the treatment. Patients underwent a full ophthalmologic examination including uncorrected distance visual acuity (UDVA), corrected distance visual acuity (CDVA), slit-lamp examination, tonometry and fundoscopy. KC was evaluated by Scheimpflug corneal tomography (Sirius C.S.O, Florence, Italy), in vivo confocal microscopy (IVCM) with the Heidelberg Retina Tomograph (HRT II,

Rostock Cornea Module, Heidelberg, Germany), anterior segment optical coherence tomography (AS-OCT, i-Vue, Optovue, Fremont, CA, USA), and endothelial cell count (I-Konan Non-Co Robot, Konan Inc., Hyogo, Japan). All patients enrolled in the treatment protocol completed the 24-month follow-up.

Inclusion criteria: stage-II keratoconus (Amsler-Krumeich's staging) [21] with a documented clinical and instrumental progression in the last 6 months of observation, expressed by an increased K max ≥1 Diopter (D), minimum corneal thickness reduction ≥10 μm; UDVA and CDVA worsening at least of +1.0 log MAR (≥0.1 decimal equivalent) or ≥0.5 Spherical equivalent. Exclusion criteria: Corneal opacities or scars, history of HSV and other infectious keratitis, autoimmune diseases, pregnancy, patients who didn't met the clinical and instrumental KC inclusion criteria. A 2-tailed paired samples Student *t* test was used to compare each baseline measurement with the respective follow-up measurement. Differences with $P < 0.05$ were considered significant. Data were collected and analysed using the *Prism* 6.0 (*Graph Pad* Software, Inc. La Jolla, CA, USA) software.

4.2.3 Surgical Technique

15 mW/cm^2 High-Irradiance Pulsed-light CXL protocol [39] at 5.4 J/cm^2 standardized Fluence was carried out under sterile operating conditions, and topical anesthesia with the application of 0.2% oxybuprocaine hydrochloride anesthetic drops was used. Topical pilocarpine 2% was administered 20 min before treatment. After application of a closed-valve eyelid speculum, corneal epithelium was removed by an epi-Bowman keratectomy performed with a disposable epi-keratome (Epi-Clear™, ORCA Surgical, Caesarea, Israel) in the central 8–9 mm area, Fig. 4.5a, b. After epithelium removal, corneal stroma was soaked for 10 min with a Riboflavin 0.1% Hydroxyl-Propyl Methyl-Cellulose (HPMC) dextran-free solution (VibeX Rapid Avedro Inc., Waltham, MA, USA), Fig. 4.5c, d. UV-A irradiation was carried out with the KXL I™ UV-A illuminator (Avedro Inc., Waltham, MS, USA) using a 15 mW/cm^2 UV-A power with pulsed-light emission (1 s ON/1 s OFF) to obtain 12 min of UV-A irradiation on balance while delivering a standard E dose of 5.4 J/cm^2, Fig. 4.5e, in a total treatment time of 22 min. After UV-A irradiation, the eye was washed with a balanced salt solution (BSS), medicated with antibiotic (moxifloxacin) and mydriatic drops (cyclopentolate), and dressed with a therapeutic soft contact lens, Fig. 4.5f. The Siena Crosslinking Center® ACXL protocol is summarized in Table 4.1.

Therapeutic contact lenses were removed 48–72 h after the treatment after biomicroscopic examination if complete epithelial healing was documented, Fig. 4.6.

Spectral Domain (SD) optical coherence tomography (OCT) corneal scan was performed 1 month after treatment to detect demarcation line depth, Fig. 4.7.

IVCM evaluation of basal corneal epithelium, sub-epithelial nerve plexus and corneal stroma keratocytes apoptosis was performed on day 3 after treatment with contact lens on and 30 days after treatment, Fig. 4.8.

Post-operative IVCM scans showed a regular epithelial healing occurring 72 h after treatment. Native epithelial cells were large with slightly defined cell borders,

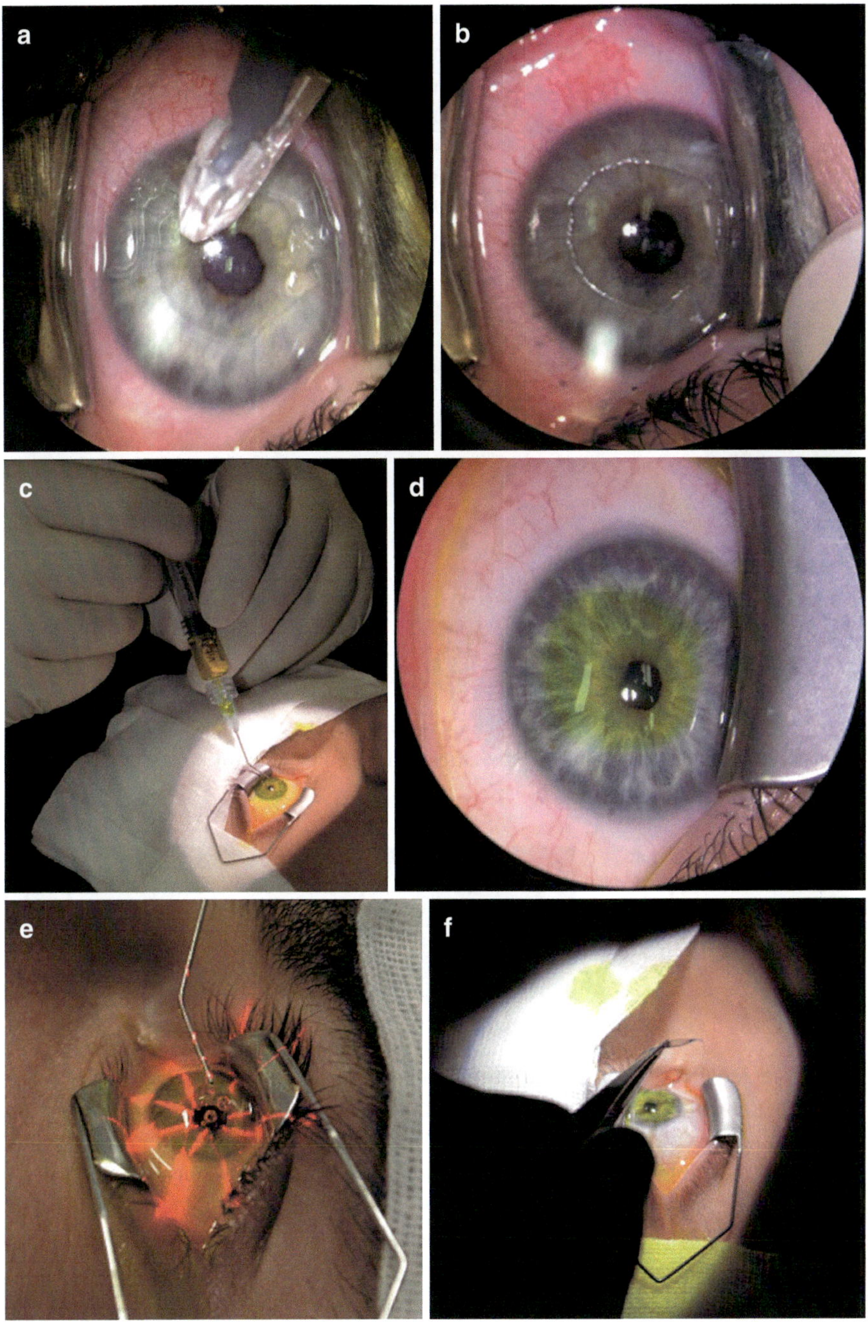

Fig. 4.5 Siena Crosslinking Center® 15 mW High Irradiance ACXL Protocol® (developed by C. Mazzotta MD, PhD according to basic laboratory studies of Krueger, Herekar and Spoerl [19])

Table 4.1 The Siena Crosslinking Center® 15 mW pulsed light ACXL protocol parameters

Soaking time	10.00 min with Riboflavin 0.1% HPMC
UV-A power setting	15 mW/cm^2
UV-A irradiation time	6.00 min
Treatment modality	Pulsed-light (1 s ON/1 s OFF)
Total UV-A exposure time	12.00 min
Total energy dose (fluence)	5.40 J/cm^2
Total treatment time	22.00 min

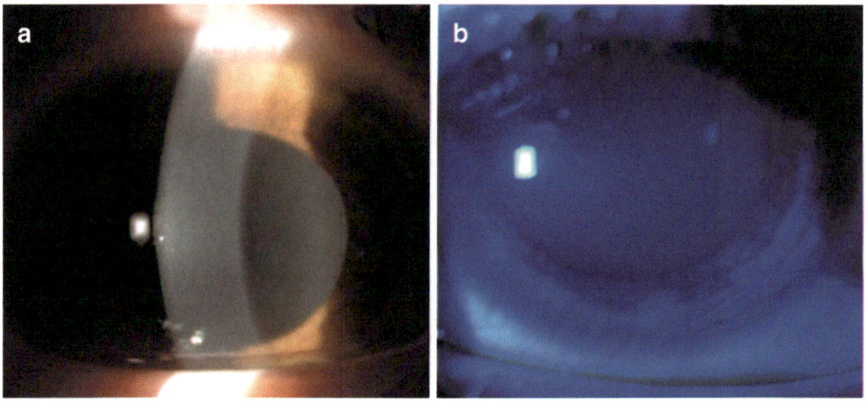

Fig. 4.6 Complete epithelial healing 48–72 h after the treatment. Biomicroscopy after therapeutic contact lens removal (**a**). Negative Riboflavin staining confirmed a fast and complete re-epithelialization (**b**)

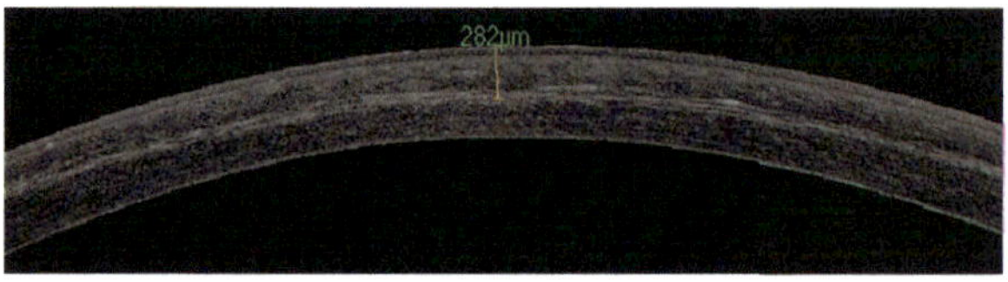

Fig. 4.7 Demarcation line 1-month after Siena Crosslinking Center 15 mW High Irradiance ACXL Protocol®

often oriented in a whorl-like fashion, Fig. 4.8a. A regular basal epithelial cells mosaic with homogeneous cellularity and clear, distinct cell borders were present 30 days after treatment, Fig. 4.8b. Sub-epithelial plexus (SEP) scans showed rarefaction and damage of SEP fibers, even not completely lost, at third day after treatment, Fig. 4.8c. SEP nerve fibers showed rapid tendency to corneal reinnervation 30 days after treatment with bright nerve fibers evident, Fig. 4.8d. 15 mW/cm^2 high-irradiance pulsed-light crosslinking induced keratocytes apoptosis in the anterior stroma associated with increased density of EC matrix, Fig. 4.8e. Lacunar corneal edema, hyperreflective trabecular mesh aspect of extracellular matrix and apoptotic bodies are well detectable, Fig. 4.8f–h. Gradual keratocytes repopulation with concomitant lacunar edema reduction and presence of activated keratocytes nuclei was recorded 30 days after contact lens removal, Fig. 4.8i. Corneal endothelium was unaltered after the treatment, Fig. 4.8j. Preoperative mean endothelial cell density was 2434

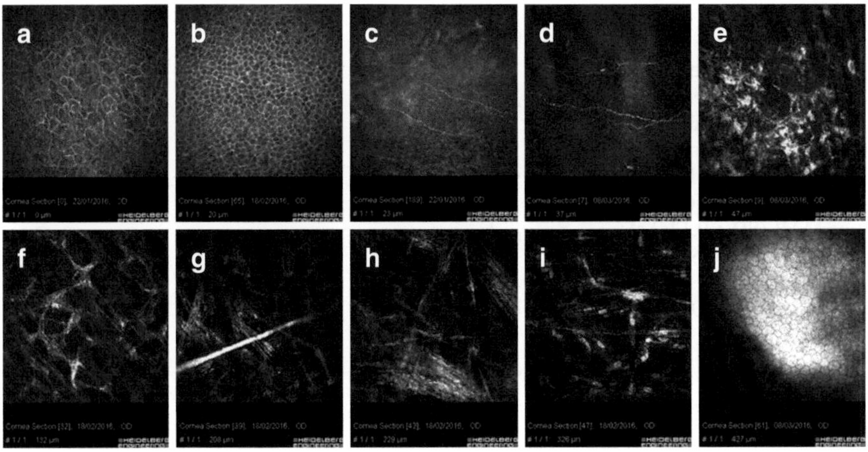

Fig. 4.8 IVCM after Siena Crosslinking Center 15 mW, 5.4 J/cm^2 High Irradiance ACXL Protocol®. Native epithelial cells were large with slightly defined cell borders oriented in a whorl-like fashion, (**a**). Regular basal epithelial cells mosaic with homogeneous cellularity and distinct cell borders 30 days after treatment (**b**). Sub-epithelial plexus (SEP) scans shows rarefaction and damage of SEP fibers, even not completely lost, at 3rd day after treatment (**c**). SEP nerve fibers showed rapid tendency to corneal reinnervation 30 days after treatment with bright nerve fibers evident, (**d**). 15 mW/cm^2 high- irradiance pulsed-light crosslinking induced keratocytes apoptosis in the anterior stroma associated with increased density of EC matrix (**e**). Lacunar corneal edema, hyperreflective trabecular mesh aspect of extracellular matrix and apoptotic bodies are well detectable (**f–h**). Gradual keratocytes repopulation with concomitant lacunar edema reduction and presence of activated keratocytes nuclei recorded 30 days after contact lens removal, (**i**). Corneal endothelium was unaltered after the treatment, (**j**)

cells/mm^2 (range 2182–2826 cells/mm^2). Post-operative endothelial cells count at 24-month was 2385 cells/mm^2 on average (range 2175–2985 cells/mm^2).

4.2.4 Results

Average Corrected Distance Visual Acuity (CDVA) showed a clinical improvement becoming statistically significant at the first postoperative month ($p = 0.0289$), from 0.27 Log MAR (SD ± 0.144) at baseline to 0.135 (SD ±0.1) at 24-month follow-up ($p = 0.0023$), Fig. 4.9.

Average K max values showed a not statistically significant reduction, from 48.33 D (SD ± 2.51 D) at baseline to 47.91 D (SD ± 1.56 D) at 24-month follow-up ($p = 0.66$), Fig. 4.10.

Average Coma values showed a statistically significant reduction since the first postoperative month ($p = 0.0004$), passing from 1.01 μm at baseline (SD ± 0.02 μm) to 0.94 μm (SD ± 0.014 μm) at 24-month follow-up ($p < 0.0001$), Fig. 4.11.

Average Minimum Corneal Thickness (MCT) showed a statistically significant value reduction from 453.3 μm at baseline (SD ± 24.01 μm) to 420 μm (SD ± 23.63 μm) ($p < 0.0001$ μm) at the first postoperative month, returning not statistically significant at the third postoperative month ($p = 0.25$ μm) maintaining a not statistically significant difference at 24-month follow-up 458.6 μm (SD ±12.83 μm) $p = 0.50$.

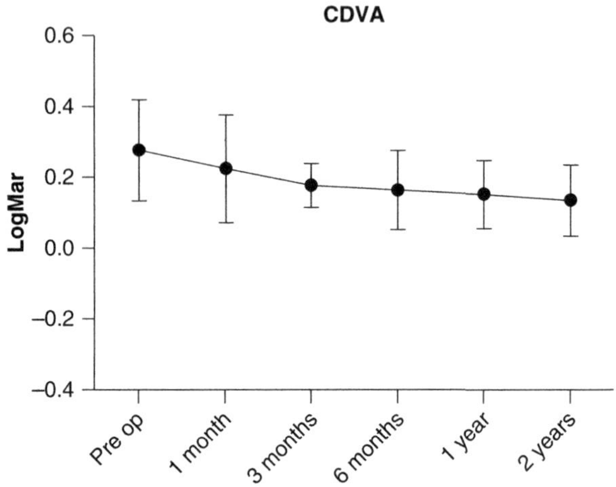

Fig. 4.9 Average Corrected Distance Visual Acuity (CDVA) showed a clinical improvement becoming statistically significant at the first postoperative month ($p = 0.0289$), from 0.27 Log MAR (SD ± 0.144) at baseline to 0.135 (SD ±0.1) at 24-month follow-up ($p = 0.0023$)

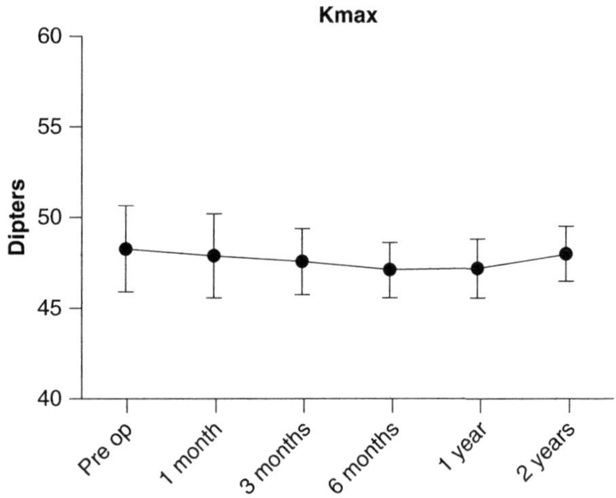

Fig. 4.10 Average K max values showed a not statistically significant reduction, from 48.33 D (SD ± 2.51 D) at baseline to 47.91 D (SD ± 1.56 D) at 24-month follow-up ($p = 0.66$)

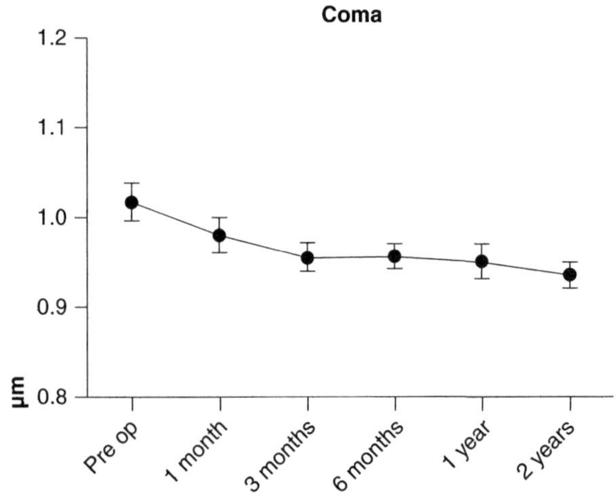

Fig. 4.11 Average Coma values showed a statistically significant reduction since the first postoperative month ($p = 0.0004$), passing from 1.01 µm at baseline (SD ± 0.02 µm) to 0.94 µm (SD ± 0.014 µm) at 24-month follow-up ($p < 0.0001$)

4.2.5 Discussion

The data tested in the laboratory study [5] performed by Krugher, Herekar and Spoerl, demonstrated that effective cross-linking requires the presence of oxygen in addition to sufficient penetration of riboflavin and UV-A exposure. It was determined that high-irradiance A-CXL was as efficacious as the conventional protocol and the better strain (elongation) test was achieved with 15 mW/cm^2 at 5.4 J/cm^2 Fluence with continuous (6 min) or pulsed (12 min, 1 s ON/1 s OFF) light UV-A exposure [5].

The Siena Crosslinking Center® high-irradiance 15 mW/5.4 J/cm^2 protocol permits a short treatment time while maintaining pulsed-light, achieving a treatment penetration comparable with conventional 3 mW CXL and 9 mW/cm^2 continuous light A-CXL [26, 27], benefiting from less SEP nerve damage, documented by the incomplete loss of nerve fibres at early postop IVCM scans as seen in Fig. 4.8. Further, contrary to conventional CXL where UDVA and CDVA often get worse in the first 3-months post op due to a variable glare disability related to stromal oedema, keratocytes loss and thin epithelium [40], the 15 mW pulsed-light high-irradiance CXL protocol at 5.4 J/cm^2 fluence showed less glare disability and not statistically significant visual acuity decay in the first three postoperative months maybe due to a lesser amount of postoperative oedema. According to our study results, the 15 mW/cm^2 pulsed-light high-irradiance CXL represents a safe and effective option to stabilize keratoconus progression, determining a statistically significant improvement of the UDVA and CDVA with a distinct tendency to a general improvement of all clinical and instrumental parameters, without adverse events and recorded complications.

As a practical consideration, we have no hesitation in accepting the opinion of Krueger, Herekar and Spoerl [5] concerning the advantages in clinical applications of high-irradiance cross-linking, not only for the reduction of treatment time, increasing patient's comfort, but also for reduced post op glare disability, reduced SEP nerves damage, no haze development and no endothelial damage with a substantially KC stabilization comparable to conventional procedure. The present study confirms the clinical safety of the Siena Crosslinking Center® 15 mW/ACXL pulsed-light treatment with epithelium removal and its efficacy in stabilizing keratoconus progression in absence of complications.

4.3 Transepithelial ACXL

4.3.1 Introduction

Trans-epithelial accelerated CXL techniques have been introduced with the aims of reducing postoperative pain, wound-related complications and infectious risk, offering the promise of CXL treatment delivery outside of the operating room [41].

There is general consensus that epi-on CXL is a safe procedure with no complications associated with the healing process but less effective that epithelium-off [41–44]. A number of enhanced riboflavin solutions [45] have been proposed for use in epi-on

CXL, including 0.01% and 0.02% benzalkonium chloride, 0.44% NaCl, TRIS, EDTA, HPMC, and hypotonic and isotonic salineas described in Chap. 2. Nonetheless, the trans-epithelial technique has three principal limitations: photo-attenuated UV-A stromal penetration, inhomogeneous penetration of riboflavin and the use of the same Fluence of standard UVA treatment (3 mW/cm^2, 5.4 J/cm^2) [46–48].

4.3.2 Iontophoresis-CXL (I-CXL)

As riboflavin is negatively charged at physiological pH and soluble in water, iontophoresis as a means of enhancing trans-epithelial absorption has been introduced [49–52] Fig. 4.12.

In vitro studies of CXL using iontophoresis-assisted delivery (I-CXL) of riboflavin 0.1% with a current of 0.5–1 mA for 5 min have been encouraging, demonstrating enhanced trans-epithelial riboflavin absorption [53]. Iontophoresis CXL (I-CXL) has been introduced in an attempt to overcome the major limitations of the original epi-on treatments (TE CXL): inhomogeneous and insufficient intrastromal riboflavin penetration and concentration and the natural shield against UV-A light penetration provided by the corneal epithelium (about 30–60% depending on UV light waveband) [43].

Iontophoresis-assisted trans-epithelial imbibition with Ricrolin + (Sooft, Montegiorgio, Italy) yielded greater and deeper riboflavin saturation compared with

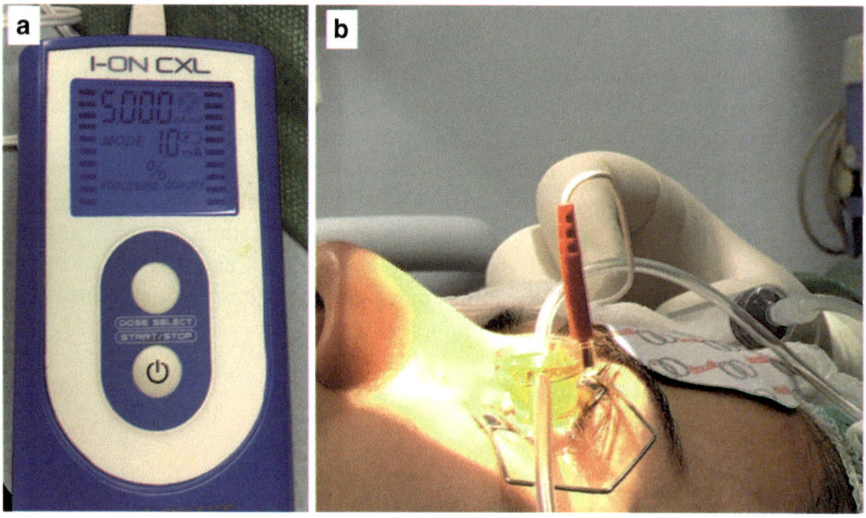

Fig. 4.12 Iontophoresis transepithelial CXL (I-CXL). The figure (**a**) shows the I-ON CXL generator and electrode-inox delivering a current of 1 mA for 5 min of corneal imbibition. Iontophoresis-assisted trans-epithelial imbibition is showed in figure (**b**) with 0.35 mL of Ricrolin + (Sooft, Montegiorgio, Italy) transfert in a 0.8 cm^2 of corneal surface, yielded greater and deeper riboflavin saturation compared with epi-on CXL with enhanced solutions (C. Mazzotta, Siena Crosslinking Center, Italy)

epi-on CXL with enhanced solutions [49, 51]. This approach also maintained the advantages of avoiding epithelial removal and shortened procedure time, but it did not reach the riboflavin concentrations obtained with standard epi-off riboflavin diffusion [44].

I-CXL has the potential to become the best possible trans-epithelial alternative for halting the progression of keratoconus and also for reducing patients' postoperative pain, reducing the risks of infection and wound-related complications, and maintaining a short treatment time. The 1-year outcomes of I-CXL were almost comparable to those with conventional epi-off CXL regarding stabilizing the progression of keratoconus [54, 55]; however, the 2-year follow-up showed less efficacy in halting keratoconus progression than conventional CXL [56, 57]. Therefore, the relative efficacy of this technique compared with standard epi-off techniques remains to be determined. There are two limitations of this method as actually used, requiring adjustments and further investigation: the halved riboflavin intrastromal concentration compared with conventional CXL, and the uneven demarcation line that is superficially visible in only 35% of eyes compared with 95% of eyes after conventional CXL [56]. At the Siena Crosslinking Center®, recently started an enhanced I-CXL protocol called SI-CXL with a customized iontophoresis epi-on treatment, calibrating the treatment fluence in relation to the UV-A light photo-attenuation provided by the corneal epithelium and Bowman's lamina according to UVA waveband, setting the UV-A power using the pulsed UV light, and calibrating the total treatment time to 17–20 min on average as showed in Fig. 4.13.

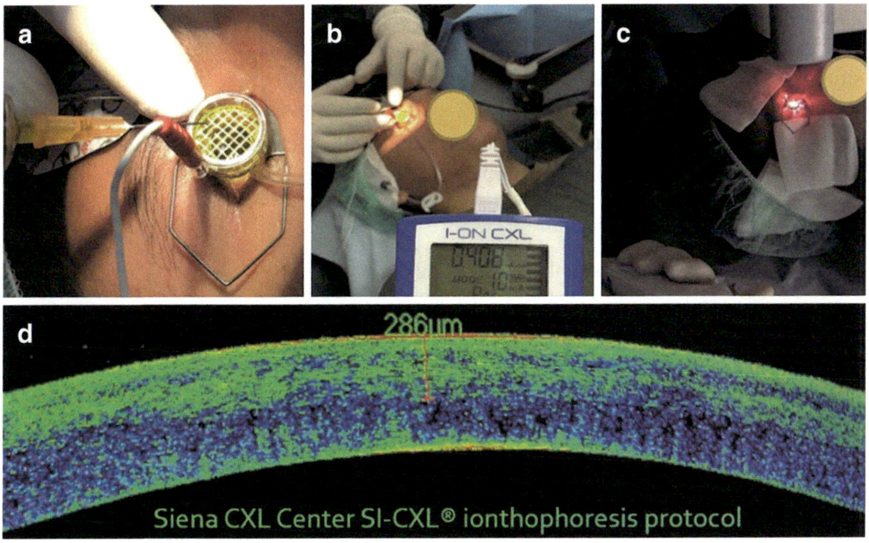

Fig. 4.13 SI-CXL Iontophoresis assisted transepithelial CXL (Mazzotta Protocol). Image (**a**) shows the corneal imbibition; image (**b**) the generator I-ON CXL. Image (**c**) shows the pulsed-light accelerated UVA irradiation (18 mW/cm^2) with enhanced Fluence of 30%. Image (**d**) shows the demarcation line observed after Mazzotta's high fluence pulsed-light I-CXL new protocol

Some studies have demonstrated that it is possible to make epithelial permeability better by modifying the standard riboflavin formula, riboflavin 5-phosphate [58].

There is laboratory evidence of riboflavin trans-epithelial stromal penetration using the preservative benzalkonium chloride (BAC), known for widening the epithelial junctures. However, when these eye drops containing BAC are chronically used, the cumulative dose can damage the corneal epithelial cells similar to the dry eye syndrome. The effects of BAC are both length and concentration dependent, and therefore it is logical that by reducing length of exposure to BAC the incidence of epithelial alterations could be reduced [59].

This was the rational for the development of the two-stage method for riboflavin application requiring a sequential application of riboflavin 0.25% with BAC (Paracel™, and riboflavin 0.25% without BAC (VibeX Xtra). A theoretical model proposed by Avedro, Inc. (Waltham, MA, USA), impregnating the cornea for 4 min with the riboflavin and BAC solution is sufficient for opening the epithelial junctions and for supplying the initial dose of riboflavin. The remaining part of the pre-soak (6 min) is completed with a solution of dextran and BAC free riboflavin (VibeX Xtra), with a consequent strong reduction of postoperative epithelial defects and pain.

Protocols for accelerated CXL have been used to shorten total treatment time for the procedure based on the Bunsen-Roscoe law are illustrated in Table 4.2.

In an epi-off procedure, an accelerated protocol using high-irradiance of 45 mW/cm^2 requires only 2 min to deliver the same dose of 5.4 J/cm^2 which is obtained in 30 min of irradiation with 3 mW/cm^2. In a transepithelial procedure, a dose of 7.2 J/cm^2 can be provided at Bowman's membrane level increasing treatment time to 2 min and 40 s, with an irradiance of 45 mW/cm^2.

Nevertheless, a higher intensity of UV-A, even if supplied with the epithelium in situ, causes slight damage to the sub-epithelial plexus nerves. In any case, stromal healing after A-CXL epi-on shows few cells in apoptosis and a sub-oedema more diffused and less lacunar as showed in confocal microscopy review studies by Mazzotta et al. [61]. A limited and irregular apoptotic effect is noticeable after

Table 4.2 Transepithelial crosslinking comparing protocols

Riboflavin formulation	Soak time (min)	UVA irradiance (mW/cm^2)	UVA time	Total energy (J/cm^2)
Ricrolin TE	30	3	30 min	5.4
Medio-Cross Te	30	3	30 min	5.4
ParaCel	15	45	2 min 40 s	7.2
Ricrolin + (with Iontophoresis)	5	10	9 min	5.4
ParaCel and VibeX Xtra (2 stage application)	4 + 6	45	2 min 40 s, continuous irradiation	7.2
ParaCel and VibeX Xtra (2 stage application)	4 + 6	45	5 min 20 s, pulsed irradiation (1 s on, 1 s off)	7.2

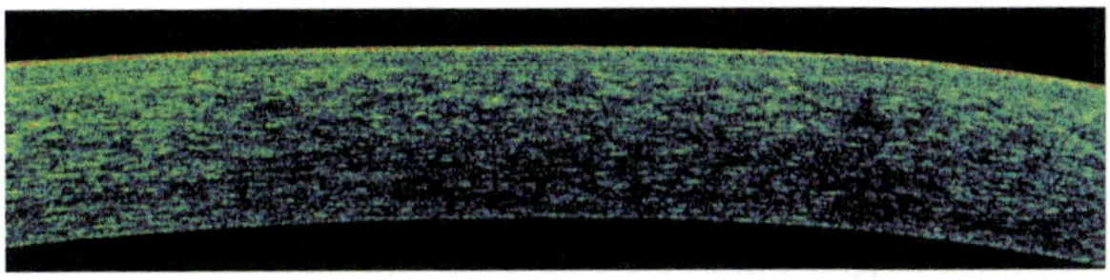

Fig. 4.14 High-Irradiance 45 mW/cm^2 transepithelial ACXL shows no evidence of demarcation line 1 month after treatment

A-CXL epi-on in the anterior stroma at an average depth of 80 μm (range 50–120 μm), Fig. 4.14, and a demarcation line is not visible at OCT scans, Fig. 4.14, confirming that the epithelium left in situ represent a barrier both for % of riboflavin and % of UV-A diffusion in the stroma inducing a superficial oxidative damage and less biomechanical effect compared with epi-off procedure.

Even in A-CXL epi-on, as in the previous transepithelial CXL procedures, the first in vivo analysis in man via confocal microscope [60] demonstrated that the presence of the corneal epithelium in situ establishes a physical barrier for UV-A radiation, reducing its penetration in the corneal stroma. The low penetration through the epithelium in A-CXL epi-on cannot biomechanically stabilize the cornea with keratoconus in a medium/long term follow-up, as demonstrated by the standard CXL trans-epithelial procedure (TE-CXL). According to most current evidences, it seems impossible to obtain sufficient riboflavin penetration in the stroma without any interruption of the epithelium. However, a compromise between efficiency and epithelial integrity should be reached. In fact, with children it could be desirable to minimize discomfort and accept inferior efficacy given the procedure can be repeated, and in very thin corneas an "aggressive" protocol could be used to maximize efficacy, having the epithelium as protection for the endothelium.

The first study with high-irradiance of 45 mW/cm^2 for 2 min and 40 s showed no significant changes in spherical equivalent, corrected distance visual acuity (CDVA) and topographical indices, but did show a significant increase in thinnest corneal thickness at 1-year and 2-year follow-up, compared with preoperative measurements in 48 eyes. The study of this protocol produced the secure and effective arrest of keratoconus progression for a follow-up period of 2 years, even if there is no valuation with a confocal microscope [61].

The other study [62] with irradiance of 30 mW/cm^2 for 3 min showed that accelerated transepithelial corneal CXL was safe and effective for progressive keratoconus over a 12-month follow-up period with a faster recovery, and a reduced rate of complications and operative and postoperative discomfort related to epithelial removal.

New methods were also introduced such as the use of pulsed light and oxygen [63] to favour UVA ray penetration in the corneal stroma, preserving the epithelium. Laboratory activity shows that additional oxygen can be supplied to the corneal surface to maximize the quantity of oxygen capable of reaching the stroma during CXL epi-on. In laboratory experiments, the combination of supplementary oxygen and pulsed light could provide substantial amplification in the CXL process. This approach can increase trans-epithelial CXL efficacy and must be evaluated in the next future.

Hence, a further, long-term follow-up is necessary to better evaluate the efficiency relative to various epi-on A-CXL protocols in the stabilization of the progression of keratoconus. A-CXL procedures, as they emerge, will be calibrated to a specific efficacy range window, with a duration of 20 min on average and a programmed treatment dose, UV-A power level and penetration depth. In the near future, the combination of sufficient stromal riboflavin uptake, adequate exposure time, increased stromal oxygenation, and calibrated UV-A fluence could lead to better efficacy of epi-on A-CXL procedures. Increasing reactive oxygen availability may increase CXL amount and efficacy of epithelium-on CXL procedures.

4.4 Thin Corneas

4.4.1 Introduction

The conventional CXL procedure, as described in the Dresden protocol [3], and the Siena protocol [13], applies to corneas with minimum stromal thickness of 400 μm and involves the removal of the central 7–9 mm of corneal epithelium followed by the instillation of isotonic riboflavin 0.1% solution in 20% dextran from 10 (Siena Protocol) to 30 min (Dresden Protocol) of stromal imbibition, UVA (370 nm) irradiation with 3 mW/cm^2 of UVA for 30 min at a fluence (E dose) of 5.4 J/cm^2 (Table 4.3).

Table 4.3 CXL in thin corneas

Author, year	No. of eyes	Surgical procedures	Follow up (months)	Endothelial loss
Kymionis 2009	2	Custom epithelial debridement	9	No
Hafezi 2009	20	Hypoosmolar riboflavin solution	6	–
Kaya 2011	2	Custom epithelial debridement	1	–
Raiskup 2011	32	Hypoosmolar riboflavin solution	12	–
Kymionis 2012	14	Conventional	12	Yes
Filippello 2012	20	Transepithelial CXL	18	No
Spadea 2012	16	Transepithelial CXL	6–12	No
Mazzotta 2014	10	Custom epithelial debridement, Epithelial Island technique	12	No
Jacob 2014	14	Contact lens-assisted	6–7	No
Wu 2014	15	Hypoosmolar riboflavin solution	12	No
Soeters 2015	13	Hypoosmolar riboflavin solution	12	No
Gu 2015	8	Hypoosmolar riboflavin solution	3	Yes

4.4.2 Hypo-osmolar Riboflavin Solution

The cornea has an inert swelling pressure [64], meaning that the stroma has the tendency to increase its volume in an isooncotic environment. The de-epithelialized cornea can swell to double its normal thickness when irrigated with a hypoosmolar solution [65]. Hafezi and his team [66] applied this method to increase corneal thickness before CXL in thin corneas. After epithelial removal, 0.1–20% dextran isoosmolar riboflavin was applied to the cornea for 30 min. They reported stabilization of ectasia in 12 patients and regression in eight patients. No clinical signs of endothelial damage or any other side effect was seen. Raiskup and Spoerl [9] published 1 year results of hypoosmolar CXL in 32 eyes. Hafezi and colleagues [67] reported a case where CXL could not stop the progression of keratoconus in a very thin cornea (minimal thickness of 268 μm after removal of the epithelium), despite the fact that swelling with hypoosmolar riboflavin solution increased the thickness to 406 μm and no adverse endothelial reaction was postoperatively observed. The authors concluded that to prevent ectasia, a minimum stromal thickness of 330 μm should be present.

Kaya et al. [68] and Soeters et al. [69, 70, 71] performed intraoperative corneal thickness measurements during CXL with hypoosmolar riboflavin solution in thin corneas. They found that the artificial swelling was significant after hypo-osmolar riboflavin application for 10 min (by 59.56 ± 29.71 μm). However, it was demonstrated that the artificial swelling effect was transient, and the thinnest pachymetric readings decreased significantly at the end of hypo-osmolar riboflavin application [69]. Other problems related to corneal expansion are the dilution of 0.1% riboflavin causing a much lower bioavailability of the photosensitizer, stromal hypotony with relative endothelial toxicity, mechanical lamellar separation and disalignment with consequent CXL amount reduction. Corneal expansion with hypo-osmolar saline riboflavin solutions could be dangerous for endothelium due to the transient effect of stromal expansion and the necessity of a constant intraoperative pachymetry check in order to be sure of the "real" stroma thickness during UVA irradiation. Thin corneas treated with unsteady expansion may have serious complications such as endothelial decompensation or endothelial-stromal hot spots and scars as showed in Fig. 4.15.

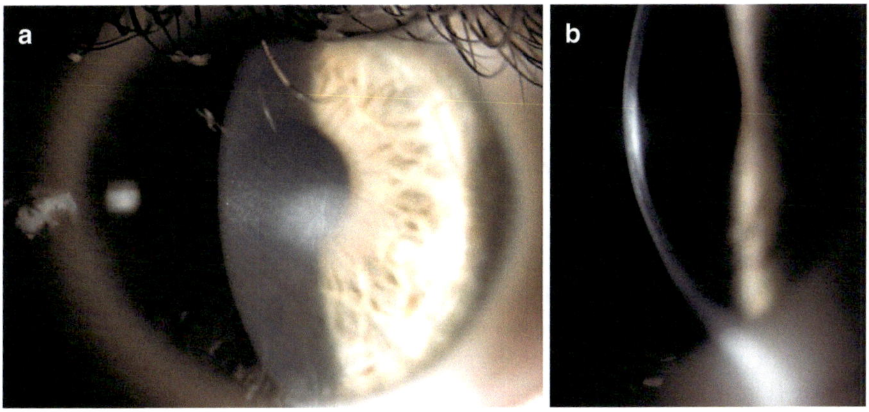

Fig. 4.15 Thin Cornea treated with corneal expansion with an hypotonic riboflavin solution. (**a**) persistent haze reducing patient's Visual Acuity. (**b**) Endothelial and stromal hot spot with a large central

It was therefore suggested that new riboflavin solutions with isooncotic properties be developed to create a stable film, which could increase the safety of CXL [71]. Moreover, lack of evaporation resistance provided by the corneal epithelium [72], and/or an increase in endothelial pump activity may also contribute to corneal thinning [73, 74]. It was proposed that removal of the lid speculum during riboflavin saturation, and use of irradiating devices with shorter irradiation time (and higher power) could be advantageous [75]. The pachymetry check should be continuous during UVA irradiation with conventional 3 mW or accelerated 9 mW/cm^2 ensuring treatment safety.

4.4.3 Transepithelial CXL

Transepithelial CXL was introduced to prevent the adverse events associated with epithelial debridement in general, as well as for its possible role in treating thinner corneas. Wollensak and Iomdina, showed a reduction of the biomechanical effect by approximately one fifth compared with standard cross linking in rabbit models [76].

Substances such as benzalkonium chloride, ethylenediaminetetraacetic acid (EDTA) and trometamol, especially when combined, enhance epithelial permeability of hydrophilic macromolecules such as riboflavin [75]. By adding the enhancers to help riboflavin penetrate to the corneal stroma through the intact epithelium, CXL can be performed without epithelial debridement (transepithelial CXL) [76].

Transepithelial CXL in 20 patients with bilateral progressive keratoconus using enhanced riboflavin solution, containing trometamol and ethylenediaminetetraacetic acid (EDTA) sodium salt, was undertaken by Filippello and his team. They reported a statistically significant improvement in visual and topographic parameters, and concluded that the treatment appeared to halt keratoconus progression [77].

Spadea and his collaborators [78], who used a similar protocol in thin corneas, confirmed its effect in stabilization of the keratoconic eyes.

Long term results by Caporossi, Mazzotta et al. [79] failed to support this technique. In their 24 month follow up they found keratoconus instability and functional regression, particularly in patients less than 18 years.

4.4.4 Customized Pachymetry Guided Epithelial Debridement

Based on the preliminary report of Kymionis et al. [80], Mazzotta and Ramovecchi [81] introduced the customized epithelium-off corneal collagen CXL technique named epithelial-island cross-linking technique (EI-CXL) in a series of ten keratoconic patients with progressive keratoconus and thin corneas, using in-vivo laser scanning confocal analysis, tomographic, and clinical evaluation in a 1-year follow-up (Fig. 4.16).

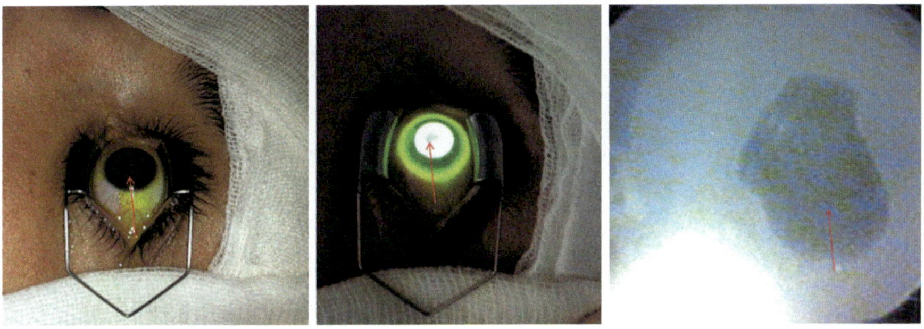

Fig. 4.16 Mazzotta Epithelial Island CXL for thin corneas (*red arrows*) during ultra violet-A exposure; the shield effect provided by epithelium in situ is well evident reducing the typical fluorescence of activated riboflavin by the UV-A illumination

The technique involves mechanically removing 8.0 mm diameter of corneal epithelium, while preserving a small localized (2–3 mm) island corresponding to the thinnest area or the area of maximum topographic steepening.

Preservation of epithelium over the thinnest area also has possible advantage of prevention of local stromal dehydration apart from blocking excessive UV radiation in this susceptible area.

Kaya and his staff [82] studied the effect of cross linking with this technique through anterior segment optical coherence tomography (ASOCT) and confocal microscopic imaging, and they reported that the CXL effect in terms of keratocyte loss and hyperreflectivity was limited to anterior 150 μm as compared to 250 μm in conventional CXL.

4.4.5 Contact Lens Assisted CXL

Jacob and his team [83] described the use of a riboflavin-soaked bandage contact lens of negligible power to artificially increase the corneal thickness for CXL, called Contact-lens Assisted CXL (CA-CXL), showed in Fig. 4.17. Both the contact lens and de-epithelialized cornea are soaked in Riboflavin 0.1% solution for 30 min, at the end of which the riboflavin soaked contact lens is applied over the cornea and collective pachymetry measured and CXL started as conventional procedure. Long-term results of this procedure are not available. Mazzotta studied in vivo confocal microscopy (IVCM) after CA-CXL in ten keratoconic eyes with thin corneas confirming the efficacy and safety of this technique useful for thin corneas between 350 and 400 μm [84].

4.4.6 Smile Assisted CXL

SMILE Assisted CXL involves the application over a thin cornea of the refractive lenticule extracted from the patients undergoing the small incision

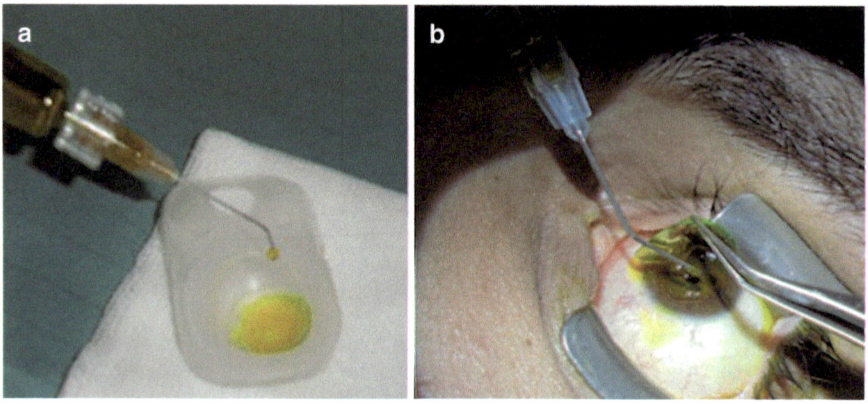

Fig. 4.17 The cornea and the contact lens are saturated with 0.1% riboflavin solution every 3 min for 30 min, at the end of which the riboflavin-soaked contact lens (**a**) is applied to the cornea. The minimum pachymetry reading of stroma and contact lens together should be above 400 μm. The riboflavin solution is instilled under the contact lens (**b**) precorneal riboflavin film, and over the contact lens (precontact lens riboflavin film). The cornea is exposed to 370 nm of UVA light and 5.4 J cm^2 for 30 min

femtosecond lenticule extraction (SMILE) procedure for myopia. Also cryopreserved lenticules are available for this use. SMILE involves the extraction of a femtosecond laser–constructed corneal lenticule through a single small incision without raising a flap [85]. The lenticular thickness depends on the refractive error of the patient. The technique hover presents some disadvantages: limited access to donor SMILE lenticule, need for donor SMILE lenticule of sufficient thickness (8D) or need to tailor according to patient and acquire correct size, storage of tissue, variability of tissue pachymetry depending on storage medium used, edema/dehydration of lenticule may cause erroneous shifts in pachymetry, intra-operative pachymetry (contact), intra-operative pachymetry in a sitting position with standard OCT pachymetry may lead to increased risk of lenticule drop.

Conclusion

Actually a safe CXL in thinner corneas can be achieved by Accelerated customized CXL treatment according to different UV-A power and exposure time [86, 87]. The usage of HPMC (Hydroxypropyl methylcellulose) riboflavin solutions avoiding intraoperative dehydration is mandatory in thin corneas management helps prevent corneal dehydration induced by dextran [88, 89]. Customized Accelerated protocol nomograms are the key in the future treatments of thin corneas according to in vivo confocal reports and OCT studies allowing to overcome the limitation of the various techniques described, obtaining a standardized method based on preoperative pachymetry, calibrated UVA power setting, exposure time and fluence [35].

References

1. Spörl E, Huhle M, Kasper M, Seiler T. Increased rigidity of the cornea caused by intrastromal cross-linking. Ophthalmologe. 1997;94(12):902–6. German.
2. Wollensak G, Spoerl E, Seiler T. Riboflavin/ultraviolet-a-induced collagen crosslinking for the treatment of keratoconus. Am J Ophthalmol. 2003;135(5):620–7.
3. Raiskup-Wolf F, Hoyer A, Spoerl E, Pillunat LE. Collagen crosslinking with riboflavin and ultraviolet-A light in keratoconus: long-term results. J Cataract Refract Surg. 2008;34(5):796–801. https://doi.org/10.1016/j.jcrs.2007.12.039.
4. Schumacher S, Oeftiger L, Mrochen M. Equivalence of biomechanical changes induced by rapid and standard corneal cross-linking, using riboflavin and ultraviolet radiation. Invest Ophthalmol Vis Sci. 2011;52(12):9048–52.
5. Krueger RR, Herekar S, Spoerl E. First proposed efficacy study of high versus standard irradiance and fractioned riboflavin/ultraviolet A cross-linking with equivalent energy exposure. Eye Contact Lens. 2014;40:353–7.
6. Wernli J, Schumacher S, Spoerl E, Mrochen M. The efficacy of corneal cross-linking shows a sudden decrease with very high intensity UV light and short treatment time. Invest Ophthalmol Vis Sci. 2013;54(2):1176–80.
7. Hammer A, Richoz O, Arba Mosquera S, Tabibian D, Hoogewoud F, Hafezi F. Corneal biomechanical properties at different corneal cross-linking (CXL) irradiances. Invest Ophthalmol Vis Sci. 2014;55(5):2881–4.
8. Ehmke T, Seiler TG, Fischinger I, Ripken T, Heisterkamp A, Frueh BE. Comparison of corneal riboflavin gradients using dextran and HPMC solutions. J Refract Surg. 2016;32(12):798–802.
9. Raiskup F, Spoerl E. Corneal cross-linking with hypo-osmolar riboflavin solution in thin keratoconic corneas. Am J Ophthalmol. 2011;152(1):28–32.
10. Seiler TG, Fischinger I, Koller T, Zapp D, Frueh BE, Seiler T. Customized corneal cross-linking: one-year results. Am J Ophthalmol. 2016;166:14–21.
11. Wittig-Silva C, Chan E, Islam FM, Wu T, Whiting M, Snibson GR. A randomized, controlled trial of corneal collagen cross-linking in progressive keratoconus: three-year results. Ophthalmology. 2014;121(4):812–21.
12. Cummings AB, McQuaid R, Naughton S, et al. Optimizing corneal cross-linking in the treatment of keratoconus: a comparison of outcomes after standard- and high-intensity protocols. Cornea. 2016;35(6):814–22.
13. Caporossi A, Mazzotta C, Baiocchi S, Caporossi T. Long-term results of riboflavin ultraviolet a corneal collagen cross-linking for keratoconus in Italy: the Siena eye cross study. Am J Ophthalmol. 2010;149(4):585–93. https://doi.org/10.1016/j.ajo.2009.10.021.
14. Greenstein SA, Shah VP, Fry KL, et al. Corneal thickness changes after corneal collagen crosslinking for keratoconus and corneal ectasia: one-year results. J Cataract Refract Surg. 2011;37(4):691–700.
15. Vinciguerra R, Romano MR, Camesasca FI, et al. Corneal cross-linking as a treatment for keratoconus: four-year morphologic and clinical outcomes with respect to patient age. Ophthalmology. 2013;120(5):908–16.
16. Grewal DS, Brar GS, Jain R, et al. Corneal collagen crosslinking using riboflavin and ultraviolet-A light for keratoconus: one-year analysis using Scheimpflug imaging. J Cataract Refract Surg. 2009;35(3):425–32.
17. Greenstein SA, Fry KL, Hersh PS. Corneal topography indices after corneal collagen crosslinking for keratoconus and corneal ectasia: one-year results. J Cataract Refract Surg. 2011;37(7):1282–90.
18. Koller T, Iseli HP, Hafezi F, et al. Scheimpflug imaging of corneas after collagen cross-linking. Cornea. 2009;28(5):510–5.
19. Raiskup F, Theuring A, Pillunat LE, Spoerl E. Corneal collagen crosslinking with riboflavin and ultraviolet-A light in progressive keratoconus: ten-year results. J Cataract Refract Surg. 2015;41(1):41–6.

20. O'Brart DP, Patel P, Lascaratos G, Wagh VK, Tam C, Lee J, O'Brart NA. Corneal cross-linking to halt the progression of keratoconus and corneal ectasia: seven-year follow-up. Am J Ophthalmol. 2015;160(6):1154–63.
21. Godefrooij DA, Gans R, Imhof SM, Wisse RP. Nationwide reduction in the number of corneal transplantations for keratoconus following the implementation of cross-linking. Acta Ophthalmol. 2016;94(7):675–8.
22. Spoerl E, Mrochen M, Sliney D, Trokel S, Seiler T. Safety of UVA-riboflavin cross-linking of the cornea. Cornea. 2007;26(4):385–9.
23. Iseli HP, Thiel MA, Hafezi F, et al. Ultraviolet A/riboflavin cross-linking for infectious keratitis associated with corneal melts. Cornea. 2008;27:590–4.
24. Tabibian D, Richoz O, Riat A, Schrenzel J, Hafezi F. Accelerated photoactivated chromophore for keratitis-corneal collagen cross-linking as a first-line and sole treatment in early fungal keratitis. J Refract Surg. 2014;30(12):855–7.
25. Tabibian D, Mazzotta C, Hafezi F. PACK-CXL: corneal cross-linking in infectious keratitis. Eye Vis (Lond). 2016;3:11.
26. Elbaz U, Shen C, Lichtinger A, et al. Accelerated (9-mW/cm2) corneal collagen crosslinking for keratoconus-A 1-year follow-up. Cornea. 2014;33(8):769–73.
27. Ulusoy DM, Göktaş E, Duru N, Özköse A, Ataş M, Yuvacı İ, Arifoğlu HB, Zararsız G. Accelerated corneal crosslinking for treatment of progressive keratoconus in pediatric patients. Eur J Ophthalmol. 2017;27(3):319–25. https://doi.org/10.5301/ejo.5000848.
28. Marino GK, Torricelli AA, Giacomin N, Santhiago MR, Espindola R, Netto MV. Accelerated corneal collagen crosslinking for postoperative LASIK ectasia: two-year outcomes. J Refract Surg. 2015;31(6):380–4.
29. Chow VW, Chan TC, Yu M, Wong VW, Jhanji V. One year outcomes of conventional and accelerated collagen crosslinking in progressive keratoconus. Sci Rep. 2015;5:14425.
30. Da Paz AC, Bersanetti PA, Salomão MQ, Ambrósio R Jr, Schor P. Theoretical basis, laboratory evidence, and clinical research of chemical surgery of the cornea: cross-linking. J Ophthalmol. 2014;2014:e890823. https://doi.org/10.1155/2014/890823.
31. Brindley GS. The Bunsen-Roscoe law for the human eye at very short durations. J Physiol. 1952;118(1):135–9.
32. Kamaev P, Friedman MD, Sherr E, Muller D. Photochemical kinetics of corneal cross-linking with riboflavin. Invest Ophthalmol Vis Sci. 2012;53(4):2360–7.
33. Mazzotta C, Traversi C, Caragiuli S, Rechichi M. Pulsed vs continuous light accelerated corneal collagen crosslinking: in vivo qualitative investigation by confocal microscopy and corneal OCT. Eye (Lond). 2014;28(10):1179–83.
34. Mazzotta C, Traversi C, Paradiso AL, Latronico ME, Rechichi M. Pulsed light accelerated crosslinking versus continuous light accelerated crosslinking: one-year results. J Ophthalmol. 2014;2014:604731.
35. Mazzotta C, Hafezi F, Kymionis G, Caragiuli S, Jacob S, Traversi C, Barabino S, Randleman JB. In vivo confocal microscopy after corneal collagen crosslinking. Ocul Surf. 2015;13(4):298–314.
36. Peyman A, Nouralishahi A, Hafezi F, Kling S, Peyman M. Stromal demarcation line in pulsed versus continuous light accelerated corneal cross-linking for keratoconus. J Refract Surg. 2016;32(3):206–8.
37. Kling S, Richoz O, Hammer A, Tabibian D, Jacob S, Agarwal A, Hafezi F. Increased biomechanical efficacy of corneal cross-linking in thin corneas due to higher oxygen availability. J Refract Surg. 2015;31(12):840–6.
38. Mazzotta C, Moramarco A, Traversi C, Baiocchi S, Iovieno A, Fontana L. Accelerated corneal collagen cross-linking using topography-guided UV-A energy emission: preliminary clinical and morphological outcomes. J Ophthalmol. 2016;2016:2031031.
39. Mazzotta C, Baiocchi S, Simone AB, MD, Fruschelli M, Alessandro M, Rechichi M. Accelerated 15 mW pulsed-light crosslinking in treatment of progressive keratoconus: Two-year clinical results. J Cataract and Refract Surg. 2017, in press.

40. Mazzotta C, Caporossi T, Denaro R, Bovone C, Sparano C, Paradiso A, Baiocchi S, Caporossi A. Morphological and functional correlations in riboflavin UV A corneal collagen cross-linking for keratoconus. Acta Ophthalmol. 2012;90(3):259–65.
41. Caporossi A, Mazzotta C, Paradiso AL, et al. Transepithelial corneal collagen crosslinking for progressive keratoconus: 24-month clinical results. J Cataract Refract Surg. 2013;39:1157–63.
42. Leccisotti A, Islam T. Transepithelial corneal collagen crosslinking in keratoconus. J Refract Surg. 2010;26:942–8.
43. Podskochy A. Protective role of corneal epithelium against ultraviolet radiation damage. Acta Ophthalmol Scand. 2004;82:714–7.
44. Magli A, Forte R, Tortori A, et al. Epithelium-off corneal collagen cross-linking versus transepithelial cross-linking for pediatric keratoconus. Cornea. 2013;32:597–601.
45. Gatzioufas Z, Raiskup F, O'Brart D, Spoerl E, Panos GD, Hafezi F. Transepithelial corneal cross-linking using an enhanced riboflavin solution. J Refract Surg. 2016;32(6):372–7.
46. Bottos KM, Schor P, Dreyfuss JL, et al. Effect of corneal epithelium on ultraviolet-A and riboflavin absorption. Arq Bras Oftalmol. 2011;74:348–51.
47. Kohlhaas M, Spoerl E, Schilde T, Unger G, Wittig C, Pillunat LE. Biomechanical evidence of the distribution of cross-links in corneas treated with riboflavin and ultraviolet A light. J Cataract Refract Surg. 2006;32(2):279–83.
48. Schumacher S, Mrochen M, Wernli J, Bueeler M, Seiler T. Optimization model for UV-riboflavin corneal cross-linking. Invest Ophthalmol Vis Sci. 2012;53(2):762–9.
49. Cassagne M, Laurent C, Rodrigues M, Galinier A, Spoerl E, Galiacy SD, Soler V, Fournié P, Malecaze F. Iontophoresis Transcorneal Delivery Technique for Transepithelial Corneal Collagen Crosslinking With Riboflavin in a Rabbit Model. Invest Ophthalmol Vis Sci. 2016;57(2):594–603.
50. Bikbova G, Bikbov M. Transepithelial corneal collagen crosslinking by iontophoresis of riboflavin. Acta Ophthalmol. 2014;92:e30–4.
51. Vinciguerra P, Mencucci R, Romano V, et al. Imaging mass spectrometry by matrix-assisted laser desorption/ionization and stress-strain measurements in iontophoresis transepithelial corneal collagen cross-linking. Biomed Res Int. 2014;2014:404587.
52. Vinciguerra P, Mencucci R, Romano V, Spoerl E, Camesasca FI, Favuzza E, Azzolini C, Mastropasqua R, Vinciguerra R. Imaging mass spectrometry by matrix-assisted laser desorption/ionization and stress-strain measurements in iontophoresis transepithelial corneal collagen cross-linking. Biomed Res Int. 2014:404587. https://doi.org/10.1155/2014/404587.
53. Mencucci R, Paladini I, Sarchielli E, et al. Transepithelial riboflavin/ultraviolet a corneal cross-linking in keratoconus: morphologic studies on human corneas. Am J Ophthalmol. 2013;156:874–84.
54. Vinciguerra P, Randleman JB, Romano V, et al. Transepithelial iontophoresis corneal collagen cross-linking for progressive keratoconus: initial clinical outcomes. J Refract Surg. 2014;30:746–53.
55. Vinciguerra P, Romano V, Rosetta P, Legrottaglie EF, Piscopo R, Fabiani C, Azzolini C, Vinciguerra R. Transepithelial iontophoresis versus standard corneal collagen cross-linking: 1-year results of a prospective clinical study. J Refract Surg. 2016;32(10):672–8. https://doi.org/10.3928/1081597X-20160629-02.
56. Jouve L, Borderie V, Sandali O, Temstet C, Basli E, Laroche L, Bouheraoua N. Conventional and iontophoresis corneal cross-linking for keratoconus: efficacy and assessment by optical coherence tomography and confocal microscopy. Cornea. 2017;36(2):153–62.
57. Bikbova G, Bikbov M. Standard corneal collagen crosslinking versus transepithelial iontophoresis-assisted corneal crosslinking, 24 months follow-up: randomized control trial. Acta Ophthalmol. 2016;94(7):e600–6. https://doi.org/10.1111/aos.13032. Epub 2016 Apr 4.
58. Raiskup F, Pinelli R, Spoerl E. Riboflavin osmolar modification for transepithelial corneal cross-linking. Curr Eye Res. 2012;37(3):234–8.
59. Cha SH, Lee JS, Oum BS, Kim CD. Corneal epithelial cellular dysfunction from benzalkonium chloride (BAC) in vitro. Clin Experiment Ophthalmol. 2004;32:180–4.

60. Mazzotta C, Paradiso AL, Baiocchi S, Caragiuli S, Caporossi A. Qualitative investigation of corneal changes after accelerated corneal collagen cross-linking (A-CXL) by in vivo confocal microscopy and corneal OCT. J Clin Exp Ophthalmol. 2013;4:313.
61. Mazzotta C, Hafezi F, Kymionis G, Caragiuli S, Jacob S, Traversi C, Barabino S, Randleman JB. In Vivo Confocal Microscopy after Corneal Collagen Crosslinking. Ocul Surf. 2015;13(4):298–314.
62. Aixinjueluo W, Usui T, Miyai T, Toyono T, Sakisaka T, Yamagami S. Accelerated transepithelial corneal cross-linking for progressive keratoconus: a prospective study of 12 months. Br J Ophthalmol. 2017. https://doi.org/10.1136/bjophthalmol-2016-309775.
63. Richoz O, Hammer A, Tabibian D, Gatzioufas Z, Hafezi F. The biomechanical effect of corneal collagen cross-linking (CXL) with riboflavin and UV-A is oxygen dependent. Transl Vis Sci Technol. 2013;2(7):6. Epub 2013 Dec 11.
64. Dohlman CH, Hedbys BO, Mishima S. The swelling pressure of the corneal stroma. Investig Ophthalmol. 1962;1:158–62.
65. Maurice DM, Giardini AA. Swelling of the cornea in vivo after the destruction of its limiting layers. Br J Ophthalmol. 1951;35:791–7. https://doi.org/10.1136/bjo.35.12.791.
66. Hafezi F, Mrochen M, Iseli HP, Seiler T. Collagen crosslinking with ultraviolet-A and hypoosmolar riboflavin solution in thin corneas. J Cataract Refract Surg. 2009;35:621–4. https://doi.org/10.1016/j.jcrs.2008.10.060.
67. Hafezi F. Limitation of collagen cross-linking with hypoosmolar riboflavin solution: failure in an extremely thin cornea. Cornea. 2011;30(8):917–9.
68. Kaya V, Utine CA, Yilmaz OF. Intraoperative corneal thickness measurements during corneal collagen cross-linking with hypoosmolar riboflavin solution in thin corneas. Cornea. 2012;31:486–90. https://doi.org/10.1097/ICO.0b013e31821e4286.
69. Soeters N, Tahzib NG. Standard and hypoosmolar corneal cross-linking in various pachymetry groups. Optom Vis Sci. 2015;92:329–36.
70. Soeters N, van Bussel E, van der Valk R, Van der Lelij A, Tahzib NG. Effect of the eyelid speculum on pachymetry during corneal collagen crosslinking in keratoconus patients. J Cataract Refract Surg. 2014;40:575–81. https://doi.org/10.1016/j.jcrs.2013.08.060.
71. Iwata S, Lemp MA, Holly FJ, Dohlman CH. Evaporation rate of water from the precorneal tear film and cornea in the rabbit. Investig Ophthalmol. 1969;8:613–9.
72. Holopainen JM, Krootila K. Transient corneal thinning in eyes undergoing corneal cross-linking. Am J Ophthalmol. 2011;152:533–6. https://doi.org/10.1016/j.ajo.2011.03.023.
73. Tahzib NG, Van der Lelij A. Pachymetry during cross-linking. Ophthalmology. 2010;117:2041. https://doi.org/10.1016/j.ophtha.2010.06.002.
74. Schmidinger G, Pachala M, Prager F. Pachymetry changes during corneal crosslinking: effect of closed eyelids and hypotonic riboflavin solution. J Cataract Refract Surg. 2013;39:1179–83. https://doi.org/10.1016/j.jcrs.2013.03.021.
75. Ozgurhan EB, Ackay BI, Kurt T, Yildrim Y, Demirok A. Accelerated corneal collagen cross-linking in thin keratoconic corneas. J Refract Surg. 2015;31:386–90.
76. Wollensak G, Iomdina E. Biomechanical and histological changes after corneal crosslinking with and without epithelial debridement. J Cataract Refract Surg. 2009;35:540–6.
77. Filippello M, Stagni E, O'Brart D. Transepithelial corneal collagen crosslinking: bilateral study. J Cataract Refract Surg. 2012;38:283–91. https://doi.org/10.1016/j.jcrs.2011.08.030.
78. Spadea L, Mencucci R. Transepithelial corneal collagen cross-linking in ultrathin keratoconic corneas. Clin Ophthalmol. 2012;6:1785–92. https://doi.org/10.2147/OPTH.S37335.
79. Caporossi A, Mazzotta C, Paradiso AL, Baiochhi S, Marigliani D, Caporossi T. Transepithelial corneal collagen crosslinking for progressive keratoconus: 24-months results. J Cataract Refract Surg. 2014;49:450–8.
80. Kymionis GD, Diakonis VF, Coskunseven E, Jankov M, Yoo SH, Pallikaris IG. Customized pachymetric guided epithelial debridement for corneal collagen cross linking. BMC Ophthalmol. 2009;9:10. https://doi.org/10.1186/1471-2415-9-10.
81. Mazzotta C, Ramovecchi V. Customized epithelial debridement for thin ectatic corneas undergoing corneal cross-linking: epithelial island cross-linking technique. Clin Ophthalmol. 2014;8:1337–43. https://doi.org/10.2147/OPTH.S66372.

82. Kaya V, Utine CA, Yilmaz OF. Efficacy of corneal collagen cross-linking using a custom epithelial debridement technique in thin corneas: a confocal microscopy study. J Refract Surg. 2011;27(6):444–50.
83. Jacob S, Kumar DA, Agarwal A, Basu S, Sinha P, Agarwal A. Contact lens-assisted collagen cross-linking (CACXL): a new technique for cross-linking thin corneas. J Refract Surg. 2014;30:366–72.
84. Mazzotta C, Jacob S, Agarwal A, Kumar DA. In vivo confocal microscopy after contact lens-assisted corneal collagen cross-linking for thin keratoconic corneas. J Refract Surg. 2016;32(5):326–31. https://doi.org/10.3928/1081597X-20160225-04.
85. Shah R, Shah S, Sengupta S. Results of small incision lenticule extraction: all-in-one femtosecond laser refractive surgery. J Cataract Refract Surg. 2011;37:127–37.
86. Wu H, Luo S, Dong N, Lin Z, Liu Z, Shang X. The clinical study of corneal cross-linking with hypo-osmolar riboflavin solution in thin keratoconic corneas. Zhonghua Yan Ke Za Zhi. 2014;50:681–6.
87. Gu SF, Fan ZS, Wang LH, Tao XC, Zhang Y, Wang CQ, et al. A short-term study of corneal collagen cross-linking with hypo-osmolar riboflavin solution in keratoconic corneas. Int J Ophthalmol. 2015;8:94–7.
88. Mazzotta C, Caragiuli S. Intraoperative corneal thickness measurement by optical coherence tomography in keratoconic patients undergoing corneal collagen cross-linking. Am J Ophthalmol. 2014;157(6):1156–62.
89. Rechichi M, Mazzotta C, Daya S, Mencucci R, Lanza M, Meduri A. Intraoperative OCT pachymetry in patients undergoing dextran-free riboflavin UVA accelerated corneal collagen crosslinking. Curr Eye Res. 2016;16:1–6.

Refractive Crosslinking: ACXL Plus

5

5.1 Crosslinking with Combined Surface Laser Ablation: STARE XL Protocol

Keratoconus is a degenerative non-inflammatory ectatic disease of the cornea characterized by biomechanical instability of stromal collagen leading to a reduction in corneal thickness, a variation in posterior and anterior corneal curvature, fluctuation and loss of visual acuity attributable to irregular astigmatism with or without a reduction in corneal transparency.

Many techniques were described for treating keratoconus but since its introduction more than 10 years ago, Riboflavin–ultraviolet A (UV-A)-induced corneal collagen cross-linking has become a well-established therapeutic approach to treat keratoconus and corneal ectasia in general.

The aim of corneal crosslinking therapy is not only a biomechanical corneal strengthening to slow down or block the progress of the disease (thus avoiding or delaying recourse to keratoplasty) but also to induce apex flattening and better corneal symmetry (corneal shape modification) that sometimes leads to a refractive improvement.

Even though the conventional and more recent Accelerated CXL (ACXL) protocols demonstrated a medium-long term improvement in visual acuity, topographic and aberrometric parameters [1], the results are highly unpredictable, and variable due to uneven collagen biological response to photodynamic reaction.

Cone location is one of the most important parameters involved in corneal flattening after CXL performed with Dresden Protocol (3 mw/cm^2, 5.4/cm^2 J energy dose). After CXL more topographic flattening occurs in eyes with centrally located cones and the least flattening effect of the cone occurs when the cone is located peripherally [2]. This cone-location effect is found in eyes with both keratoconus and ectasia with an average difference of more than two diopters. Many factors are involved to explain this behavior but in addition to the biomechanically different properties of central and peripheral cornea, the radiation beam pattern of CXL device plays a decisive role. The flat irradiation beam delivered by older CXL machines does not fit well with curvilinear corneal shape. Studies conducted on

C. Mazzotta et al., *Management of Early Progressive Corneal Ectasia*,
DOI 10.1007/978-3-319-61137-2_5

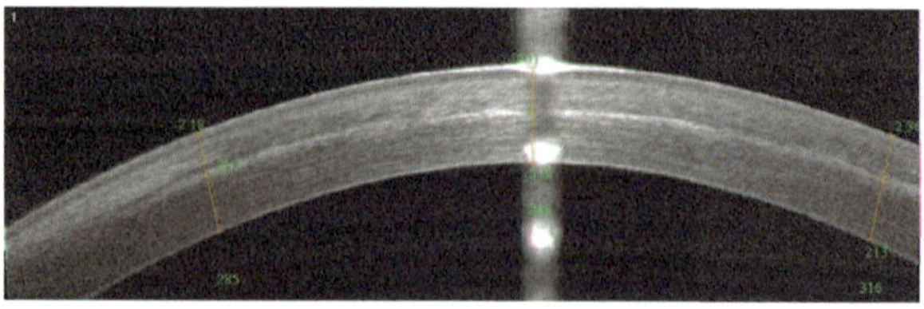

Fig. 5.1 Demarcation line 30 days after ACXL 15 mW cm², 5.4 J Fluence irradiation profile results in a line depth substantially equal from center to periphery

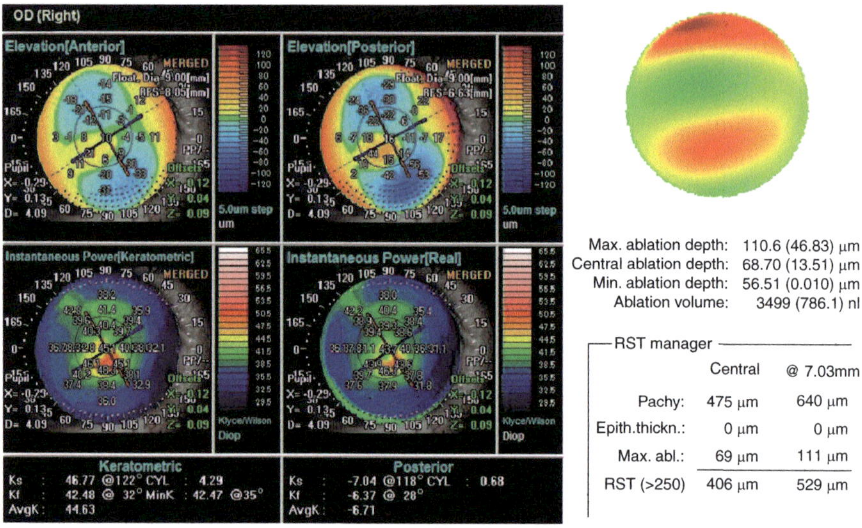

Fig. 5.2 Preoperative corneal tomography. Central posterior elevation cone (more than 50 within central 3 mm)

energy absorption profile demonstrated a significant difference (more than 4 J) between central and peripheral cornea creating a very uneven energy delivery profile (Fig. 5.1, **top left**). First of all if a flat beam profile irradiate a convex surface (the cornea) the central part will absorbs more energy because is closer to energy source respect to periphery. The other issue is that cone apex location in keratoconus is most located in paracentral and peripheral cornea (2–3 mm out of from corneal center). The result is that CXL procedure performed with older machines centered on the cornea will produce more crosslinking effect (and by the time a flattening effect) on the central cornea rather than cone apex. The uneven energy delivery can be easily understood looking at demarcation line depth that could be appreciated since 10–15 days after cxl. The line is deeper in the center and gradually becomes superficial going towards periphery (smile profile).

Top-hat or umbrella-like beam produced by newer CXL devices significantly improved energy management delivering a more even amount of radiation from center to periphery improving the crosslinking effect in the apex zone (Fig. 5.1). By the way the opinion of the authors is anyway to center the beam on the posterior elevation apex protecting the limbus. The results is that demarcation line depth is even from center to periphery (Fig. 5.2).

A customized and cone-centered irradiation profile will lead to better CXL effect, more flattening in the apex zone and finally better chance to aim to better refractive effect.

5.1.1 Basic Concepts

CXL alone represents an optimal solution for progressive early ectasia (better if central stage I-II disease) in which our aim is to "freeze" for life the condition of these patients that generally have a good best spectacle corrected visual acuity and few high order aberrations, preserving them from corneal transplant.

The real challenge today is the management of the keratoconus in patients with more advanced or decentered ectasia, intolerant to rigid gas permeable contact lenses and poor spectacles corrected visual acuity. The refraction of these patient is always difficult because spectacle correction is unable to correct high order aberration and irregular astigmatism, especially in peripheral cones, and a comfortable contact lens fitting sometimes is hard to reach or not possible at all and could cause corneal itself corneal scarring of infection. These patients become the natural candidates to lamellar or penetrating keratoplasty. We strongly believe that, before keratoplasty, a conservative way to improve patients visual acuity and quality of life must be tried.

This new and modern therapeutic paradigm is represented by corneal reshaping techniques associated with accelerated corneal collagen CXL customized protocol.

In other words the target is to regularize as much as possible the corneal shape (geometry) in the central 4 mm zone aiming to reduce vertical asymmetry and high order aberrations (especially the coma-like aberration) induced by ectasia.

Many invasive or semi-invasive surgical techniques were described in the past for corneal reshaping in ectasic disorders. Intra-corneal rings (ICRS) were an effective method for corneal reshaping but not free of complication (corneal reactions, ring extrusion, infections), also with femtosecond-assisted tunnel creation. Corneal reshaping is anyway not so predictable leaving the ectatic cornea structure remain unaltered. Moreover in complicated cases, the ICRS removal becomes difficult resulting in irreversible irregularities (removable but not reversible procedure).

The treatment of corneas with keratoconus using excimer laser machine was historically considered not appropriate because of further corneal thinning and possible weakening of corneal microstructure followed by iatrogenic ectasia worsening. Recent advances in technology led to development of topography-guided and wave-front-guided treatments that changed the quality of laser treatment introducing the concept of "customized treatments". The target of customized ablation is to improve the quality of visual acuity reducing the lower and the higher-order aberrations with partial or total treatment of corneal irregular astigmatism. Wave-front-guided ablation takes in account the aberration of full eye while topography-guided treatment consider only the corneal aberration.

Many authors [3–15] described several approaches combining different corneal collagen crosslinking and refractive surgery protocols performed at the same time (same-day) or in two surgical step.

The thinnest corneal thickness (measured with epithelium) considered for residual stromal bed in these papers varied from 300 to 450 μm. The common opinion of the Authors is to consider 50 μm as maximum stromal ablation depth.

The benefit of combined CXL plus refractive surgery (CXL Plus procedure) is to directly reshape (regularize) the ectatic cornea and reinforce the reshaped cornea with CXL procedure that will further flatten the cornea in the following months.

To achieve this goal two Italian researchers developed an adjustable personalized protocol called **STARE-XL**: *Selective Trans-epithelial Ablation for Regularization of Ectasia and simultaneous Cross-linking.*

5.1.2 STARE-XL: Selective Transepithelial Ablation for Regularization of Ectasia and Simultaneous Cross-Linking

Developed in 2015 by Miguel Rechichi MD, PhD and Cosimo Mazzotta MD, PhD, the ***STARE XL (Selective Transepithelial Ablation for Regularization of Ectasia and simultaneous Cross-linking)*** protocol was to combine the best technology in refractive surgery and cxl actually available to obtain a great improvement of higher order aberration in ectatic cornea. We started our experience with this protocol more than 2 years ago combining a transepithelial topoguided ablation treatment with Amaris Laser Platform (Schwind Eye tech-Solution) and Accelerated CXL performed with Avedro's (Waltham, MA) KXL I cross-linker.

The inclusion criteria for patient selection were: Age ≥ 21 years, Mild Ectasia (Stage I-II), necessity of visual quality improvement, HRGP lens Intolerance or altered fitting, CDVA ≤20/40 or ≤0.6 Snellen Lines, K average ≤ 48 Diopters or K maximum ≤55 Diopters, Optical Thinnest Point pachymetry: **400 μm ≥ T-PTK** (minimum 350 stromal), maximum stromal ablation ≤50 μm, minimum residual stromal bed ≥350 μm. The exclusion criteria were: Ocular Infections, History of Interstitial Keratitis, HSV or other autoimmune diseases, presence of corneal scars.

5.1.3 The STARE-XL Protocol

5.1.3.1 First Step: Excimer Laser Corneal Regularization

Laser Platform: ***Schwind Amaris*** platform linked with Anterior segment Scheimpflug Tomography with integrated placido topography and pupillometry (Sirius, CSO, Florence, Italy). We start from subjective refraction before consider topography-based Trans-epithelial All Surface Laser Ablation (TASLA). The procedure consists of Single step corneal topo-guided TRANS-PRK 7 mm optical zone **(OZ)** plus 0.6 mm transition zone (TZ) for central cone or 6.5 OZ plus TZ 0.5 mm for peripheral cone.

Treatment strategy for CENTRAL Kc > 50% within 3 mm on posterior elevation map: high negative Q factor with high myopic refractive error.

Trans-PRK with planning of partial refractive correction is influenced by pachymetry and spherical equivalent value. We can apply a partial refractive correction planning spherical refraction between −2 or zero and focusing on irregular astigmatism we will preserve the asphericity reducing the Q value to a less negative value. The most suitable patients for this treatment are those with spherical equivalent <5 D and pachymetry over 450 μm.

Treatment strategy for PERIPHERAL Kc >50% out of 3 mm on posterior elevation tangential map, have less negative or positive Q value and lower myopia.

These are the most complex case. The risk is to induce a significant negative Q value, resulting a myopic shift. In order to compensate this overshot we can apply a refractive correction planning zero as spherical refraction and focusing just on irregular astigmatism and coma aberration, correcting 50% of subjective cylinder refraction keeping always max ablation under 50 μm.

The algorithm for laser epithelium removal of Amaris consists in ablation of 55 μm in the center that gradually reach 65 μm at the edge of optical zone. The epithelium removal is trimmed on each case computing the thickness of central cornea and a paracentral point that is calculated half-way between OZ boundary and center.

In the keratoconic cornea the epithelium is normally thinner on the cone apex acting as masking agent smoothing the elevation irregularities. We have to consider this important findings because if conventional thickness value in paracentral zone are computed in the planning the ablation in keratoconic cornea we will always ablate much more stromal tissue on the steeper corneal meridian respect to the flatter one. Anyway often the refraction and the corneal asymmetry will improve per se because more stromal tissue will be removed around the corneal apex flattening.

To limit the stromal ablation under the cone apex in the STARE-X protocol we computed in the algorithm the central thickness value and the paracentral value corresponding to the thinnest point located on the cone apex, creating a customized epithelium removal ablation. More than this the depth saving mode is always used. This is useful because the limited cylinder correction will be shifted toward the peripheral and thicker cornea. The target is to reduce stromal ablation under the cone during epithelium removal preserving always a RST ≥ 350 μm. Previous studies showed an average thinning of 10–13 μm at 1.2 mm from corneal vertex between normal and keratoconic eyes. This means that a 60 μm epithelial ablation in the apex zone will remove about 15–18 μm of stromal tissue. This is a crucial information to be considered especially if we plan a further topo-guided stromal regularization to not exceed the ablation depth target.

5.1.3.2 Second Step: Customized Energy Accelerated Collagen Crosslinking

The target RST planned before laser excimer corneal ablation will guide decision about UV-A irradiation power and dose that will be adopted for crosslinking just after the first step [16]. The protocol includes the Siena CXL Center Protocol with 15 mW pulsed light UV-A irradiation (12 min, 15 mw/cm^2, 5.4 J Fluence) if the RST is >400 μm and pulsed UVA irradiation (8 min, 30 mw/cm^2, 7.2 J dose energy) if the RST < 400 μm. The beam is carefully centered on posterior elevation cone for all the treatment.

The Riboflavin solution used in both treatment groups is composed of dextran-free riboflavin 0.1% with hydroxyl, propyl, methyl, and cellulose (VibeX Rapid, Avedro Inc., Waltham, MS, USA), with 10 min of corneal soaking. After treatment, eyes are dressed by a soft contact lens bandage for 3–4 days and medicated with antibiotic, non-steroidal anti-inflammatory and lubricants eye drops 4 times/day. The application of these protocols will produce a demarcation line between 250 and 280 μm that is ideal for a cornea with a RST > 350 μm.

Figures 5.3 and 5.4 shows 1 years results of 30 keratoconic eyes treated with stare protocol divided in two groups: group 1 (G1) was 15 central cones (apex

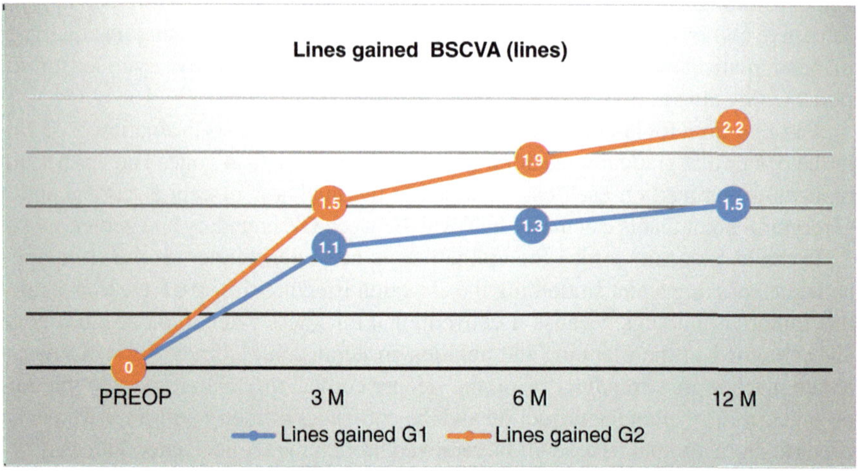

Fig. 5.3 G1 Central cones. G2 Peripheral cones. G2 group gained an average of 0.7 lines more than G1 1 year after STARE XL protocol

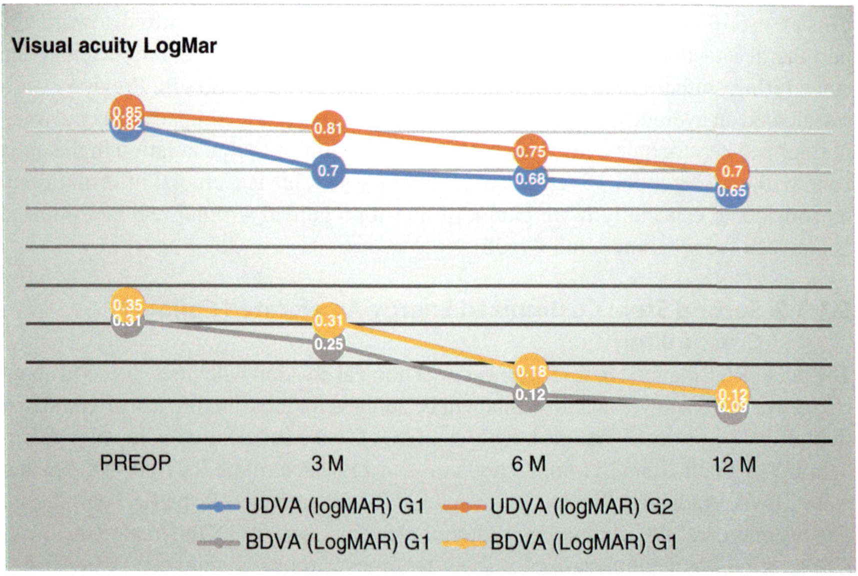

Fig. 5.4 Visual acuity. G1 group gained a better final visual acuity but G2 had the more recently improvement

within 3 mm from corneal vertex), group 2 (G2) was peripheral cone (apex outside 3 mm from corneal vertex). A marked improvement in UDVA and BDVA was observed in both group. A better improvement in lines gained was observed in G2 nevertheless the G1 was better in terms of visual acuity.

5.1.4 Clinic Case 1

- Male, 28 stable KC, Central pachymetry 475 μm, thinnest point 456 μm
- BSCVA Right Eye 20/60, ref. sph + 0.50 cyl<> −4.25 (70°)
- BSCVA Left Eye 20/20, ref. cyl −0.75 (90°)
- CL intolerance
- Right Eye: Partial correction −3 cyl (70°) by spectacle because of anisometropia complaints)
- Corneal tomography: Central posterior elevation cone (more than 50 within central 3 mm). Fig. 5.5 **left.**

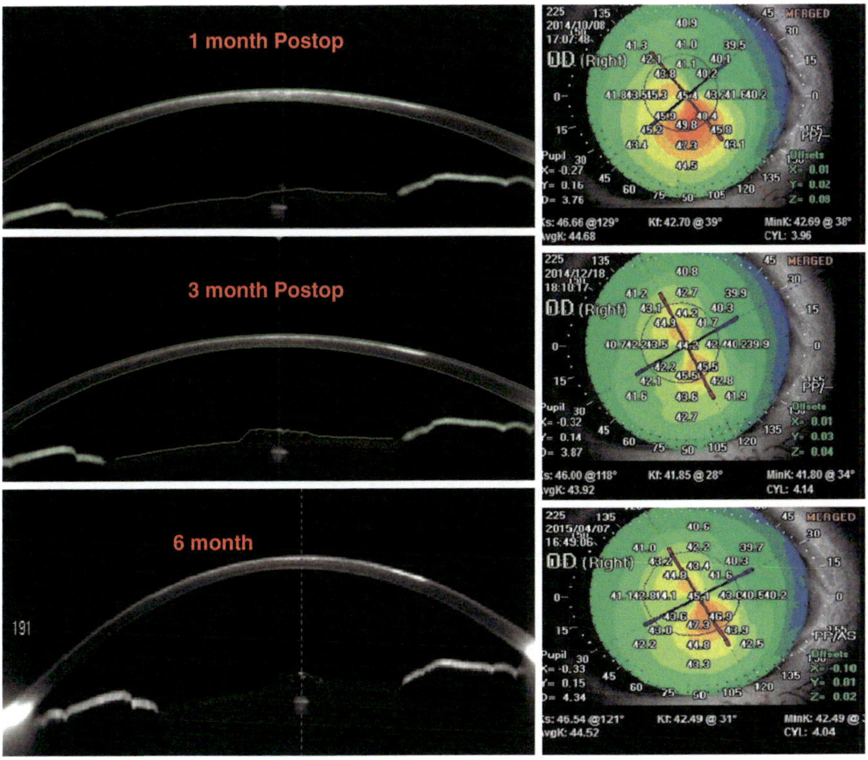

Fig. 5.5 Stare-X postoperative result. *Left*: Corneal tomography: 1 month is notable the typical cxl-induced corneal hyperreflectivity that gradually vanish after 6 months. *Right*: Axial Map topography. After 6 month the topography shows a marked reduction in corneal asymmetry

Treatment Strategy: 6.5 OZ plus TZ 0.5 mm. Topo-guided ablation, depth save algorithm, optimization for coma reduction, partial refractive correction with Q compensation (respecting 50 μm max depth ablation): sp. −1<> cyl −1.50 (70) Fig. 5.5 **right**. Excimer laser treatment is followed by pulsed accelerated CXL (16 min, 15 mw/cm^2, 7.2 J dose energy). The patient recovered preop visual acuity after 15 days and after 6 months the reshaped cornea improved the best spectacle corrected visual acuity (BSCVA) up to 20/20 with a refraction of sp. −1<> cyl −2.50 (30) (Fig. 4). No adverse effect was observed.

5.1.5 Conclusion

The Stare –X protocol, as part of combined refractive and CXL treatments (CXL plus) is a safe and effective procedure for the treatment of corneal ectatic disorders. Corneal regularization improve BSCVA, giving to the patient an opportunity to be less dependent on contact lens improving the quality of life.

CXL-plus procedure seems to be the present and future for minimally invasive treatment of corneal ectasia. CXL plus may be the way of the future for appropriate candidates, a combined procedure that might represent an actual treatment for most of the cases of corneal ectatic disorders.

5.2 Topography-Guided Accelerated Corneal Collagen Crosslinking

5.2.1 Introduction

Conventional riboflavin UVA corneal crosslinking (CXL) actually represents an evolving therapy for the conservative treatment of progressive keratoconus (KC) [17, 18] and secondary corneal ectasia [19, 20] due to its capacity to increase the corneal biomechanical resistance and anti-collagenase activity. The physiochemical basis of conventional CXL lies in the photodynamic type I-II reactions induced by the interaction between riboflavin molecules, absorbed in corneal tissue, and UVA rays delivered at 3 mW/cm^2 for 30 min (5.4 J/cm^2 energy dose), that releases reactive oxygen species capable to mediate cross-link formation between and within collagen fibers and within proteoglycan core proteins in the inter-fibrillary space [21, 26].

Conventional CXL with epithelium removal (epithelium-off) represents an evidence based and scientifically well supported treatment, with documented long-term efficacy in stabilizing progressive keratoconus and secondary ectasia as reported in a series of non-randomized and randomized clinical trials [22, 23]. Since conventional CXL procedure requires long treatment time (1 h approximately) [24], accelerated crosslinking (ACXL) treatment protocols have been proposed with the purpose of shortening treatment time, improving patient's comfort and reducing hospital waiting lists.

Topography-guided ACXL was proposed as a potential approach to improve optical predictability of CXL and maximizing corneal regularization in a patient specific computational modeling study of keratoconus progression and differential responses to CXL [25] In simulations comparing broad-zone CXL treatments to focal, cone-localized treatment, much greater reductions in cone curvature and higher order aberrations (HOA) were observed with cone-localized patterns for a variety of patient tomographies [25]. Given that corneal ectasia is driven by focal rather than generalized weakness [26], focal stiffening of the cone region may promote a more favorable material property redistribution with compensatory steepening of surrounding areas, thereby enhancing topographic normalization [51].

5.2.2 Materials and Methods

The first topography guided ACXL study performed in Italy was conducted at the Siena Crosslinking Center® and at the Ophthalmic Unit of the Arcispedale Santa Maria Nuova of Reggio Emilia according to the ethical principles stated in the Helsinki Declaration as renewed in 2013. Preoperatively and postoperatively at 1, 3, 6, 12 months, patients underwent a full ophthalmologic examination including uncorrected distance visual acuity (UDVA) logMAR, corrected distance visual acuity (CDVA) logMAR, refraction, slit lamp evaluation, tonometry and fundoscopy. At the same time intervals patients were investigated by using Scheimpflug corneal tomography (Pentacam™ HR, Oculus, Arlington, WA, USA), in vivo confocal microscopy (IVCM) with the Heidelberg Retina Tomograph II (HRTII) (Rostock Cornea Module, Heidelberg, Germany) and anterior segment optical coherence tomography (AS-OCT) (Zeiss, Jena, Germany). All patients included for this analysis completed the 1-year follow-up visit.

5.2.3 Surgical Technique

Topography-guided ACXL procedures were carried out under sterile operating conditions and topical anesthesia with the application of 4% lidocaine and 0.2% oxybuprocaine hydrochloride anesthetic drops. Topical pilocarpine 2% was administered 10 min before treatment. After application of a closed valves lid speculum, the corneal epithelium was removed by a blunt metal spatula in the central 9 mm area. Corneal stroma was soaked for 10 min with a Riboflavin 0.1% Hydroxyl-Propyl Methyl-Cellulose (HPMC) dextran-free solution (VibeX Rapid Avedro Inc., Waltham, MS, USA). Topography-guided ACXL were carried out with the KXL II™ UVA illuminator (Avedro Inc., Waltham, MS, USA) using a 30 mW/cm^2 UV-A power with pulsed light emission (1 s on/1 s off). Treatments were individually planned by using a dedicated software (Avedro Mosaic System version 1.0, Avedro Inc., Waltham, MS, USA), according to the preoperative topography data. The 30 mW/cm^2 customized, topography based,

ACXL treatments, consisted in a differentiated energy dose release according to the different corneal curvatures showed by each keratoconus. The entry level energy dose of 7.2 J/cm^2 was delivered the in the flattest peripheral cone area under 48 diopters (D) of maximum corneal curvature (Kmax), by using 30 mW/cm^2 (1 s on/1 s off) pulsed (or fractionated) light illumination for 8 min of UV-A exposure time. Ectatic areas with corneal curvature over 48 D and under 52 D were treated with an energy dose of 10 J/cm^2 maintaining the same UV-A power of 30 mW/cm^2 prolonging the exposure time of 3 min in order to reach the programmed dose of 10 J/cm^2 (11 min of total exposure time). If present, the steepest areas of corneal curvature over 52 D were treated by extending further the exposure time, until reaching the maximum energy dose of 15 J/cm^2 with a total UV-A treatment time of 16 min on balance. The treatment planning was established by using semi-meridians K values on Pentacam maps. Total treatment time was 8 min for keratoconus under or equal to 48 D of maximum K values, 11 min for keratoconus including simulated K values over 48 and under 52 D in the steepest areas, extending the exposure time to 16 min for keratoconus showing curvatures over 52 D in the steepest areas. The treatment starts from a baseline broad beam illumination including the flattest peripheral areas (48 D and under) at 7.2 J/cm^2; then after the first 8 min, these areas are masked and the steepest zones illumination is further extended until the final energy dose of 10 J or 15 J/cm^2 is delivered according to maximum curvature values. The thinnest point and the area of major posterior elevation were included within the highest dose treatment zone. The irradiation patterns shapes included arc, circular, oval and combined patterns according to keratoconus tomography and shape. The irradiation pattern was aligned by using a direct real time visualization of the cornea, maintaining a perfect centration by the eye-tracking system provided by the machine.

After UV-A irradiation, the cornea was washed with sterile balanced salt solution (BSS), medicated with antibiotics (moxifloxacin), cyclopentolate eye drops and dressed with a therapeutic soft contact lens that was removed after 4 days. Inclusion criteria and treatment protocol are listed in Table 5.1.

Statistical analysis was performed using the Wilcoxon test. All analyses were performed using the IBM SPSS Statistics version 16.0 (Armonk, USA). A p value of $\leq$0.05 was considered statistically significant.

Table 5.1 Inclusion criteria and topography-guided ACXL treatment protocol

Keratoconus progression criteria	Increased Sim K max ≥1 D; pachymetry reduction ≥10 μm
Procedure	Epithelium removal, 10 min soaking with VibeX Rapid 0.1 riboflavin, saline, HPMC solution applied every 90 s
Irradiance	30 mW/cm^2 pulsed or fractionated UVA light exposure (1 s on/1 s off).
Energy	From 7.2 J/cm^2 up to 15 J/cm^2 total energy dose.
Patterns	Arc patterns for "peripheral cones" (apex distance ≥3 mm from the pupillary center); Circular patterns for "central cones".
Thickness	Minimum stromal thickness 400 μm.

5.2.4 Results

Twenty-one eyes of 20 patients, 16 males and 4 females, mean age 28.9 ± 5.8 years (range 22–34 years) with progressive keratoconus were included in the study. One patient underwent a bilateral treatment. Mean UDVA and CDVA respectively changed from preoperative 0.55 ± 0.2 logMAR and 0.21 ± 0.1 logMAR, to 0.36 ± 0.1 logMAR ($p = 0.65$) and 0.10 ± 0.1 logMAR at 12 months ($p = 0.10$). The mean preoperative topographic astigmatism improved from −4.61 ± 0.74 diopters (D) to −3.20 ± 0.81 D at 12-month follow-up ($p = 0.048$). The 12th month difference from preoperative topographic astigmatism was −1.41 D. Visual acuity and topographic astigmatism are reported for each time interval in Fig. 5.6.

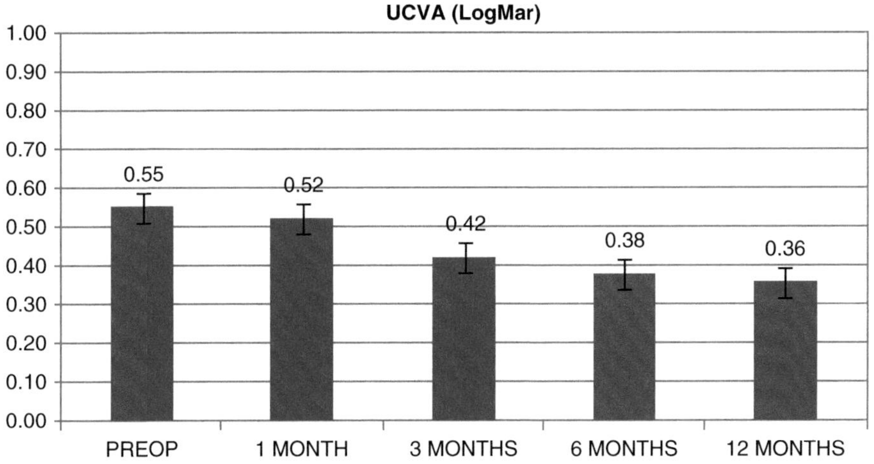

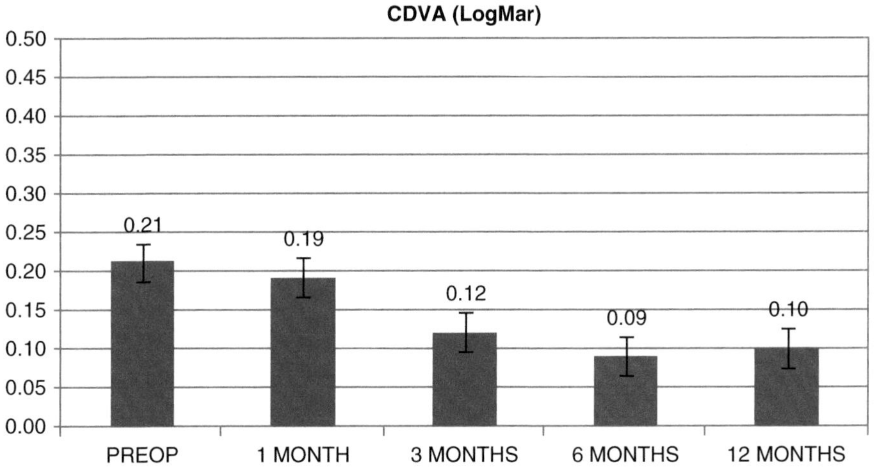

Fig. 5.6 LogMAR Average UDVA (*top*), CDVA (*middle*), and topographic astigmatism (*bottom*) values after high-irradiance topography-guided CXL. 1-year follow-up mean topographic astigmatism value significantly improved from −4.61 Diopters (D) to −3.20 D ($p < 0.05$)

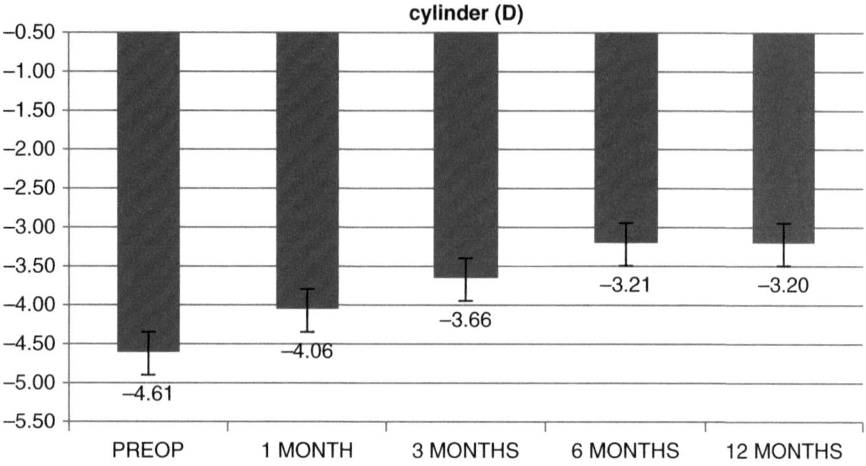

Fig. 5.6 (continued)

Mean preoperative K max, K min and K average values outlined at 3 mm, were 47.50 ± 1.14D, 45.21 ± 0.67D and 47.44 ± 0.99D respectively; values changed to 46.50 ± 1.81D ($p = 0.088$), 45.70 ± 0.7D ($p = 0.055$) and 47.98 ± 1.42D ($p = 0.077$) at 12 months follow-up respectively. Topography K values are reported for each time interval in Fig. 5.7.

Mean preoperative coma, RMS and spherical aberration values were respectively 0.95 ± 0.03 μm, 2.09 ± 0.01 μm and 0.02 ± 0.01 μm; values changed to 0.88 ± 0.04 μm ($p = 0.049$), 1.89 ± 0.03 μm (p 0.58) and 0.00 ± 0.01 (0.068) μm at the 12 months follow-up. The 1 year change from baseline in coma was statistically significant ($p = 0.049$). High order aberrations values are reported for each time interval in Fig. 5.8.

Mean preoperative minimum pachymetry values varied from 462.20 ± 10 μm at baseline, to 466.29 ± 8.2 μm ($p = 0.087$) at 6 months and to 460.01 ± 12.1 μm ($p = 0.079$) at 12-months follow-up. Mean endothelial cell density changed from 2490 ± 17 cells/mm^2 at baseline to 2469 ± 31 cells/mm^2 at 1 month ($p = 0.66$), to 2475 ± 28 cells/mm^2 at 3 months ($p = 0.65$), to 2482 ± 23 cells/mm^2 at 6 months ($p = 0.65$) and to 2488 ± 37 cells/mm^2 at 12-month follow-up ($p = 0.67$).

5.2.5 Anterior Segment OCT Analysis

Corneal OCT scan (Fig. 5.9a) showed a double demarcation line according to the different energy doses delivered in the corneal tissue and different exposure times. Treatment irradiation patterns combined a peripheral single arc illumination (7.2 J) followed by a central circular irradiation pattern (10 J), Fig. 5.9b. The corresponding treatment planning is showed in Fig. 5.9c based on corneal curvatures. After

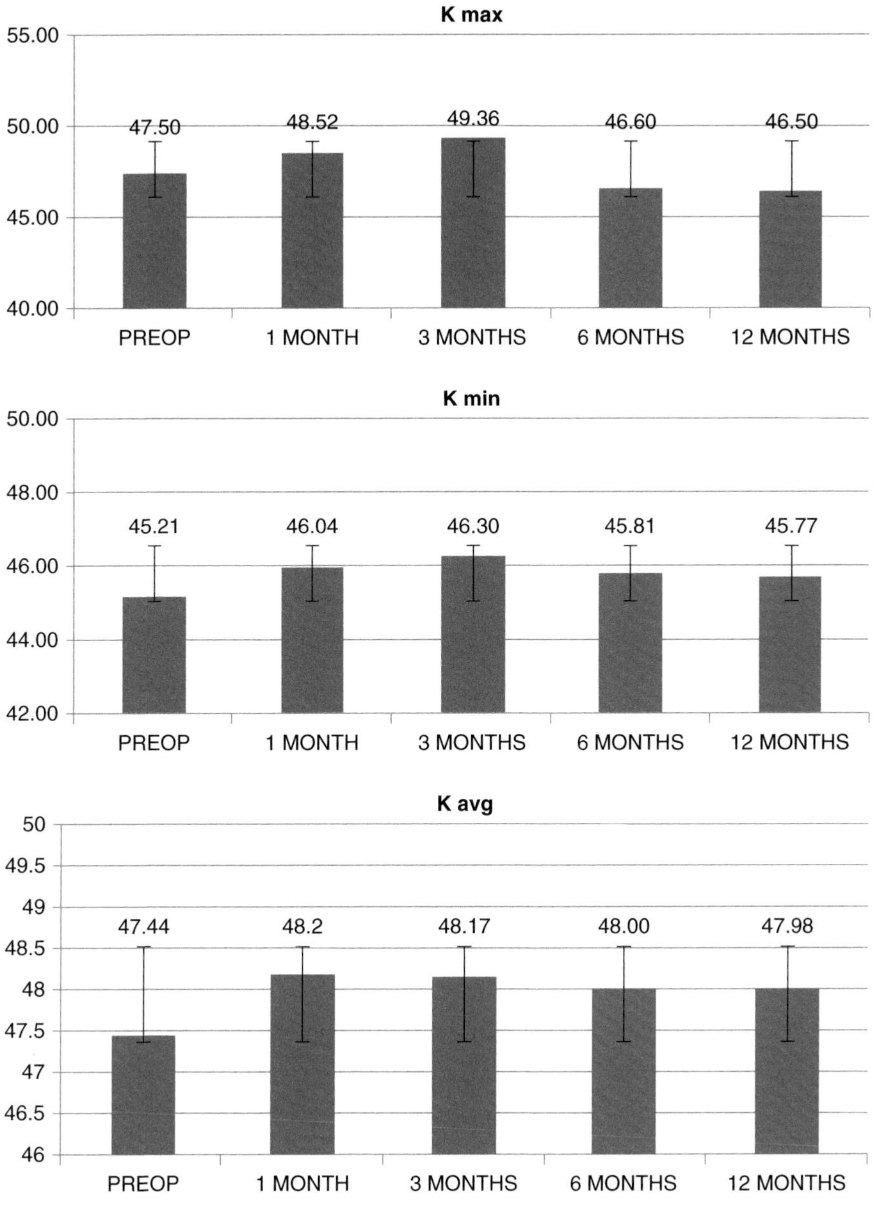

Fig. 5.7 K max, K min and K average after high-irradiance topography-guided CXL. 1-year follow-up of simulated K readings tangential algorithm values data showed that K max changed from 47.50 ± 1.14 D to 46.50 ± 1.81 D ($p > 0.05$), while K min value increased from 45.21 ± 0.67 D to 47.7 ± 0.91 D ($p < 0.05$). K average values passed from 47.44 ± 0.99 D to 47.98 ± 1.42 D ($p > 0.05$)

8 min of UV-A exposure time at 30 mW/cm^2 power with pulsed light illumination (1 s on/1 s off) to deliver 7.2 J/cm^2 in the peripheral flattest area, the average depth of demarcation line, measured from epithelial surface, was 150 ± 18 μm SD in the flatter corneal area and 300 ± 37 μm SD in the steeper corneal area treated at 10 J/cm^2 as shown in Fig. 5.9a by the deeper demarcation line. The greater depth of the demarcation line in the paracentral area was correlated with the prolonged exposure time (11 min) and higher energy dose delivered in the central steepest zone (10 J). The hyper-reflectivity of the stroma corresponded to the central area treated with the highest energy dose. Differential Corneal topography between preoperative (Fig. 5.9e) and postoperative acquisition, Fig. 5.9d, at 6 months show a clear

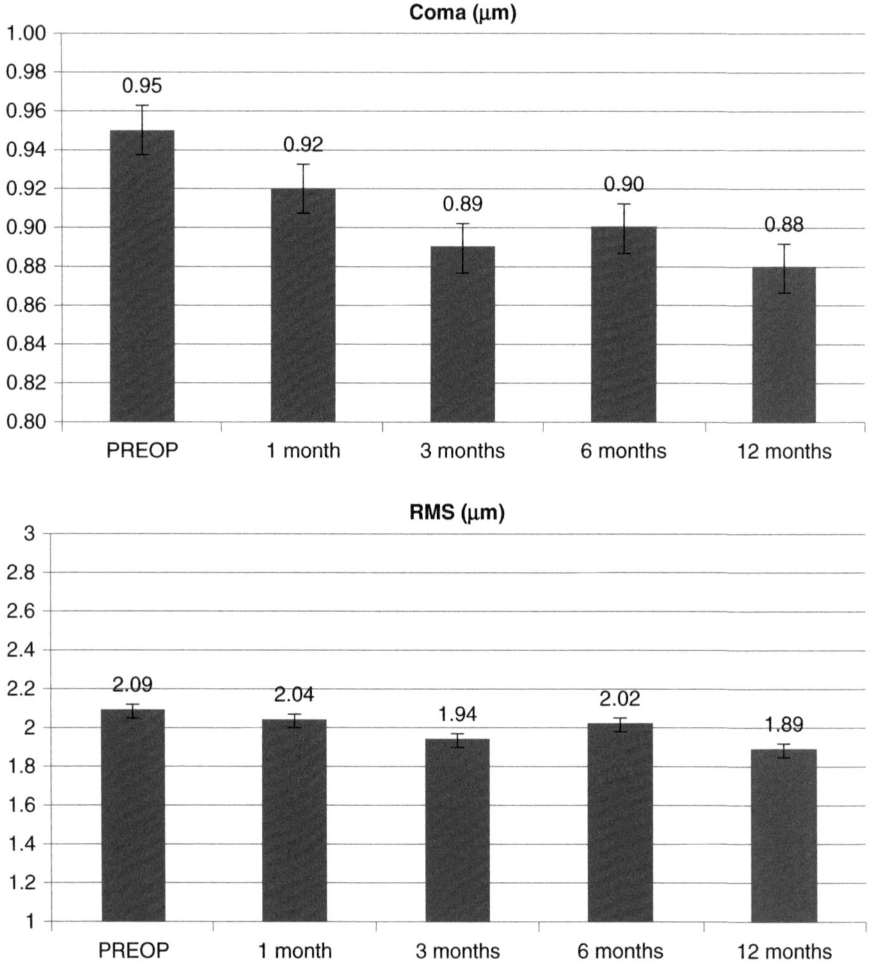

Fig. 5.8 Coma, RMS and spherical aberration values after high-irradiance topography-guided CXL. 1-year follow-up aberrometry data showed a statistically significant Coma value reduction ($p < 0.05$). No statistically significant changes were recorded for RMS and spherical aberrations

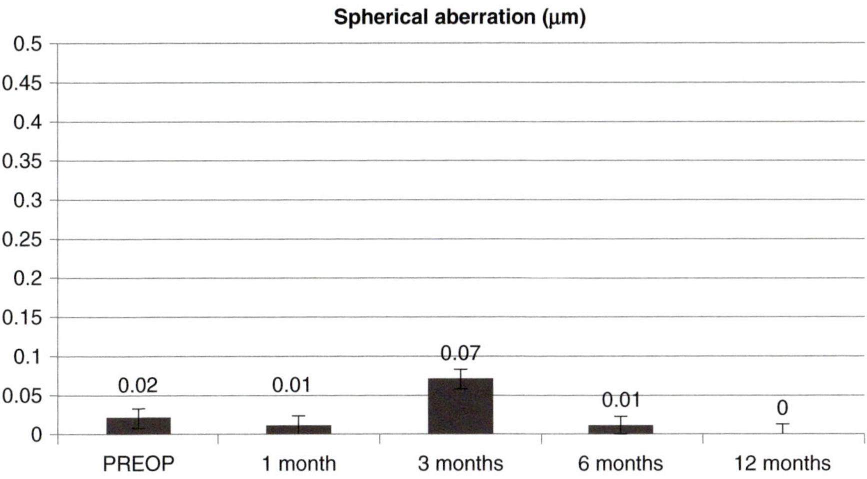

Fig. 5.8 (continued)

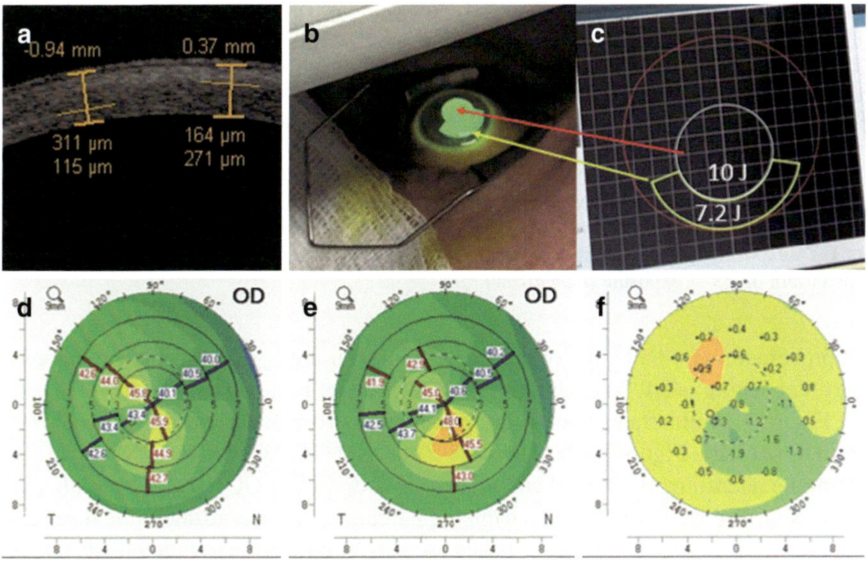

Fig. 5.9 Corneal OCT following high-irradiance topography-guided CXL. At 3rd postoperative month (scan **a**), multiple demarcation lines due to the different energy doses delivered according to the topography-guided CXL protocol were evident. Image **b** illustrates the topography-guided treatment in progress. Image **c** shows the topo-guided treatment planning with programmed double energy dose: 7.2 J/cm^2 in the flattest area under 48D (*yellow arrow*) with arc-step pattern, and 10 J/cm^2 in the steepest central area over 48D (*red arrow*) with circular pattern. Image **d** show the 12th month postoperative flattening compared with preoperative tomography (image **e**), followed by compensatory steepening of the flattest superior cornea documented in differential corneal tomography (image **f**)

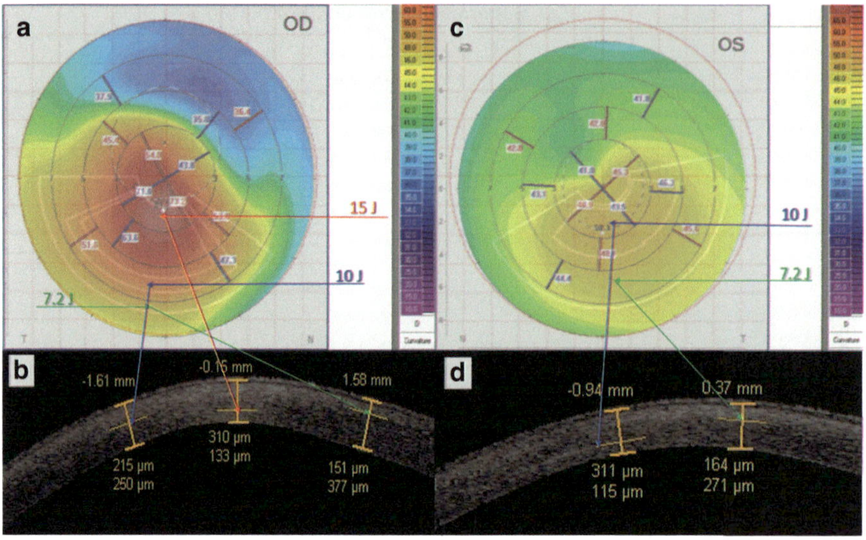

Fig. 5.10 Topography-Guided ACXL treatment programs according to different KC severity. (**a**) Shows a 3-Zone topography guided ACXL treatment planning according to corneal curvatures. Post-operative OCT scans 1 month after treatment, (**b**) revealed a triple demarcation line according to the three different exposure times and energy doses: 7.2 J/cm^2 in the peripheral KC flattest area 48 D and under (depth 151 μm), *green arrows* (8 min UV-A exposure); 10 J/cm^2 in the intermediate area between 48 and 52 D (depth 215 μm), *blue arrows* (11 min UV-A exposure); 15 J/cm^2 in the steepest area (depth 310 μm), *red arrows* (16 min UV-A Exposure). (**c**) Shows a 2-Zone topography guided ACXL treatment with 7.2 (*green arrows*) and 10 J/cm^2 (*blue arrows*) E doses treatment planning. OCT scan performed 1 month after treatment, (**d**) revealed a double demarcation line according to the different exposure times and doses delivered according to corneal curvatures, reaching a demarcation line depth of 164 μm in the peripheral area treated with 7.2 J/cm^2 for 8 min of UVA exposure (*green arrow*) and 311 μm in the steeper paracentral area treated with 10 J/cm^2 for 11 min of UV-A exposure (*blue arrow*)

improvement with flattening of the steepest inferior area (−1.9 D) and a compensatory steepening (+0.9 D) of the superior flatter zone, Fig. 5.9f.

Figure 5.10 illustrates two different treatment programs according to the different KC severity. Figure 5.10a shows a 3-Zone topography guided ACXL treatment planning according to corneal curvatures. Post-operative OCT scans 1 month after treatment, Fig. 5.10b, revealed a triple demarcation line according to the three different exposure times and energy doses used: 7.2 J/cm^2 in the peripheral KC flattest area 48 D and under (depth 151 μm), green arrows; 10 J/cm^2 in the intermediate area between 48 and 52 D (depth 215 μm), blue arrows; 15 J/cm^2 in the steepest area indicated by the red arrows (depth 310 μm). Figure 5.10c shows a 2-Zone topography guided ACXL treatment with 7.2 (green arrows) and 10 J/cm^2 (blue arrows) E doses treatment planning. OCT scan performed 1 month after treatment, Fig. 5.10d, revealed a double demarcation line according to different exposure times and doses delivered according to the corneal curvature reaching a demarcation line depth of 164 μm in the peripheral area treated with 7.2 J for 8 min of UVA exposure (green arrow) and 311 μm in the steeper paracentral area treated with 10 J (blue arrow).

5.2.6 IVCM Outcomes

Different demarcation lines were also documented with IVCM at 150 μm ± 28 μm SD depth in the flattest areas (48D and under), irradiated at 7.2 J/cm^2 (Fig. 5.11a–c), at 250 μm ± 22 μm SD depth in the areas (> 48 D and ≤52 D) irradiated at 10 J/cm^2 energy dose, (Fig. 5.11d), and 300 μm ± 31 μm SD depth in the steepest corneal areas (> 52 D) irradiated at 15 J/cm^2 energy dose (Fig. 5.11e).

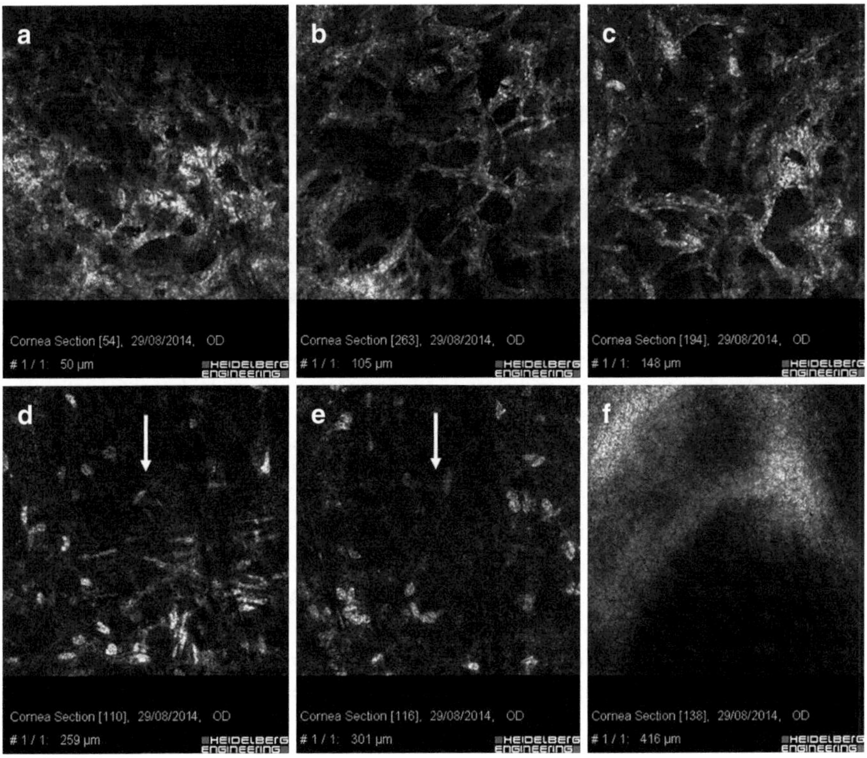

Fig. 5.11 IVCM scans in the first month after high-irradiance topography-guided CXL. Different demarcation lines were documented at 150 μm depth in the flattest areas (48D and under) irradiated at 7.2 J/cm^2 (scans **a**–**c**); at 250 μm depth in the area (>48D and ≤52 D) irradiated at 10 J/cm^2 E dose (scan **d**); at 300 μm depth in the steepest cone area (>52D) irradiated at 15 J/cm^2 E dose (scan **e**). IVCM also showed hyper-reflectivity of corneal tissue and keratocytes apoptosis associated with dense trabecular patterned lacunar edema and nerve disappearance (scans **a**–**c**). No endothelial damage was documented (scan **f**)

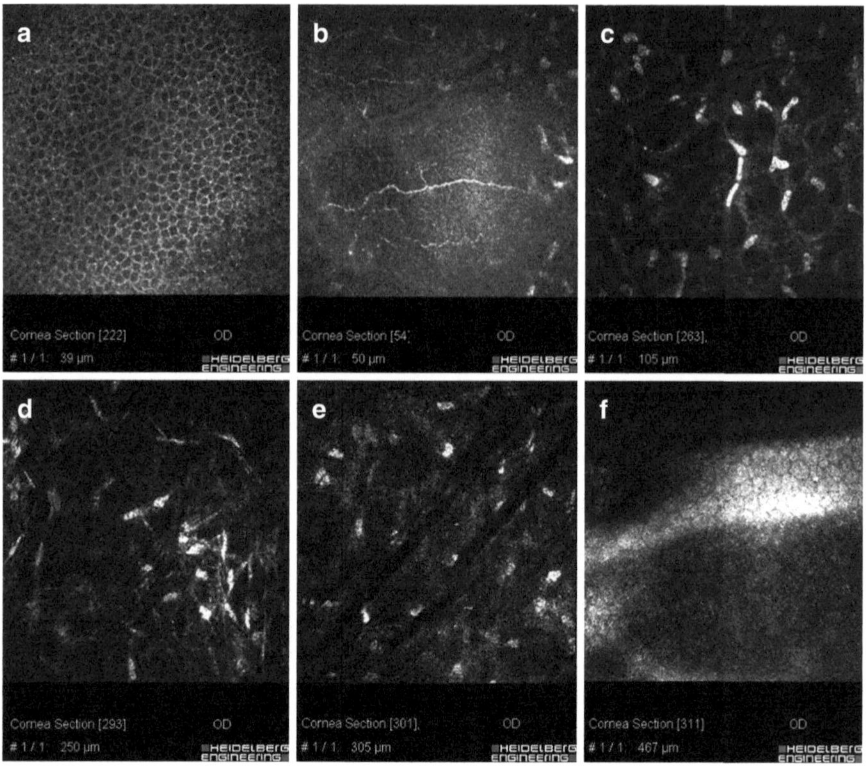

Fig. 5.12 IVCM scans 6 months after high-irradiance topography-guided CXL Regular epithelium (scan **a**) and regenerated sub-epithelial plexus nerves (scan **b**) were evident at 6 months. The hyper-reflectivity of extracellular matrix and the lacunar edema gradually disappeared with progressive keratocytes repopulation (scans **c**–**e**). Oblique dark micro-striations are visible (scans **d** and **e**) in absence of endothelial micro-morphological alterations (scan **f**)

IVCM scans were performed in the central corneal areas, paracentral areas and peripheral one by a direct real time control view of the acquisition zone by the same operator and controlled by a second expert observer. An average of repeated measurements was reported. IVCM scans performed in the first postoperative 3 months showed hyper-reflectivity of corneal tissue and keratocytes loss were associated with marked stromal lacunar edema and nerve disappearance in the treated areas (Fig. 5.12a–c).

The intensity of stromal reflectivity and the depth of keratocytes apoptosis was correlated with the increasing energy dose delivered in the tissue. The higher the dose, the higher the reflectivity detected in the first 3 months. The depth of keratocytes apoptosis well correlated with exposure times and energy doses delivered to the different areas of corneal tissue analyzed by IVCM. No endothelial damage was documented (Fig. 5.12f). After the 3rd postoperative month, epithelium appeared healthy and sub-epithelial plexus fibers reappeared (Fig. 5.12a, b). The hyper-reflectivity of extracellular tissue was progressively reduced, lacunar edema gradually disappeared with keratocytes repopulation, similar to all conventional and accelerated epi-off CXL procedures (Fig. 5.12c–e). Twelve months after treatment IVCM analysis showed diffuse keratocytes repopulation with no endothelial micro-morphological alterations (Fig. 5.12f).

5.2.7 Conclusion

The preliminary evaluations documented that the topography-guided ACXL was safe and effective in halting keratoconus progression, improving corneal topography at 12-months. Interestingly, regional effects on keratocyte stromal reflectivity and corneal nerves, as well as multiple stromal demarcation lines, indirectly demonstrated the effectiveness of topography guided treatment planning according to different E doses and UV-A exposure time.

Recently, accelerated cross-linking protocols have been investigated in several studies. Bunsen-Roscoe's law [27] established that photochemical reactions, including CXL, depend on the absorbed UVA energy (E) and their biological effect is proportional to the total energy dose delivered to the tissue [28, 29]. According to the so called "equal-dose" physical principle [23, 24]. The clinical results of high-irradiance 30 mW/cm^2 ACXL protocol with continuous and pulsed UV-A light exposure [30, 31] and 18 mW/cm^2 demonstrated keratoconus stability, endothelial safety but less anterior corneal flattening effect compared to conventional CXL [32] On the other hand, a recent review [33] on laser scanning in vivo confocal microscopy (IVCM) of the cornea after conventional and accelerated CXL protocol, documented less intrastromal penetration using 30 mW/cm^2 UVA irradiance compared with standard 3 mW/cm^2 CXL [34, 35]. The safety of conventional CXL and ACXL riboflavin UVA-induced corneal collagen cross-linking in the conservative treatment of keratoconus was evaluated and confirmed in vivo in humans by laser scanning in vivo confocal microscopy (IVCM) of the cornea [36, 37]. IVCM allowed for a detailed, high magnification in vivo micro-morphological analysis of corneal layers, enabling the assessment of early and late corneal changes induced by these treatments with much greater axial resolution (1 μm) than traditional bio-microscopy and corneal optical coherence tomography (OCT), both in progressive keratoconus and secondary corneal ectasias [36, 48].

CXL is known to be an effective mean for stabilizing keratoconus over extended follow-up periods. Even though conventional broad-beam CXL and ACXL protocols induce improvements in visual acuity and topographic and aberrometric parameters in many patients, these optical outcomes vary from case to case due to patient-specific factors and inhomogeneous responses to the intrinsic photodynamic reaction and its stiffening effects [38, 50].

In order to improve patient's quality of vision, while maintaining keratoconus stability, we have investigated this novel topography-guided accelerated CXL protocol with customized energy dose release according to corneal curvatures. In this pilot study we have observed a statistically significant reduction of the mean topographic cylinder magnitude along with a decrease in coma aberration. Patients corneal topographies were characterized by the flattening of the steeper KC areas associated with a compensatory steepening on the flattest areas resulting in an improved corneal symmetry. All functional parameters (UDVA and CDVA, K max and K average) tended to improve, and we recorded a flattening of the central cone area as showed in Fig. 5.9d compared with preoperative tomography (Fig. 5.9e), followed by compensatory steepening of the flattest superior cornea documented in differential corneal tomography map (Fig. 5.9f).

The micro-structural corneal analysis performed by IVCM showed that in the topography guided ACXL protocol using energy doses higher than conventional 5.4 J/cm^2 (from 7.2 up to 15 J/cm^2), keratocytes apoptosis was detected between 250 (10 J/cm^2) and 300 μm (15 J/cm^2). As showed by corneal OCT scans we revealed multiple demarcation lines underlying the different energy doses and UV-A exposure times used according to the topography-guided ACXL principle, Fig. 5.10b, d.

These preliminary observations allow us to formulate the hypothesis that CXL induced biodynamic interaction and CXL treatment volume is not only related to the UV-A power and relative exposure time, but also to energy dose delivered to the corneal tissue. In conventional 5.4 J/cm^2 energy dose CXL, we demonstrated with IVCM analysis that CXL stromal penetration (i.e. cell apoptosis) appeared to be inversely proportional to UV-A power and directly proportional to exposure time. The same basic concepts were applicable to 7.2 J/cm^2 energy dose. After high-irradiance, fractionated ACXL with 7.2 J/cm^2 our previously published IVCM data showed an increased hyper-reflectivity of stromal tissue surrounding keratocytes compared to 5.4 J/cm^2 Energy dose [33, 35]. After topography guided high-irradiance pulsed light CXL, IVCM showed that by using energy doses over 7.2 J/cm^2 (10 J/cm^2 and 15 J/cm^2) we can achieve higher penetration (i.e. cell apoptosis) with reduced exposure time and increased UV power compared to conventional epithelium-off CXL.

The possibility to have a topography guided ACXL treatment capable of improving patient's quality of vision, with reduced corneal aberrations and astigmatism, by mean of a non-ablative, non-incisional surgery, should be highly desirable in reducing the need of combined procedures for CXL refractive empowerment [61–63].

Current study not only address the potentiality of CXL customization through a customized energy dose release according to corneal curvature, but rather a customized irradiation time (at the same irradiance, which also implies a higher energy dose). Mazzotta et al. [30] and remore recently Peyman et al. [39] have shown that pulsed-light CXL induces a deeper demarcation line than continuous-light CXL maintaining the same irradiance and the same energy, potentially because pulsed-light CXL has a longer overall irradiation time. In the same line, Kling et al. [40] have shown that the biomechanical effect of continuous and pulsed-light CXL (different energies and irradiances, but same overall irradiation time) is equivalent. Therefore, the deeper demarcation line in the "high energy" zone and the observed reduction of astigmatism may result from the longer irradiation time. However, considering that the depth of conventional CXL (C-CXL) with 5.4 J/cm^2 E dose and 30 min of total UV-A exposure time reached 300 μm of depth on average [34], the Topography guided accelerated CXL reach a comparable treatment penetration in

18 min instead of 30 min and in this contest the higher dose may be a possible explanation of the increased treatment penetration beyond the exposure time.

Topography-guided ACXL results, in our preliminary experience, reduced some degree of corneal aberrations and topographic cylinder value with improvement in patient's quality of vision that was recorded since the first postoperative month. However, the overall 1-year results of this pilot study showed no better clinical outcomes compared with literature data reported in conventional broad beam epithelium off CXL [17, 18, 22, 41]. Of interest, all treated patient's reported a faster improvement in their quality of vision without the typical glare disability reported in the first 1–3 months after conventional epithelium-off treatment.

Conventional broad-beam epithelium-off CXL and ACXL remain a safe and efficient solution to delay or halt corneal ectasia progression in progressive keratoconus, for which the primary aim is to stabilize the disease. Topography-guided ACXL may represent an adjunctive option for visual rehabilitation, both for patients with early ectasia with acceptable best spectacle corrected visual acuity and low high order aberrations, as well as for patients with more advanced irregular or decentered cones.

5.3 Intracorneal Rings and Other Associated Procedures

The intrastromal ring implant in the deep layers of the stroma in the paracentral area of the cornea was originally developed as a method for surgical correction of high degree myopia and myopic astigmatism thanks to its ability to change refraction in the central zone of the cornea due to its peripheral-only effect [42–48].

Experimental clinical studies have repeatedly modified the surgical technique, the model of the implant, position, depth, and materials. With this methodology, it has been possible to obtain better results in refraction change and a significant increase in correct distance (CDVA) and uncorrect distance visual acuity (UDVA). Advantages of the "additive" method are: absence of the necessity to resection (weakening) corneal tissue, maintenance of optical cornea zone integrity, and partial reversibility of the surgery.

The results have shown that the refractive effect of this surgery is directly proportional to the thickness of the implant, and inversely proportional to its internal diameter.

The refractive effect increases with the number of implants, and with their positioning at the centre of the cornea. Stabilization comes generally in the 3rd postoperative month (3–6 months). Implants with a smaller diameter have less reactivity, and cause a lower percentage of extrusion due to the implant being deeper [47–96].

With an increase in diameter of the rings the depth of the implant has less influence on the flattening of the central zone. After surgery, a flattening effect takes place not only in the central zone of the cornea, but there is also a reduction in curvature in the peripheral area [54, 97–100]. Varying the length of the implant, its height and position in the tunnel in respect to the optical centre of the cornea and the ectasic zone, it is possible to prearrange refraction modification.

Table 5.2 Selection criteria for ICRS implant in ectatic corneas

Criteria for patient selection for ICRS: Intra Corneal Rings Segments
1. Absence of corneal opacity
2. Intolerance for contact lenses and spectacles
3. Minimum corneal thickness in the central zone >400 μm
4. Keratometry <65D
5. Elevation of the anterior surface /BFS from 26 to 65 μm
6. Elevation of the posterior surface /BFS from 40 to 89 μm

The best material for intracorneal implants has proven to be polymethylmethacrylate (PMMA) thanks to its bio-compatibility with cornea tissue, low inertia, refraction index being near that of the cornea and with sufficient density, as well as its flexibility and ease to work with [57, 59–62, 95], Table 5.2 shows the selection criteria for ICRS implant.

The rings were first proposed for treating keratoconus in 1995 by Paulo Ferrara [57]. They were made of PMMA, they had a triangular cross-sectional shape with different internal and external diameters, 6.2 mm, and 5.6 mm respectively.

The length of the implant at 60° has a base thickness of 600 μm, a radius of curvature of 2.5 mm, whereas the height varies from 150 to 350 μm with a pace of 50 μm.

The first surgeries were carried out in patients with keratoconus who could not tolerate rigid gas permeable contact lenses, and in candidates with penetrating keratoplasty. The recommendations for the surgery were for a transparent cornea with a central thickness of at least 400 μm, and an endothelial cell density (ECD) of >1.800 cells/mm^2. The ring implants were inserted mechanically with local topical anaesthesia. In all cases, 2 segments were implanted on both sides from the curved meridian, 5–7 mm from the centre of the cornea to avoid creating peripheral vision obstacles. The depth of the insertion was 50–80% of corneal thickness in the implant zone.

The analysis of the literature results showed around a five-time decrease of the spherical defect (from −10.2 ± 5.98 to −2.02 ± 2.02 dioptres), and the cylindrical error by two times (from −4.09 ± 2.42 to 1.89 ± 1.31 dioptres). At the same time, an almost three-time increase of the UDVA, from 0.07 ± 0.08 to 0.3 ± 0.21, and two-time increase of the CDVA (from 0.37 ± 0.25 to 0.60 ± 0.17 decimal equivalents). However, preservation of corneal asphericity was observed. Sensitivity to contrast improved, like the increase of corneal topographic regularity and the reduction of its supero-inferior asymmetry, Table 5.3.

The histological exam revealed complete absence of inflammatory reactions in the cornea, and a pronounced compression of the collagen fibres [64, 75, 80, 99–104].

The advantages of this method are: micro-invasiveness, no-tissue subtraction, short rehabilitation time, flattening of the ectatic area, increase of UDVA and

Table 5.3 ICRS literature results

Five-time decrease of the Spherical defect (from −10.2 ± 5.98 to −2.02 ± 2.02 Dioptres)
Two times decreased Cylindrical error (from −4.09 ± 2.42 to 1.89 ± 1.31 Dioptres)
Three-times increase of the UDVA, from 0.07 ± 0.08 to 0.3 ± 0.21 decimal equivalents)
Two-times increase of the CDVA (from 0.37 ± 0.25 to 0.60 ± 0.17 decimal equivalent)
Increase of Topographic Corneal Surface Regularity Index (SRI)
Reduction of Superior-Inferior corneal asymmetry (SI)

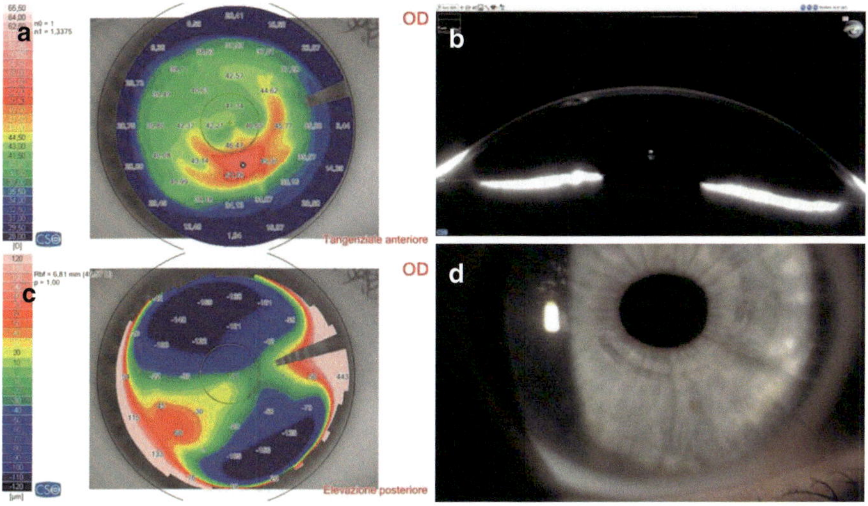

Fig. 5.13 KeraRing™. Tangential map (**a**) and posterior elevation map (**c**) show an extremely decentered KC with very poor functional result of triangular ICRS documented by Scheimpflug camera (**b**) and Biomicroscopy

CDVA. Another notable advantage of the method is its reversibility. Thus, at the confirmation of hypo or hypercorrection or in case of complication, the segments can be removed if or replaced with another of a higher or lower height [80, 99, 100, 103–108].

In the worldwide clinical model, there are mainly three different kinds of intrastromal PMMA rings used: the KeraRing™ (Mediphacos, Brasil), Intacs (Addition Technology, USA), and MyoRing™ (Dioptex, Austria). The KeraRing™ intrastromal rings have a triangular cross section with an internal diameter of 5.0, 5.5, 6.0 mm and an external diameter of 6.2 mm, a height of 150–350 (±50) µm, and the length of the arch at 90°, 120°, 150°, 160°, 210° with a rounded border, Fig. 5.13.

The Intacs™ rings have a hexagonal cross section an external diameter of 8.1 mm and an internal diameter of 6.8 mm, height of 150–450(±50) µm, with an arch-length of 150° with a squared border, Fig. 5.14.

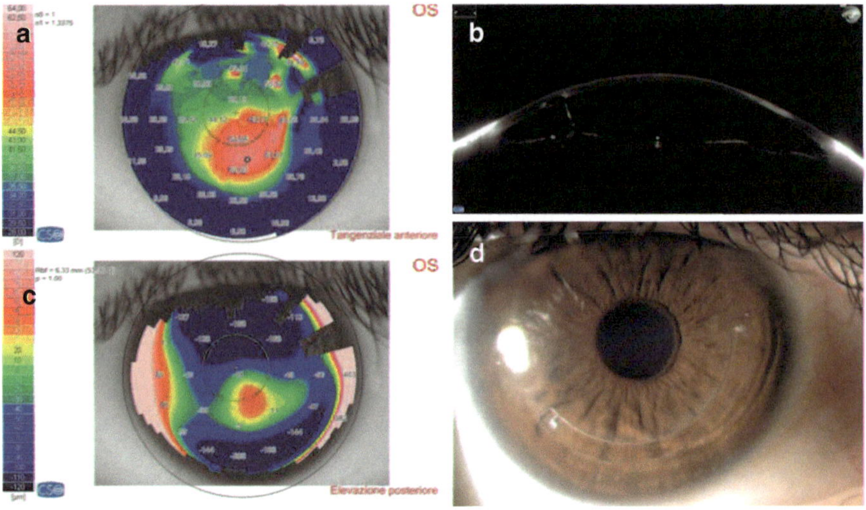

Fig. 5.14 Intacs™. Tangential map (**a**); Scheipflug image showing the esagonal profile of the ICRS. Posterior elevation (**c**); Biomicroscopy (**d**) showing the inferior ring segment (the superior one was removed for an extrusion)

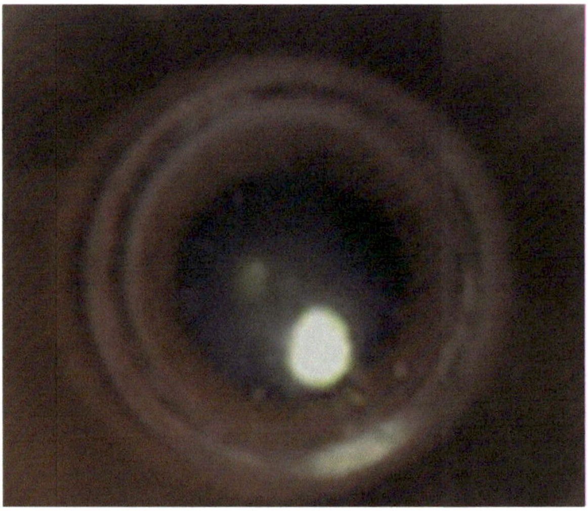

Fig. 5.15 MyoRing™ (Dioptex, Austria)

The Myoring™ rings have a circular form with a sickle-cell like shape of the cross-section and an internal diameter of 5, 6, 7 and 8 mm, a height of 150–350(±50) µm, it is a 360° ring, Fig. 5.15.

Per many Researchers, the strategy is based on corneal reshaping and new limbus creation. The mechanism of intrastromal implants is based on the concept that the corneal collagen fibres build a frame of support, stretching from limbus to limbus.

During the formation of the intrastromal tunnels (mechanical and femtolaser assisted), a break in the fibrillar stroma occurs leading to a concentration of the damaged fibres towards the limbus, which is on the edge of the cornea in the border area of the tunnel and the intact zone. A marked thickening happens, and in the central area a flattening of the rest of the frame occurs which is under the pulling action of the freed fibrils. The implanted rings form a frame that acts as a "second limbus", and put direct pressure towards the outside area of the corneal curvature; the result is a flattening of the apex of the cone, and the cornea returns to a more natural shape, clinically shown by the reduction of the spherical component of the refraction value [53, 109–113].

In clinical practice, today there are different possible modifications of the segments (in height, length, curvature radius and shape in the cross-section), and multiple options both in the depth of the implant and the number of segments, as well as in the position of the corneal incision on the strong or weak meridian.

The efficiency of the ICRS implant in primary keratoconus eyes is advanced and clear-cut. In most cases a stable result is reached with a small decrease of risk of further progression of the disease, significant reduction of the degree of irregular astigmatism, and an increase of visual acuity with or without contact lenses [114–119].

Nonetheless, despite the evident advantages of this method, in some cases possible complications can occur: perforation of the cornea in the formation of the tunnel (1–3%), further thinning of the stroma and ring extrusion (5–19%) or their decentralization, moving and asymmetrical positioning (2.7–13%), formation of neovessels (1–2%), keratitis (2.7–3%), and disappearance of deposits in the corneal tunnel (10–25%). Most complications are due to a superficial positioning of the rings, at a depth of 50–70% of the cornea [44–46, 58, 80, 84, 85, 89, 91, 120], Table 5.4.

Multiple authors claim that to reach the best results of the implant it is necessary to position the widest segment (height) in the inferior part of the cornea. Since the refractive effect and the positioning of the segment in the tunnel depend on the depth of the implant, it is recommended that the segment be implanted at a depth of 80% of the thickness of the cornea to reduce the risk of extrusion of the segment, and to use preferably rings with rounded borders, Fig. 5.13.

Table 5.4 ICRS complications and limits

Perforation of the cornea in the tunnel dissection (1–3%) in mechanical technique
Further thinning of the stroma and EXTRUSION (5–19%)
Decentralization and asymmetrical positioning (2.7–13%)
Neovascularization (1–2%)
Infectious and non-infectious keratitis (2.7–3%)
Deposits in the corneal tunnel (10–25%)
Less results in Central-inferior KC
Less pronounced flattening in Peripheral KC

In the case of central-inferior keratoconus or decentered peripheral kones, the UDVA and CDVA results are not statistically different or get worse as showed in Fig. 5.13. However, in the case of central keratoconus the data of postoperative astigmatism, spherical equivalent and refractive cylinder are better.

This is explained by the fact that in the case of central keratoconus the thinning of the cornea occurs exactly in the centre, while the edge maintains a structure closer to normal. Hence, this kind or initial "symmetrical thinning" of the cornea, contributes to further flattening when the segment is implanted. When keratoconus is paracentral the corneal thickness in the inferior segment is thinner than the superior one, and so the ability of the cornea to flatten is less pronounced. Further, the thin ectasia of the cornea in the inferior segment, corresponding to the top of the paracentral keratoconus, is unable to completely support the segment implanted in the correct position, thus the effect of the superior and inferior semi-ring is irregular [71, 80, 107, 121–128].

Presently, in the case of progressive keratoconus the ring implants are used in conjunction with Riboflavin UVA- crosslinking, in both single or multiple procedures.

In the combined treatment, regardless of surgery time, UDVA and CDVA, the average spherical equivalent and keratometric data are significantly better than monotherapy.

Current data from various studies demonstrate that in the case of progressive keratoconus, the combined treatment is more efficient: the first phase is the rings implant, the second the execution of UVA- crosslinking with a 6-month interval between the two allowing an improvement in the clinical-functional data and contemporary increase in the rigidity of the cornea, stabilizing ectasia progression.

This information has been clarified through the study of the biomechanical properties of the cornea, both with the ocular response analyser (ORA) as well as confocal microscopy. The ocular response analyser (ORA) shows that the most pronounced increase of the corneal hysteresis (CH) is observed in cases of the ICRS implant and the subsequent execution of the CXL. The CH before combined treatment, on average, was 7.18 ± 0.13 mmHg, and after 1 year around 9.71 ± 0.13 mmHg, thus 35.2% above initial values. When the CXL treatment proceeds, the ICRS implant a minor increase up to 9.35 ± 0.12 mm Hg is detected, more than 29.1% compared to the initial levels. The ORA studies of the corneal resistance factor (CRF) further demonstrate that with patients who underwent the combined treatment in the ICRS + CXL sequence, an increase of 42.1% of the CRF was observed after 1 year compared to the baseline level (from 6.10 ± 0.14 to 8.67 ± 0.14 mmHg), while when CXL was the first step in the combined treatment the CRF resulted as slightly inferior (39.2%, up to 8.42 ± 0.17 mm Hg). The sequence can also be inverted (CXL first as stabilization treatment, ICRS after as refractive empowerment treatment), at least 6–12 months after the CXL procedure without complications but with less functional efficacy reasonably due to CXL induced corneal rigidity that reduce the flattening power of rings.

The micro-morphological analysis of the cornea with confocal microscopy after femtosecond laser assisted ICRS implant, shows that the biggest reaction observed in the area surrounding the implant, is a fibrosis with the presence of activated keratocytes (hyper-reflective nuclei) and irregular hyper-reflective extracellular matrix. These alterations are due to micro-traumas caused by exposition to the "shock energy" from the femtolaser. In the area above the implant, intact fibres of the sub-epithelial and stromal plexus are seen. Six months after the ICRS implant with femtolaser, a flattening of the posterior stroma and a decrease in the quantity of creases compared to the pre-operative data is observed. The endothelium remains at a constant density and morphology. At 6 months from the ICRS implant, the intensity of the fibroblastic reaction diminishes in such a way that the CXL treatment can be performed in a corneal area of 5–6 mm of diameter, avoiding the irradiation of the fibrotoc area surrounding the implants preventing the "second energy shock" on keratocyters driving to further stromal scarring. In 23.2% of the cases, intrastromal lipids are also revealed in the area adjacent to the implants after 11–12-months post-surgery. Perhaps these deposits are the result of changes in the biosynthesis of lipids and metabolism of keratocytes, compared to their activation during the micro-traumas caused by the femtosecond laser at the time of the implant. The comparative analysis of the average values variations of UDVA, CDVA, keratometry, the spherical and cylindrical components of refraction show that the best clinical and functional results can be obtained with combined treatment: Phase 1—the ICRS implant with femtosecond laser, Phase 2 (6 months after) the CXL to stabilize the ectasia increasing the flattening effect. The rings implant contributes to the reduction of refraction in the cornea in the optical zone thanks to the flattening of the anterior surface, and moving the apex of the cone from a paracentral to a central zone without affecting the transparent optical centre, as revealed with corneal topography. The stabilization of clinical and functional parameters is verified 6 months after surgical intervention, but the main changes happen in the first 3 months. The execution of the second phase (crosslinking) contributes to a consolidation of the obtained results. Successively, further flattening of the cornea is verified as well as improvement of the clinical and functional parameters [17, 125, 129–137].

When the combined treatment is carried out, but in inverted sequence (Phase 1—crosslinking, Phase 2—ICRS implant), the density and rigidity of the corneal tissue is increased due to the CXL effect, for this the ICRS implant is unable to completely change the corneal curvature and therefore optimize visual acuity.

The use of ICRS-only offers outstanding functional results. The rings significantly contribute to the flattening of the anterior surface of the cornea and in the optical zone, tending towards an improvement in visual acuity and refraction. The ICRS implant can be used independently when we are facing a refractive stationary keratoconus. Must be used together if we are working on a progressive disease. The application of rings is limited to those keratoconic eyes with poor spectacles CDVA, not suitable or intolerant to contact lenses. Therefore, to obtain ectasia stabilization increasing the biomechanical strength of the cornea, as well as a significant improvement of the functional results, the combined treatment (femtolaser assisted ICRS first) [65, 68, 69, 72, 88].

5.3.1 IOL Pseudo-phakic (Toric and Non toric) in Ectasia Treatment

The first implants of the toric IOL to correct high ametropia in the keratoconus were carried out during the phacoemulsification of the cataract after penetrating keratoplasty. Comparing the results of the implant of these toric lenses with that of spherical ones, better results are observed, thanks to the capacity of simultaneous correction of the spherical and cylindrical components of the refractive error [42, 48, 63, 93, 138–144]. The toric IOL are mono-focal and have an optical component that concedes astigmatism correction of 1.0° or more. The main function of the toric IOL lens is based on the variation of optical strength of the lens along an axis, obtained by modifying the form of the anterior surface. The radius of and optical axis of a toric lens is thereby increased by the radius of another axis (R1 > R2). Thus, an IOL combines the properties of two lenses—spherical and cylindrical. For ease of positioning the toric lens on the anterior surface there are marks that must be set with precision during the operation based on the necessary axis of the cornea.

At the moment, there are different models of pseudo-Phakic toric lenses: toric AcrySof™, Tflex™ AsphericToric, Envista™ Toric, AT Torbi™, Tecnis™ Toric Aspheric, Staar NanoFlex™ and others.

Presently, cataract surgery, indeed phacoemulsification, with the toric IOL is considered an effective and secure correction of ametropia in keratoconus patients, Fig. 5.16. Nonetheless, patient selection for this kind of surgery is complex, because compared to the general population, the cataract in thick keratoconus is diagnosed at a young age and the rehabilitation of the patients requires special attention. At the same time, it is necessary to consider not only the age of the patient, but also their activity, and the status of the other eye. On the other hand, the correct strategy of treatment is necessary: begin with the correction of the ametropia due to ectasia or cataract treatment (Table 5.5).

The correction of the ametropia in eyes with stable keratoconus of the 1st or 2nd stage (Amsler-Krumeich staging system) and of the cataract, an intervention of

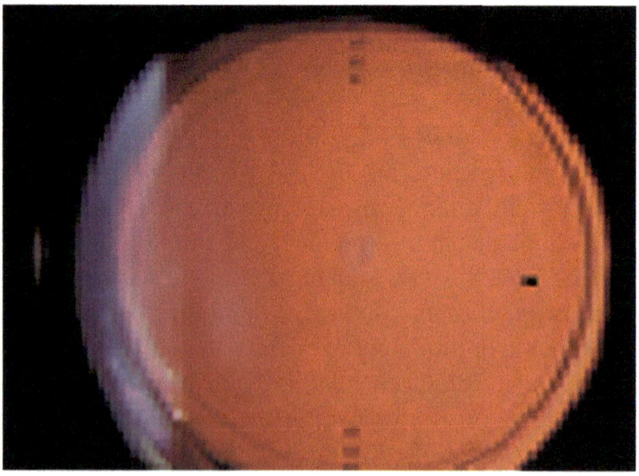

Fig. 5.16 Toric-intraocular lens

Table 5.5 Criteria for KC patient selection for PHACO + IOL

Criteria for patient selection for PHACO + IOL
1. Cataract diagnosis;
2. Stable Keratoconus;
3. Patients after intrastromal ring implant and or CXL
4. Absence of opacity in the central zone of the cornea

phacoemulsification is performed and the pseudo-phakic toric lens is implanted. This operation leads to a reduction in the cylindrical component of 60–70% and a UCVA and BCVA increase of 10% and 50–60%, respectively. In all eyes a faint hyper-metropical refraction is detected, on average 1.5 ± 0.3° and an IOL rotation inside of 5.5–7.4° [86, 93, 145].

There are currently multiple approaches for cataract treatment in progressive keratoconus eyes: (1) ICRS implants, and after 3-months phacoemulsification cataract surgery, after 3 months a mono-focal toric IOL implant targeting emmetropia is put in. (2) only phacoemulsification with a mono-focal toric IOL implant. (3) Simultaneous execution of PRK and CXL in instable cornea following the "Athens" protocol, suggested by Kanellopoulos, thus, after keratotopographic stabilization in 4–18 months the phacoemulsification with mono-focal lens or mono-focal toric IOL is performed. The values of the astigmatism can be decreased up to 70–75%. The question of the calculation of the optical power of the IOL remains. The main requirements of a toric lens should be its rotational stability in the capsular bag, which depends in turn on the "haptic elements" design. Thus, if the haptic elements have a "C" form a post-operational rotation of >10° in 41% of the cases is detected [70, 79, 146]. The best method for preoperatively marking the axis is considered marking under the slit-lamp. Today, to calculate optic strength of the toric IOL various techniques and formulas are used. At the same time, there are two principal classes of formula: empirical (of regression) SRK II, and the third-generation mixed formulas (Holladay, SRK/T, Hoffer Q, Haigis). Despite the great variety of formulas to calculate toric IOL optic strength, there is still high difficulty for the calculation of keratoconus patients and the biometric surprise is often present in the postoperative requiring IOL exchange. The keratometric parameters cannot be trusted due to their variability, which is based on from whence and how the measurement came, and for the fact that the visual axis in keratoconus eyes as well as others with ectasias is not located on the corneal apex but towards the cone. Further, the software used for the toric IOL optic strength calculation is calibrated and controlled on eyes without keratoconus, and with a regular astigmatism where the corneal apex coincides with the visual axis. Therefore, the keratometric data used for the calculations of toric IOL are generally inaccurate. Further, factors like irregular astigmatism, aberrations, etc. can notably influence refractive results after the intervention [147, 148].

Also, the question regarding the correction of the ametropic residue after complete treatment with multifocal toric lenses remains open. According to various authors the postoperative results in these patients are lower compared to those with the mono-focal toric lenses, and this could lead to an increase in the quantity of aberrations [147, 148].

One method exists which proposes implanting a spherical, not toric lens, which offers more expected results with shorter rehabilitation time. This method includes the creation of preventive tunnels, simultaneous phacoemulsification and the implant of mono-focal not toric IOL (objective refraction—2.0–3.0° of myopia), then ICRS implants are put in, (on average after 1.2 weeks) and CXL performed. The second phase permits not only the stabilization of the keratoconus but also gains further correction of corneal astigmatism. Implanting mono-focal IOL with null or negative sphericity does not further complicate eventual surgical treatment of keratoconus in the case of eventual future progression. The authors of this method explain that with the toric lens implant we can obtain a programmed, high complex astigmatism, but any successive transplant of the cornea is complicated due to the need to substitute the IOL.

5.3.2 Phakic IOLs

Currently, one of the most promising and rapidly developing methods of correction of high ametropia is the implantation of a toric IOL in phakic eyes. Today this kind of intraocular correction is becoming ever more popular among surgeons who perform surgical correction of high myopia and myopic astigmatism. From their point of view, the precision, predictability, stability of visual function, as well as short rehabilitation time provides a significant increase in quality of life and quick recovery of operated patients [43, 66, 70].

Actually there are various models of phakic intraocular lenses (pIOLs), that differ from one another depending on their position in the eye (in the anterior or posterior chamber) and the kind of fixation. The models inserted in the anterior chamber consist of lenses with the fixation in the anterior chamber angle (angle-supported) (AcrySof Cachet™, Alcon) and the lens with fixation on the iris (iris-fixated), unfoldables Artisan Ophtec, Verisyse™ Abbot Medical Optics (AMO), and foldables Artiflex™ Ophtec, Veriflex™ AMO, Fig. 5.17.

For the posterior chamber lens the position of the optical device is placed in the ciliary sulcus, Implantable Collamer Lenses (ICL), STAAR Surgical, Fig. 5.18, and Phakic Refractive Lenses (PRL), Carl Zeiss Meditec [43, 70, 79, 92, 146, 149].

The first publications regarding intraocular ametropia correction with a pIOL for keratoconus after deep penetrating keratoplasty describe the results of the pIOL ZSAL-4 (Morcher) implant in the anterior chamber, and pIOL Artisan (Ophtec AMO) in the posterior chamber. The follow up period was 6–12 months. In all cases an increase of the UCVA up to 8–10/10 was observed thanks to a notable reduction of the spherical and cylindrical components of refraction. The results permitted the authors to conclude that there are prospects for the use of toric pIOL for ametropia correction in operated keratoconic eyes [83, 150, 151].

With the development and improvement of modern methods to treat keratoconus (Riboflavin UVA Cross-linking and ICRS), the toric pIOL implant is used most frequently as a final stage in the algorithm of keratectasia treatment (KC and

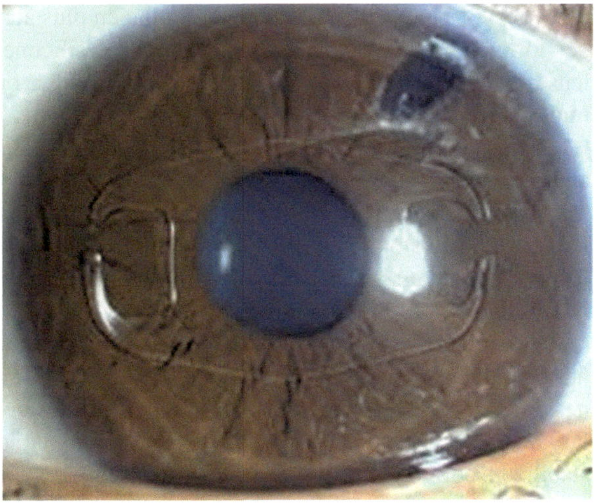

Fig. 5.17 Iris-fixated anterior chamber pIOL

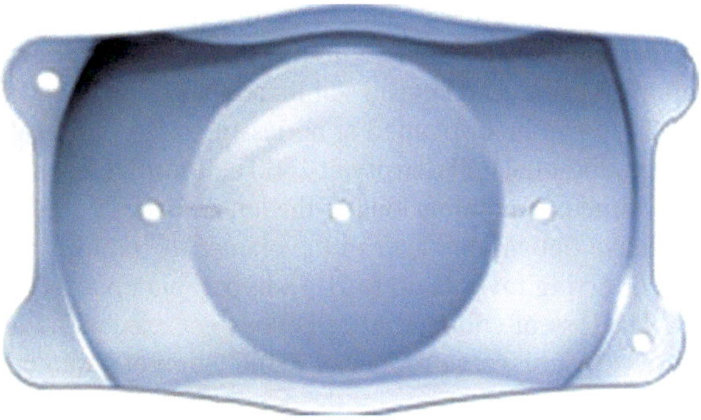

Fig. 5.18 Posterior chamber Implantable Collamer Lens (Visian™ ICL, STAAR)

Pellucid Marginal Degeneration), secondary CXL-stabilized ectasias. Nonetheless, with the latest clinical data it seems that the pIOL can trigger the onset of side effects like cataracts, oval pupils, the loss of corneal endothelial cells, induced astigmatism, secondary glaucoma, iridocyclitis, etc. The adequate choice of pIOL model per case following accurate preoperative diagnostic evaluation including refraction, UDVA, CDVA assessment, applanation tonometry, biomicroscopy, corneal tomography, pachymetry, dynamic pupillometry, anterior segment OCT and UBM to measure the anterior chamber depth, the white to white (WTW) diameter, the angle to angle (ATA) distance, the sulcus to sulcus distance (STS), biometry and ocular fundus examination are mandatory. Most authors prefer to use on-line calculators to calculate the optical power of toric pIOL which are directly provided by the manufacturers of the pIOL [56].

According to the literature, the most used models of toric pIOL to correct residual ametropia in keratoconic eyes are the posterior chamber "Visian™ Toric-ICL"

(STAAR) of biocompatible collamer (collagen plus acrylic) and the anterior chamber toric Artiflex/Veryflex foldable lenses of silicone with PMMA aptic. These lenses can be used after ICRS implants, after ACXL or in combination in triple or multiple procedures.

Some authors prefer the Artiflex pIOL in the anterior chamber, fixated by its aptic elements to the medial part of the iris stroma, providing a good stability of the iris in absence of restriction for pupil dilation and reduction. This fact, in their opinion, prevents postoperative pseudo-phacodonesis, vaulting, and reduces risk of lens de-contraction; and, above all, permits fixation in any position: horizontal, vertical oroblique.

Implanting these pIOLs, the IOL sizing is fundamental, so we recommend to have an anterior chamber depth (ACD) of at least 3.2 mm in the centre, with a corneal thickness of 450 μm, endothelial cell count at more than 2200 cells/mm^2, pupillary diameter < 6.5 mm, WTW > 11 mm, stable axial length, stable or CXL/ACXL stabilized corneal ectasia. The Artiflex can correct the spherical component of refraction in the interval from −1.0 D up to −13.5D and the cylindrical component from −1.0 to −7.0 D. The loss of endothelial cells within a year after the surgery does not exceed 3.29% [74, 93, 152].

Despite all the advantages of the Artiflex anterior chamber lens, 64% of the actual implants are done with a soft, elastic posterior chamber ICL (STAAR) lens after CXL induced ectasia stabilization, Fig. 5.19 and 5.20.

They can be implanted at no less than 2.8 mm of depth in the anterior chamber and endothelial cell density at 1800 cell/mm^2. Depending on horizontal diameter of the cornea, the dimensions of the lenses vary in diameter, 12.2–13.7 mm, and their effective optical diameter in the plan of the pupil is 6–6.8 mm. The lens is capable of correcting myopia up to 20 D, hyperopia up to 10 D and astigmatism up to −6.0 D. The loss of endothelial cells does not exceed 3.2%. The essential condition for correct residual ametropia is a stabilization of keratoconus for at least 1 year. As far as the recommendations for the combined treatment go the paradigm is always "cornea first" (ICRS, CXL, CXL Plus All Surface Laser minimal Aablation for corneal regularization, pIOLs), this treatment remains reserved for very selected clinical cases of keratoconus. Thus, the ICRS can approximately correct 7.0D with an

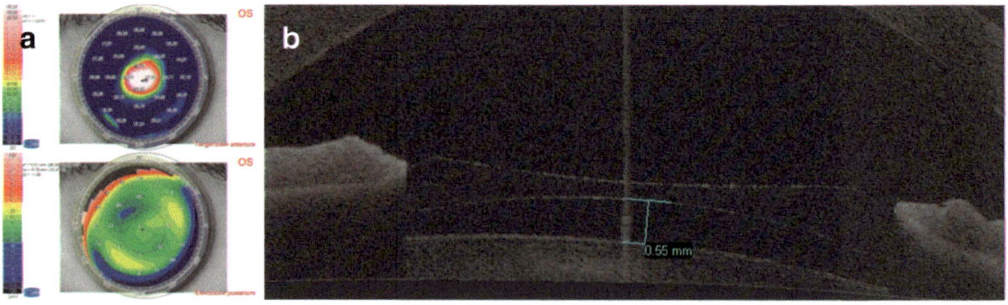

Fig. 5.19 KC (**a**) in a 27 years old patients intolerant to spectacles and contact lenses, treated by combined CXL and Visian™ Toric ICL. Preoperative data −10 myopia, 3 cylinder 90° at Department of Ophthalmology, Siena University, Italy

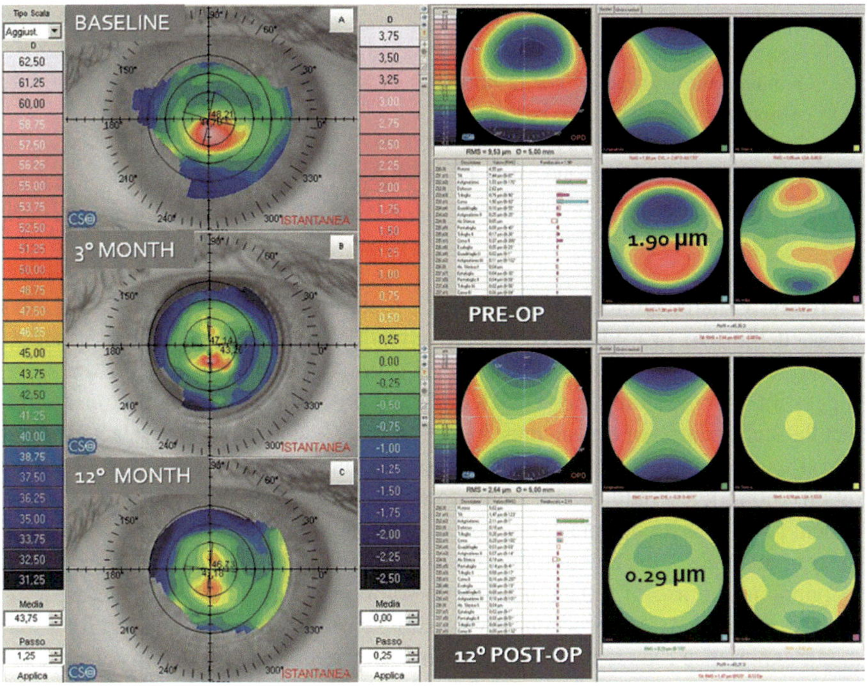

Fig. 5.20 CXL Plus All surface laser ablation. Evident KC regularization and symmetry after 3 and 12-months follow-up. The coma value passed from 1.90 μm at baseline to 0.29 μm over a year follow-up. The 15 mW sequential CXL protocol with pulsed light and 5.4 J/cm^2 was used to stabilize the cornea (C. Mazzotta, Siena Crosslinking Center, Italy)

improvement in CDVA; CXL can further reduce 2.0D of corneal irregularity with an improvement in flat, steep, and mean K values; and pIOL can decrease the spherical component up to 20.0D and cylindrical up to 6 D increasing the UCVA.

5.3.3 Trans-PRK

The combined approach of ectasia treatment consists of various steps including both ICRS implants, CXL to stabilize the pathological process with consequential correction of residual ametropia with the help of toric IOL and/or transepithelial PTK or PRK. Considering recovery of visual function after ectasia stabilization, frequent complications are the appearance of irregular astigmatisms. According to various authors the PRK could be successfully used in sequential same-day treatment or postponed after 6–12 months after CXL induced stabilization. The PRK allows correction of the coma aberration and small amount (1/3 or more of the sphero-cylindrical component of refraction). The aim is not to eliminate the necessity of spectacles correction in patient intolerant to contact lenses, but to regularize the corneal surface increasing the optical performance of spectacle correction, Fig. 5.20.

Patient selection for Trans-PRK and CXL	
1.	Age > 21 years
2.	Simultaneously (same-day) or 12 months after CXL-induced KC stabilization
3.	Absence of corneal and lens opacities
4.	Minimal Residual Stromal pachymetry >400 μm
5.	Keratometry <55.0 D; no more than di 63 D in K max value
6.	Contact lens and spectacle intolerance
7.	KC asymmetry or anisometropia

Today a shared protocol does not exist regarding the time that needs to pass between the two procedures (CXL and trans-PRK) [133] but a lot of protocols already exists with long-term over 5-years follow-ups. At present, there are some suggestions for the simultaneous PRK and CXL procedure (CXL Plus). Considering that the stabilization of ectasia must be well established in these very selected cases. The aim is to ablate the small amount of tissue reducing ectasia related corneal aberrations (coma); it would be also useful to reduce the spherical and cylindrical component for a 30% ametropia correction minimizing depth ablation in any case. The maximum depth of the ablation mustn't exceed 50 μm of corneal stroma. We do not recommend the use of 0.02% mitomycin solution in ectatic corneas, and recommend associated ACXL procedures with shorter irradiation times, pulsed light that in our experience reduce the potentiality of haze development. There is an accelerated impregnation of the stroma thanks to the removal of the Bowmann lamina due to ablation, and therefore riboflavin soaking time is reduced [73, 114, 153–155], see Sect. 5.1 of the book, STARE X protocol.

In our opinion, the advantage of simultaneous (same-day) surgery is that it is only one step, and so the visual recovery is faster. Nonetheless, other studies have shown that there is some difficulty in obtaining predicted refraction to obtain deferred stabilization of keratometry after CXL. Added to this, there is a risk of overcorrection (hypermetropic refraction) in the case of a slight initial ametropia.

It would be opportune to further study the effect of the combination of ablation and UV-exposition on the cornea. Studies exist that compare simultaneous surgery with that done 6 months after. The data demonstrated that the average value of the sub-epithelial fibroplasia (Durrie classification) in the case of sequential execution (first CXL and then PRK) is 1.20, and in the case of the simultaneous surgery it is 0.50. Based on the Durrie classification, 1.0 corresponds to "minimal density opacity, that does not influence the refraction of the patient", and 0.5° is "single but not sufficient traces of opacity". The average reparative response in Durrie's opinion corresponds to the degree of haze manifestation, which is 0.5 and 1.0. Thus, the data would show that there is no important difference in the intensity of the fibroplasia in both interventions [77]. The literature describes the formation of corneal opacity in the deep stroma after the execution of the simultaneous intervention PRK + CXL. Confocal microscopy data observe this opacity 1 month after the procedure in 46.42% of the cases, and within 12 months a change in opacity towards the anterior part of the stroma with a reduction in the intensity [82]. Some authors believe that haze formation in the combined procedure, and in the sequential

6-month interval, could be linked to an incompletion of the reparation processes of the corneal stroma after CXL, and an added effect from the ablation. In the case of the CXL and PRK sequence we recommend to wait at least 12 months to regain a proper stromal restoration reducing cell reactivity and potentiality of haze development.

References

1. Mazzotta C, Traversi C, Paradiso AL, Latronico ME, Rechichi M. Pulsed light accelerated crosslinking versus continuous light accelerated crosslinking: one-year results. J Ophthalmol. 2014;2014:604731.
2. Greenstein SA, Fry KL, Hersh PS. Effect of topographic cone location on outcomes of corneal collagen cross-linking for keratoconus and corneal ectasia. J Refract Surg. 2012;28(6):397–405.
3. Kymionis GD, Grentzelos MA, Portaliou DM, Kankariya VP, Randleman JB. Corneal collagen cross-linking (CXL) combined with refractive procedures for the treatment of corneal ectatic disorders: CXL plus. J Refract Surg. 2014;30(8):566–76.
4. Shetty R, D'Souza S, Srivastava S, Ashwini R. Topography-guided custom ablation treatment for treatment of keratoconus. Indian J Ophthalmol. 2013;61(8):445–50. https://doi.org/10.4103/0301-4738.116067. PubMed PMID: 23925335; PubMedCentral PMCID: PMC3775085
5. Kanellopoulos AJ, Asimellis G. Keratoconus management: long-term stability of topography-guided normalization combined with high-fluence CXL stabilization (the Athens protocol). J Refract Surg. 2014;30:88–93.
6. Krueger RR, Kanellopoulos AJ. Stability of simultaneous to- pography-guided photorefractive keratectomy and riboflavin/ UVA cross-linking for progressive keratoconus: case reports. J Refract Surg. 2010;26:S827–32.
7. Stojanovic A, Zhang J, Chen X, Nitter TA, Chen S, Wang Q. Topography-guided transepithelial surface ablation followed by corneal collagen cross-linking performed in a single combined procedure for the treatment of keratoconus and pellucid marginal degeneration. J Refract Surg. 2010;26:145–52.
8. Kymionis GD, Portaliou DM, Diakonis VF, et al. Management of post laser in situ keratomileusis ectasia with simultaneous topography guided photorefractive keratectomy and collagen cross-linking. Open Ophthalmol J. 2011;5:11–3.
9. Kymionis GD, Portaliou DM, Kounis GA, et al. Simultaneous topography-guided photorefractive keratectomy followed by corneal collagen cross-linking for keratoconus. Am J Ophthalmol. 2011;152:748–55.
10. Tuwairqi WS, Sinjab MM. Safety and efficacy of simultaneous corneal collagen cross-linking with topography-guided PRK in managing low-grade keratoconus: 1-year follow-up. J Refract Surg. 2012;28:341–5.
11. Lin DT, Holland S, Tan JC, Moloney G. Clinical results of topography-based customized ablations in highly aberrated eyes and keratoconus/ectasia with cross-linking. J Refract Surg. 2012;28:S841–8.
12. Alessio G, L'abbate M, Sborgia C, La Tegola MG. Photorefractive keratectomy followed by cross-linking versus cross-linking alone for management of progressive keratoconus: two-year follow-up. Am J Ophthalmol. 2013;155:54–65.
13. Kymionis GD, Grentzelos MA, Karavitaki AE, et al. Transepithelial phototherapeutic keratectomy using a 213-nm solid-state laser system followed by corneal collagen cross-linking with riboflavin and UVA irradiation. J Ophthalmol. 2010;2010:146543.
14. Kymionis GD, Grentzelos MA, Kounis GA, Diakonis VF, Lim- nopoulou AN, Panagopoulou SI. Combined transepithelial phototherapeutic keratectomy and corneal collagen cross-linking for progressive keratoconus. Ophthalmology. 2012;119:1777–84.

15. Kymionis GD, Grentzelos MA, Kankariya VP, Pallikaris IG. Combined transepithelial phototherapeutic keratectomy and corneal collagen crosslinking for ectatic disorders: Cretan protocol. J Cataract Refract Surg. 2013;39:1939.
16. Mazzotta C, Baiocchi S, Simone AB, MD, Fruschelli M, Alessandro M, Rechichi M. Accelerated 15 mW pulsed-light crosslinking in treatment of progressive keratoconus: Two-year clinical results. J Cataract Refract Surg. 2017, in press.
17. Wollensak G, Spoerl E, Seiler T. Riboflavin/ultraviolet-a-induced collagen crosslinking for the treatment of keratoconus. Am J Ophthalmol. 2003;135(5):620–7.
18. Caporossi A, Baiocchi S, Mazzotta C, Traversi C, Caporossi T. Parasurgical therapy for keratoconus by riboflavin-ultraviolet type A rays induced cross-linking of corneal collagen: preliminary refractive results in an Italian study. J Cataract Refract Surg. 2006;32(5):837–45.
19. Hafezi F, Kanellopoulos J, Wiltfang R, Seiler T. Corneal collagen crosslinking with riboflavin and ultraviolet A to treat induced keratectasia after laser in situ keratomileusis. J Cataract Refract Surg. 2007;33(12):2035–40.
20. Mazzotta C, Baiocchi S, Denaro R, Tosi GM, Caporossi T. Corneal collagen cross-linking to stop corneal ectasia exacerbated by radial keratotomy. Cornea. 2011;30(2):225–8.
21. Spoerl E, Seiler T. Techniques for stiffening the cornea. J Refract Surg Thorofare NJ 1995. 1999;15(6):711–3.
22. Raiskup-Wolf F, Hoyer A, Spoerl E, Pillunat LE. Collagen crosslinking with riboflavin and ultraviolet-A light in keratoconus: long-term results. J Cataract Refract Surg. 2008;34(5):796–801.
23. Raiskup F, Theuring A, Pillunat LE, Spoerl E. Corneal collagen crosslinking with riboflavin and ultraviolet-A light in progressive keratoconus: ten-year results. J Cataract Refract Surg. 2015;41(1):41–6.
24. Spoerl E, Mrochen M, Sliney D, Trokel S, Seiler T. Safety of UVA-riboflavin cross-linking of the cornea. Cornea. 2007;26(4):385–9.
25. Roy AS, Dupps WJ Jr. Patient-specific computational modeling of keratoconus progression and differential responses to collagen cross-linking. Invest Ophthalmol Vis Sci. 2011;52(12):9174–87.
26. Roberts CJ, Dupps WJ Jr. Biomechanics of corneal ectasia and biomechanical treatments. J Cataract Refract Surg. 2014;40(6):991–8.
27. Brindley G. The Bunsen-Roscoe law for the human eye at very short durations. J Physiol. 1952;118(1):135–9.
28. Schumacher S, Oeftiger L, Mrochen M. Equivalence of biomechanical changes induced by rapid and standard corneal cross-linking, using riboflavin and ultraviolet radiation. Invest Ophthalmol Vis Sci. 2011;52(12):9048–52.
29. Wernli J, Schumacher S, Spoerl E, Mrochen M. The efficacy of corneal cross-linking shows a sudden decrease with very high intensity UV light and short treatment time. Invest Ophthalmol Vis Sci. 2013;54(2):1176–80.
30. Mazzotta C, Traversi C, Caragiuli S, Rechichi M. Pulsed vs continuous light accelerated corneal collagen crosslinking: in vivo qualitative investigation by confocal microscopy and corneal OCT. Eye (Lond). 2014;28(10):1179–83.
31. Mita M, Waring GO, Tomita M. High-irradiance accelerated collagen crosslinking for the treatment of keratoconus: six-month results. J Cataract Refract Surg. 2014;40(6):1032–40.
32. Chow VW, Chan TC, Yu M, Wong VW, Jhanji V. One-year outcomes of conventional and accelerated collagen crosslinking in progressive keratoconus. Sci Rep. 2015;5:14425. https://doi.org/10.1038/srep14425.
33. Mazzotta C, Hafezi F, Kymionis G, Caragiuli S, Jacob S, Traversi C, Barabino S, Randleman B. In vivo confocal microscopy after corneal collagen cross-linking. Ocul Surf. 2015;13(4):298–314.
34. Mazzotta C, Balestrazzi A, Traversi C, et al. Treatment of progressive keratoconus by riboflavin-UVA-induced cross-linking of corneal collagen: ultrastructural analysis by Heidelberg Retinal Tomograph II in vivo confocal microscopy in humans. Cornea. 2007;26(4):390–7.

35. Mazzotta C, Paradiso AL, Baiocchi S, Caragiuli S, Caporossi A. Qualitative investigation of corneal changes after accelerated corneal collagen cross-linking (A-CXL) by in vivo confocal microscopy and corneal OCT. J Clin Exp Ophthalmol. 2013;4:313.
36. Mazzotta C, Traversi C, Baiocchi S, et al. Corneal healing after riboflavin ultraviolet-A collagen cross-linking determined by confocal laser scanning microscopy in vivo: early and late modifications. Am J Ophthalmol. 2008;146(4):527–33.
37. Croxatto JO, Tytiun AE, Argento CJ. Sequential in vivo confocal microscopy study of corneal wound healing after cross-linking in patients with keratoconus. J Refract Surg Thorofare NJ 1995. 2010;26(9):638–45.
38. Mazzotta C, Caporossi T, Denaro R, et al. Morphological and functional correlations in riboflavin UV A corneal collagen cross-linking for keratoconus. Acta Ophthalmol. 2012;90(3):259–65.
39. Peyman A, Nouralishahi A, Hafezi F, Kling S, Peyman M. Stromal demarcation line in pulsed versus continuous light accelerated corneal cross-linking for keratoconus. J Refract Surg. 2016;32(3):206–8.
40. Kling S, Richoz O, Hammer A, Tabibian D, Jacob S, Agarwal A, Hafezi F. Increased biomechanical efficacy of corneal cross-linking in thin corneas due to higher oxygen availability. J Refract Surg. 2015;31(12):840–6.
41. Caporossi A, Mazzotta C, Baiocchi S, Caporossi T. Long-term results of riboflavin ultraviolet a corneal collagen cross-linking for keratoconus in Italy: the Siena eye cross study. Am J Ophthalmol. 2010;149(4):585–93.
42. Alfonso JF, Fernandez-Vega L, Lisa C, Fernandes P, Gonzalez-Meijome JM, Montes-Mico R. Collagen copolymer toric posterior chamber phakic intraocular lens in eyes with keratoconus. J Cataract Refract Surg. 2010;36(6):906–16.
43. Alio JL. Advances in phakic intraocular lenses: indications, efficacy, safety, and new designs. Curr Opin Ophthalmol. 2004;15(4):350–7.
44. Alio J. Analysis of results related to good and bad outcomes of lntacs implantation for keratoconus correction. J Cataract Refract Surg. 2006;32(5):756–61.
45. Alio J, Pinero D, Sogutlu E, Kubaloglu A. Implantation of new intracorneal ring segments after segment explantation for unsuccessful outcomes in eye with keratoconus. J Cataract RefractSurg. 2010;36:1303–10.
46. Alio J, Shabayek MH. Intracorneal asymmetrical rings for keratoconus: where should the thicker segment be implanted? J Refract Surg. 2006;22(3):307–9.
47. Alio JL, Shabayek MH, Artola A. Intracorneal ring segments for keratoconus correction: long-term follow-up. J Cataract Refract Surg. 2006;32(6):978–85.
48. Alio JL, Agdeppa MC, Pongo VC, El Kady B. Microincision cataract surgery with toric intraocular lens implantation for correcting moderate and high astigmatism: pilot study. J Cataract Refract Surg. 2010;36(1):44–52.
49. Alio JL, Artola A, Hassanein A. One or two Intacs segments for the correction of keratoconus. J Cataract Refract Surg. 2005;31(5):943–53.
50. Amsler M. Keratoconus. Bull De Sos Beige d'ophthalm. 1961;129:331–6.
51. Davis LJ. Collaborative Longitudinal Evaluation of Keratoconus (CLEK) Study Group. Longitudinal changes in visual acuity in keratoconus. Invest. Ophthalmol Vis Sci. 2006;47(2): 489–500.
52. Daxer A. Intracorneal continuous ring implantation for keratoconus: one year follow-up. J Cataract Refract Surg. 2010;36:1296–302.
53. Daxer A, Fratzl P. Collagen fibrill orientation in human corneal stroma and its implication in keratoconus. Invest Ophthalmol Vis Sci. 1997;38(1):121–9.
54. De-Cunda DA, Woodward EG. Measurement of corneal topography in keratoconus. Ophthalmic Physiol Opt. 1993;13(4):377–82.
55. Dohlman CH. Syntetic polymers I corneal surgery. I. Glyceryl mehacrylate. Arch Ophthalmol. 1967;77(2):252–7.
56. Ertan A, Ozkilic E. Effect of age on outcomes in patients with keratoconus treated by Intacs using a femtosecond laser. J Refract Surg. 2008;24(7):690–5.
57. Ferrara de A, Cunha P. Tecnica cirurgica para correçao de miopia; Anel corneano intraestromal. Rev Bras Oftalmol. 1995;54:577–88.

58. Ferrer C, Alió JL, Montañés AU, Pérez-Santonja JJ, del Rio MA, de Toledo JA, Teus MA, Javaloy J. Causes of intrastromal corneal ring segment explantation: clinicopathologic correlation analysis. J Cataract Refract Surg. 2010;36(6):970–7.
59. Fleming JF. The intrastromal corneal ring-two cases in rabbits. J Refract Surg. 1987;3(6):227–32.
60. Fleming JF, Wan WL, Schanzlin DJ. The theory of corneal curvature change with the intrastromal corneal ring. CLAO J. 1989;15:146–50.
61. Fujimori E. Cross-linking and fluorescence changes of collagen by glycation and oxidation. Biochim Biophys Acta. 1989;998:105110.
62. Gefen A. Biochemical analysis of the keratoconic cornea. J Mech Behav Biomed Mater. 2009;2:224–36.
63. Gills JP. Piggyback minus-power lens implantation in keratoconus. J Cataract Refract Surg. 1998;24(4):566–8.
64. Gonzalez JM. Ferrara ring implant better for advanced keratoconus. Ocular Surg News Europe/Asia-Pacific. 2002;13(4):7–8.
65. Hersh PS, Greenstein SA, Fry KL. Corneal collagen crosslinking for keratoconus and corneal ectasia: One-year results. J Cataract Refract Surg. 2011;37(1):149–60.
66. Hoffmann PC, Auel S, Hutz WW. Results of higher power toric intraocular lens implantation. J Cataract Refract Surg. 2011;37(8):1411–8.
67. Holland E, Lane S, Horn JD, Ernest P, Arleo R, Miller KM. The AcryS of Toric intraocular lens in subjects with cataracts and corneal astigmatism: a randomized, subject-masked, parallel-group, 1-year study. Ophthalmology. 2007;117(11):2104–11.
68. Hollingsworth JG, Bonshek RE, Efron N. Correlation of the appearance of the keratoconic cornea in vivo by confocal microscopy and in vitro by light microscopy. Cornea. 2005;24(4):397–405.
69. Hollingsworth J, Efron N, Tullo A. In vivo corneal confocal microscopy in keratoconus. Ophthalmic Physiol Opt. 2005;25(3):254–60.
70. Huang D, Schallhorn SC, Sugar A, Farjo AA, Majmudar PA, Trattler WB, Tanzer DJ. Phakic intraocular lens implantation for the correction of myopia: a report by the American Academy of Ophthalmology. Ophthalmology. 2009;116(11):2244–58.
71. Hwang DG. The intrastromal corneal ring segment: current status and review of US phase II clinical results. Ophthalmol Clin. 1997;10:591–7.
72. Imre L, Resch M, Nagymihály A. In vivo confocal corneal microscopy after keratoplasty. Ophthalmologe. 2005;102(2):140–6.
73. Iovieno A, Légaré ME, Rootman DB, Yeung SN, Kim P, Rootman DS. Intracorneal ring segments implantation followed by same-day photorefractive keratectomy and corneal collagen cross-linking in keratoconus. J Refract Surg. 2011;27(12):915–8.
74. Izquierdo L Jr, Henriquez MA, McCarthy M. Artiflex phakic intraocular lens implantation after corneal collagen cross-linking in keratoconic eyes. J Refract Surg. 2011; 27(7):482–7.
75. Izmailova SV Sistema medico-tecnologica del trattamento chirurgico dell'ectasie progressive di varie genesi.//Tesi per il grado di Dottore in Scienze Mediche. 2014.
76. Kamiya K, Shimizu K, Ando W, Asato Y, Fujisawa T. Phakic toric Implantable Collamer Lens implantation for the correction of high myopic astigmatism in eyes with keratoconus. J Refract Surg. 2008;24(8):840–2.
77. Kanellopoulos AJ, Pe LH, Perry HD, Donnenfeld ED. Modified intracorneal ring segment implantations (INTACS) for the management of moderate to advanced keratoconus: efficacy and complications. Cornea. 2006;25:29–33. KeraVision Inc, phase III protocol summary, USA
78. Kanellopoulos AJ, Binder PS. Collagen cross-linking (CCL) with sequential topography-guided PRK: a temporizing alternative for keratoconus to penetrating keratoplasty. Cornea. 2007;26:891–5.
79. Kohnen T, Knorz MC, Cochener B, Gerl RH, Arne JL, Colin J, Alio JL, Bellucci R, Marinho A. AcrySof phakic angle-supported intraocular lens for the correction of moderate-to-high

myopia: one-year results of a multicenter European study. Ophthalmology. 2009;116(7):1314–21. 1321 e1-3
80. Kwitko S, Severo NS. Ferrara intracorneal ring segments for keratoconus. J Cataract Refract Surg. 2004;30(8):12–20.
81. Kymionis GD, Bouzoukis DI, Portaliou DM, Pallikaris IG. New INTACS SK implantation in patients with post-laser in situ keratomileusis corneal ectasia. Cornea. 2010;29(2):214–6.
82. Kymionis GD, Diakonis VF, Kalyvianaki M, et al. One-year follow-up of corneal confocal microscopy after corneal cross-linking in patients with post laser in situ keratosmileusis ectasia and keratoconus. Am J Ophthalmol. 2009;147(5):774–8.
83. Leccisotti A, Fields SV. Angle-supported phakic intraocular lenses in eyes with keratoconus and myopia. J Cataract Refract Surg. 2003;29(8):1530.
84. Levy J, Lifshit T. Keratitis after implantation of intrastromal corneal ring segments (Intacs) aided by femtosecond laser for keratoconus correction: case report and description of the literature. Eur J Ophthalmol. 2010;20(4):780–4.
85. Lim L. Late onset post-keratoplasty astigmatism in patients with keratoconus. Br J Ophthalmol. 2004;88(3):371–6.
86. Maslova N. Cheratoplastica intrastromale con laser a femtosecondi con l'impianto di segmenti corneali nei pazienti con cheratocono.//Tesi per il grado di Candidato delle scienze mediche 2012.
87. Mahmood H, Venkateswaran RS, Daxer A. Implantation of a complete corneal ring in an intrastromal pocket for keratoconus. J Refract Surg. 2011;27:63–8.
88. Mazzotta C, Balestrazzi A, Baiocchi S, Traversi C, Caporossi A. Stromal haze after combined riboflavin-UVA corneal collagen cross-linking in keratoconus: in vivo confocal microscopic evaluation. Clin Experiment Ophthalmol. 2007;35(6):580–2.
89. McAlister JC, Ardjomand N, Hari L, Mengher LS. Keratitis after intracorneal ring segment insertion for keratoconus. J Cataract Refract Surg. 2006;32:676–8.
90. Morris E, et al. Corneal endothelial specular microscopy following deep lamellar keratoplasty with lyophilised tissue. Eye. 1998;12:619–22.
91. Mortensen J, Carlsson K, Ohrstrom A. Excimer laser surgery for keratoconus. J Cataract Refract Surg. 1998;24(7):893–8.
92. Moshirfar M, Barsam CA, Parker JW. Implantation of an Artisan phakic intraocular lens for the correction of high myopia after penetrating keratoplasty. J Cataract Refract Surg. 2004;30(7):1578–81.
93. Visser N, Gast ST, Bauer NJ, Nuijts RM. Cataract surgery with toric IOL implantation in keratoconus Case report. Cornea. 2011;30(6):720–3.
94. Nose W, Neves RA. Intrastromal corneal ring – 1-year results of first implants in humans: a preliminary nonfunctional eye study. Refract Corneal Surg. 1993;9(6):452–8.
95. Nose W, Neves RA. Intrastromal corneal ring: 12-month sighted myopic eyes. J Refract Surg. 1996;12(1):20–8.
96. Pershin KB, Gurmizov EP. Cataract and progressing keratoconus. Ophthalmology in Russia. 2015;12(3):36–43.
97. Ambrosio RJ, Klyce SD, Wilson SE. Corneal topographic and pachymetric screening of keratorefractive patients. J Refract Surg. 2003;19(1):24–9.
98. Andreassen TT, Simonsen AH, Oxlund H. Biomechanical properties of keratoconus and normal corneas. Exp Eye Res. 1980;31:435–41.
99. Burris TE, Ayer CT, Evensen DA, Davenport JM. Effects of Instrastromal corneal ring size and thickness on corneal flattening in human eyes. Refract Corneal Surg. 1991;7(1):46–50.
100. Burris TE, Baker PC, Ayer CT, Loomas BE, Mathis L, Silvestrini T. Flattening of central corneal curvature with intrastromal corneal ring of increasing thickness: an eye bank eye study. J Cataract Refract Surg. 1992;Suppl:182–7.
101. Asbel PA, Uçakhan OO. Intrastromal corneal ring segments: reversibility of refractive effect. J Refract Surg. 2001;17(1):25–31.
102. Burris TE. Intrastromall corneal ring technology: results and indications. Curr Opin Ophthalmol. 1998;9(4):9–14.

103. Colin J, Ertan A. Intracorneal ring segments and alternative treatments for corneal ectatic diseases. Ankara: Kudert Eye Hospital; 2007.
104. Colin J, Velou S. Current surgical options for keratoconus. J Cataract Refract Surg. 2003;29(2):379–86.
105. Boxer Wachler BS. Intacs for keratoconus. Ophthalmology. 2003;110(5):1031–40.
106. Colin J, Cochener B. INTACS inserts for treating keratoconus: one-year results. Ophthalmalogy. 2001;108(8):1409–14.
107. Colin J, Cochner B, Savary G. Correcting keratoconus with intracorneal rings. J Cataract Refract Surg. 2000;26:1117–22.
108. D'Hermies F, Hartmann C, von Ey F. Biocompatibility of a refractive intracorneal PMMA ring. Forschr Ophthalmol. 1991;88:790–3.
109. Chan CC, Sharma M, Wachler BS. Effect of inferior-segment Intacs with and without C3-R on keratoconus. J Cataract Refract Surg. 2007;33(1):75–80.
110. Chan CC. Intrastromal corneal ring segments as treatment of keratoconus an active area of research. Eurotimes 2006 Jul; 35.
111. Ertan A, Karacal H, Kamburoğlu G. Refractive and topographic results of transepithelial cross-linking treatment in eyes with intacs. Cornea. 2009;28(7):719–23.
112. Radner W, Zehemayer M, Skorpik C, Mallinger R. Altered organization of collagen in apex of keratoconus corneas. Ophthalmic Res. 1998;30:327–32.
113. Spoerl E. Increased rigidity of the cornea caused by intrastromal crosslinking. Ophthalmologe. 1997;94(2):902–6.
114. Baiocchi S, Mazzotta C, Cerretani D, Caporossi T, Caporossi A. Corneal crosslinking: riboflavin concentration in corneal stroma exposed with and without epithelium. J Cataract Refract Surg. 2009;35(5):893–9.
115. Belin MW, Khachikian SS, Ambrosio R Jr. Elevation based corneal tomography. 2nd ed. New Delhi: Jaypee-Highlights Medical Publishers, Inc; 2011.
116. Colin J. Intacs safe and viable long-term treatment for keratoconus. Eurotimes 2009 Feb; 16.
117. Samimi S, Leger F, Touboul D, Colin J. Histopathological findings after intracorneal ring segment implantation in keratoconic human corneas. J Cataract Refract Surg. 2007;33(2):247–53.
118. Sansanayudh W, Bahar I, Kumar NL, Shehadeh-Mashour R, Ritenour R, Singal N, Rootman DS. Intrastromal corneal ring segment SK implantation for moderate to severe keratoconus. J Cataract Refract Surg. 2010;36(1):110–3.
119. Smolek MK, Beekhuis WH. Collagen fibril orientation in the human corneal stroma and itsimplications in keratoconus. Invest Ophthalmol Vis Sci. 1997;38(7):1289–90.
120. Al-Torbak A, Al-Amri A, Wagoner MD. Deep corneal neovascularization after implantation with intrastromal corneal ring segments. Am J Ophthalmol. 2005;140(5):926–7.
121. Colin J, Malet FJ. Intacs for the correction of keratoconus: two-year follow-up. J Cataract Refract Surg. 2007;33(1):69–74.
122. Colin J, Chan CK. Intrastromal corneal ring segments as treatment of keratoconus an active area of research. EuroTimes 2009 Mar; 1112.
123. Colin J, Velou S. Implantation of Intacs and a refractive intraocular lens to correct keratoconus. J Cataract Refract Surg. 2003;29:832–4.
124. Coskunseven E. Toric phakic IOL enhances astigmatic correction of ring segments in eyes with keratoconus. Eurotimes 2007 Jun; 38.
125. Rabinowitz YS. Keratoconus. Surv Ophthalmol. 1998;42(4):297–319.
126. Siganos CS. Management of keratoconus with Intacs. Am J Ophthalmol. 2003;135(1):64–70.
127. Siganos D, Ferrara P. Ferrara intrastromal corneal rings for the correction of keratoconus. J Cataract Refract Surg. 2002;28(11):1947–51.
128. Ucakhan OO, Kanpolat A, Ozdemir O. Contact lens fitting for keratoconus after Intacs placement. Eye Contact Lens. 2006;32:75–7.
129. Coskunseven E, Kymionis GD, Bouzoukis DI, Aslan E, Pallikaris I. Single intrastromal corneal ring segment implantation using the femtosecond laser after radial keratotomy in a keratoconic patient. J Cataract Refract Surg. 2009;35:197–9.

130. Coskunseven E, Kymionis GD. Intrastromal corneal ring segment implantation with the femtosecond laser in a post-keratoplasty patient with recurrent keratoconus. J Cataract Refract Surg. 2007;33:1808–10.
131. Coskunseven E. Channel creation for Intacs with Intralase v. s. mechanical technique for keratoconus. XXII Congress of the ESCRS, Abstract. - Lisbon, 2005.
132. Dauwe C, Touboul D, Roberts CJ, Mahmoud AM, Kérautret J, Fournier P, Malecaze F, Colin J. Biomechanical and morphological corneal response to placement of intrastromal corneal ring segments for keratoconus. J Cataract Refract Surg. 2009;35(10):1761–7.
133. Rabinowitz YS. Intacs for keratoconus using the femtosecond (Intralase) laser. XXII Congress of the ESCRS, Abstract. - Paris, 2004.
134. Ruckhofer J. Confocal microscopy after implantation of intrastromal corneal ring segments. Ophthalmology. 2000;107(12):2144–51.
135. Somodi S, Hahnel C, Slowik C, Richter A, Weiss DG, Guthoff R. Confocal in vivo microscopy and confocal laser-scanning fluorescence microscopy in keratoconus. Ger J Ophthalmol. 1996;5(6):518–25.
136. Wollensak G. Crosslinking treatment of progressive keratoconus: new hope. Curr Opin Ophthalmol. 2006;17:356–60.
137. Yeung S, Low AS, Ku J, et al. Transepithelial phototerapeutic keratectomy combined with intrastromal corneal ring segment and collagen crosslinking in keratoconus. J Cataract Refract Surg. 2013;39:1152–6.
138. Budo C, Bartels MC, van Rij G. Implantation of Artisan toric phakic intraocular lenses for the correction of astigmatism and spherical errors in patients with keratoconus. J Refract Surg. 2005;21:218–22.
139. Chun YS, Park IK, Lee HI, Lee JH, Kim JC. Iris and trabecular meshwork pigment changes after posterior chamber phakic intraocular lens implantation. J Cataract Refract Surg. 2006;32(9):1452–8.
140. Chung TY, Park SC, Lee MO, Ahn K, Chung ES. Changes in iridocorneal angle structure and trabecular pigmentation with STAAR implantable collamer lens during 2 years. J Refract Surg. 2009;25(3):251–8.
141. Donnenfeld ED, Kontos MA, Fry LL, Masket S, Raviv T, Safran SG, Stein R, Steinert RF. Cataract surgery in the keratoconic patient. Cataract and Refractive Surgery Today 2011 May; 20.
142. Pitault G, Leboeuf C, Leroux Les Jardins S, Auclin F, Chong-Sit D, Baudouin C. Ultrasound biomicroscopy of posterior chamber phakic intraocular lenses: a comparative study between ICL and PRL models. J Fr Ophtalmol. 2005;28(9):914–23.
143. Sun XY, Vicary D, Montgomery P, Griffiths M. Toric intraocular lenses for correcting astigmatism in 130 eyes. Ophthalmology. 2000;107(9):1776–81. discussion 1781-2
144. Thebpatiphat N, Hammersmith KM, Rapuano CJ, et al. Cataract surgery in keratoconus. Eye Contact Lens. 2007;33:244–6.
145. Shimizu K, Misawa A, Suzuki Y. Toric intraocular lenses: correcting astigmatism while controlling axis shift. J Cataract Refract Surg. 1994;20(5):523–6.
146. Tahzib NG, Cheng YY, Nuijts RM. Three-year follow-up analysis of Artisan toric lens implantation for correction of postkeratoplasty ametropia in phakic and pseudophakic eyes. Ophthalmology. 2006;113(6):976–84.
147. Parikakis EA, Chatziralli IP, Peponis VG, David G, Chalkiadakis S, Mitropoulos PG. Toric intraocular lens implantation for correction of astigmatism in cataract patients with corneal ectasia. Case Rep Ophthalmol. 2013;4:219–28.
148. Lee SJ, Kwon HS, Koh IH. Sequential intrastromal corneal ring implantation and cataract surgery in a severe keratoconus patient with cataract. Korean J Ophthalmol. 2012; 26(3):226–9.
149. Sedaghat M, Ansari-Astaneh MR, Zarei-Ghanavati M, Davis SW, Sikder S. Artisan iris-supported phakic IOL implantation in patients with keratoconus: a review of 16 eyes. J Refract Surg. 2011;27(7):489–93.
150. Sauder G, Jonas JB. Treatment of keratoconus by toric foldable intraocular lenses. Eur J Ophthalmol. 2003;13(6):577–9.

151. Tehrani M, Dick HB. Implantation of an ARTISANtrade mark toric phakic intraocular lens to correct high astigmatism after penetrating keratoplasty. Klin Monatsbl Augenheilkd. 2002;219(3):159–63.
152. El-Raggal TM, Abdel Fattah AA. Sequential Intacs and Verisyse phakic intraocular lens for refractive improvement in keratoconic eyes. J Cataract Refract Surg. 2007;33(6):966–70.
153. Bilgihan K. Results of photorefractive keratectomy in keratoconus suspects at 4 years. J Refract Surg. 2000;16(4):438–43.
154. Braun E, Kanellopoulos J, Pe L, Jankov M. Riboflavin/ultraviolet-A induced collagen cross-linking in the management of keratoconus. ARVO 2005; www.iovs.org 4964/B167.
155. Caporossi A, Baiocchi S, Mazzotta C, Traversi C, Caporossi T. Parasurgical therapy for keratoconus by riboflavin-ultraviolet type A - rays induced cross-linking of corneal collagen: preliminary refractive results in an Italian study. J Cataract Refract Surg. 2006;32(5):83745.

ACXL Beyond Keratoconus: Post-LASIK Ectasia, Post-RK Ectasia and Pellucid Marginal Degeneration

6

6.1 Other Ectasias: Introduction

Corneal ectasia remains one of the most insidious complications encountered after refractive surgery including laser in situ keratomileusis (LASIK), radial keratotomy (RK) and photorefractve- keratectomy (PRK) and more recently small incision lenticule extraction (SMILE). Ectasia after refractive surgery is a progressive increase in myopic defect, with or without irregular astigmatism, associated with fast keratometric steeping and topographic asymmetric inferior corneal steeping. Over time, there can be associated thinning of the central and paracentral ectatic corneal tissue. Normally this it come to patient's clinical attention when there is associated loss of uncorrect distance visual acuity (UDVC) [1, 2].

Since the first report by Seiler and colleagues [3, 4] in 1998, fewer that 150 cases have been reported in literature, although this number is likely under-representation of the actual incidence [5, 6]. Actually there are over 300 cases of CXL-managed post-LASIK ectasia in literature. The major part of the trials are retrospective case series and some prospective studies and the follow-up is comprised between 12 and 62 months.

6.1.1 Conventional Crosslinking in Post-LASIK Ectasia

Traditional treatment for ectasia after excimer laser refractive surgery included rigid gas permeable contact lenses, intracorneal ring segments (ICRS) and corneal transplant. The two first options did not seem to be effective in arresting the progression of keratectasia and anterior lamellar and penetrating keratoplasty represent a last hope for its invasive nature and its possible complications, especially considering that this dramatic condition involves patients, often healthy, who were looking for a solution to an unpleasant situation such as myopic refractive error and find themselves in a worse condition with a progressive pathologic profile. Since

C. Mazzotta et al., *Management of Early Progressive Corneal Ectasia*,
DOI 10.1007/978-3-319-61137-2_6

post-refractive surgery keratectasia is characterised by weakened corneal biomechanics, caused by the tissue removal from the stromal bed, which can lead to a progressive focal corneal steepening, centrally or inferiorly [7], corneal collagen crosslinking (CXL) has been proposed as an option to take on this complication for its demonstrated ability to increase the corneal biomechanical stability by inducing chemical covalent bonds, bridging amino groups of stromal collagen fibrils, thereby increasing their intra- and interfibrillar rigidity [8–10].

The studies repost an average K max flattening of—2 Dioptres and CDVA improvement of 1 Snellen line or more, documenting the safety and efficacy of conventional CXL in stopping post-LASIK iatrogenic keratectasia (Table 6.1).

The stiffening effect induced by CXL on ectatic corneas is correlated with corneal collagen photolymerization and its additional strengthening on extracellular matrix named "*Glue Effect*" by Mazzotta C. It consists of a modification of biomechanical resistance and cohesive forces of extracellular matrix on proteoglycans and reduction of collagenase activity [20] (Figs. 6.1 and 6.2).

Table 6.1 Literature studies in post-lasik ectasia and CXL

Author	Country	Study design	No. of eyes	Follow-up (months)	Topography	Visual acuity
Kohlhaas et al. [11]	Germany	Case report	2	18	Kmax stable	Not recorded
Hafezi et al. [12]	Switzerland, Greece	Retrospective, case series	10	12–25	Kmax decreased in all cases	BCVA improved in 90%, stable in 10%
Vinciguerra et al. [13]	Italy	Retrospective, case series	13	12	Kmax decreased by 2.02D	BCVA improved by 0.1 logMAR
Salgado et al. [14]	Germany	Prospective, nonrandomized	22	12	Kmax changes were not statistically significant	BCVA improvement was not statistically significant
Hersh et al. [15]	USA	Prospective, randomized, controlled trial	22	12	Kmax decreased by 1.0D	CDVA improved significantly
Li et al. [16]	China	Prospective, nonrandomized, single-centre study	20	12	The maximum K showed a statistically significant improvement of 1.50 D	CDVA improvement of 0.07 and 0.13 logMAR

Table 6.1 (continued)

Author	Country	Study design	No. of eyes	Follow-up (months)	Topography	Visual acuity
Richoz et al. [17]	Switzerland	Retrospective, interventional cases series	26	12–62	Kmax decreased by 2.0D (statistically significant)	CDVA improved to a mean of 0.3 logMAR units
Yildirim et al. [18]	Turkey	Retrospective case series study	20	42	The maximum K value decreased from 46.0 ± 4.4 diopters (D) to 45.6 ± 3.8 D	CDVA improved significantly from 0.27 ± 0.23 logMAR to 0.19 ± 0.13 logMAR
Marino et al. [19]	Switzerland	A prospective, single-center case series	40	24	Kmax decreased in a statistically significant way ($P = 0.956$)	BCVA improvement was not statistically significant
Kanellopoulos et al. [12]	Greece	Consecutive randomized prospective comparative study	65	24	The steep K was 38.38 D at 2 year from 45.15 D pre-op	Not recorded

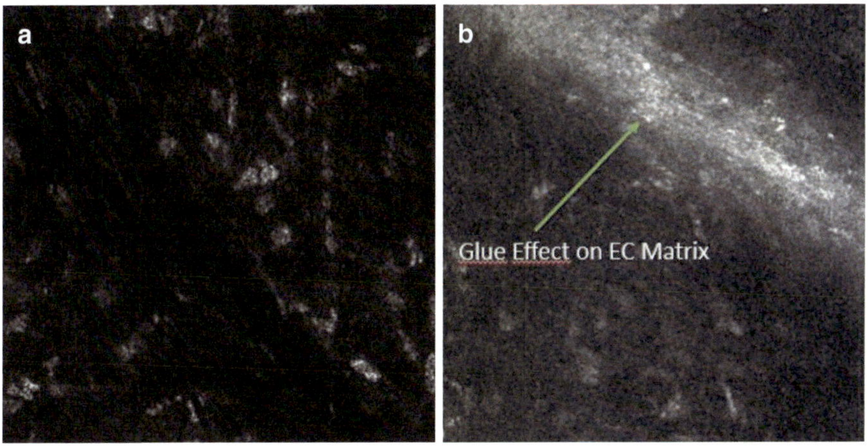

Fig. 6.1 "Glue Effect" of CXL demonstrated by in vivo confocal microscopy in a patient with corneal ectasia exacerbated by radial keratotomy (C. Mazzotta, personal observation)

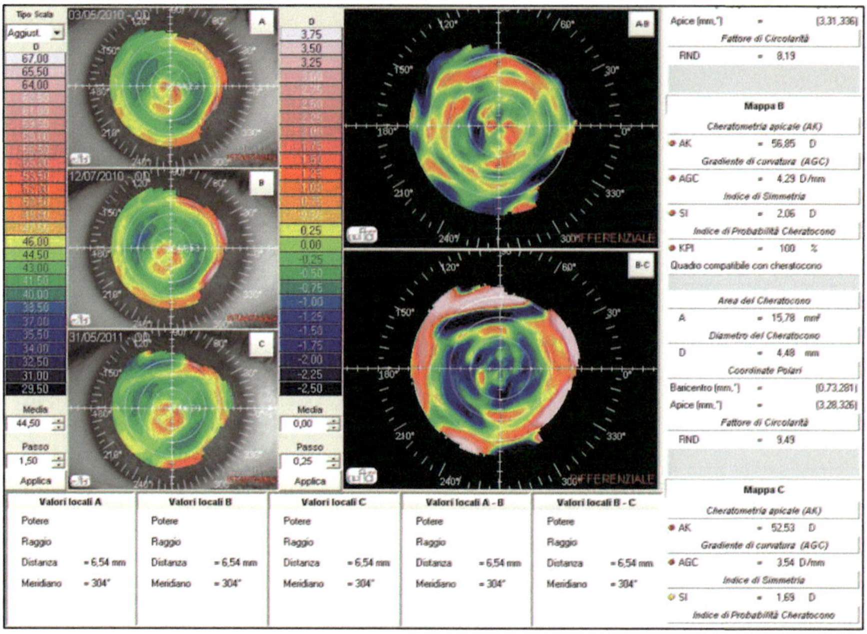

Fig. 6.2 Post-Lasik ectasia regression after conventional 3 mW/cm² Epi-Off CXL. One-year follow-up is showed by differential topography (C.S.O. EyeTop, Florence, Italy)

6.1.2 Clinical Trials

The recent literature produced many evidences about safety and efficacy of corneal collagen cross linking in arresting the progression of post refractive surgery ectasias as showed in Table 6.1. The first report to CXL for post-LASIK keratectasia was described by Kohlhaas et al. in 2005, when a female patient who developed keratectasia in both eyes 4 weeks after LASIK was treated with riboflavin/UVA cross-linking and gained a stabilization of the postoperative refraction and corneal topography during a follow up of 18 months [11].

Several studies followed this first attempt to stop progression of iatrogenic corneal ectasia by the use of CXL and reported that post-refractive surgery corneal ectasia can be successfully treated by this technique, indicating that it may be a useful option for treating a lot of these progressing iatrogenic diseases. In 2007 Hafezi et al. enrolled for CXL treatment ten contact lens-intolerant eyes with formerly undiagnosed forme fruste keratoconus or pellucid marginal corneal degeneration (PMD) who had laser in situ keratomileusis for myopic astigmatism and subsequently developed iatrogenic keratectasia. They showed how in five cases it was possible to arrest the progression of keratectasia and partially reverse it in the other five cases, after a postoperative follow-up of up to 25 months, as demonstrated by preoperative and postoperative corneal topography and a reduction in maximum keratometric readings [12].

An in vivo confocal microscopy analysis of five patients (five eyes) with iatrogenic keratectasia after LASIK and five patients (five eyes) with progressive keratoconus was performed by Kymionis et al. in 2008, demonstrating that corneal alterations after corneal cross-linking, such as keratocyte disappearance in the anterior and intermediate corneal stroma for the first 3 months after CXL, were similar in both keratoconic and post-LASIK corneal ectasia eyes [21]. In 2010, Vinciguerra et al. described a case series of 13 eyes of 9 consecutive patients who developed unstable corneal ectasia after refractive surgical procedures (both PRK or LASIK) and were selected to undergo CXL. The 1-year follow-up findings of the study were that best spectable-corrected visual acuity improvement, mean spherical equivalent refraction and mean refractive sphere reduction were statistically significant, 6 months after surgery, with a mean pupil center pachymetry and corneal thickness at 0 and 2 mm from the thinnest corneal point decreasing significantly [13].

Some other studies published in 2011 reported promising data about CXL for treatment of post-operative keratectasia. Salgado et al. selected a study cohort composed by 22 eyes of 15 patients followed up preoperatively 1, 3, 6 and 12 months after crosslinking evaluating uncorrected visual acuity (UCVA), best-corrected visual acuity (BCVA), slit-lamp examination, pachymetry and topography. The stabilisation of VA and of the corneal curvature, and in some cases even an improvement in VA and reversal of the corneal ectasia, correlated well with the results published by Kohlhaas and Hafezi [14].

A prospective randomized controlled clinical trial was published in the same year by Hersch et al. [15] The purpose of the study was to evaluate the 1-year outcomes of corneal collagen crosslinking (CXL) for treatment of keratoconus and corneal ectasia. Seventy-one eyes of 58 patients had CXL and were followed for 1 year. Of the eyes, 49 were in the keratoconus subgroup and 22 in the post-LASIK ectasia subgroup. The treatment group results were compared with the ones of a shame control group and a fellow eye control group, concluding that collagen cross-linking was effective in improving UDVA, CDVA, the maximum K value, and the average K value. Keratoconus patients had more improvement in topographic measurements than patients with ectasia. Both CDVA and maximum K value worsened between baseline and 1 month, followed by improvement between 1, 3, and 6 months and stabilization thereafter [15]. A long-term follow-up study was conducted by Kissner at al. and presented at the ARVO Annual Meeting in 2011. 10 eyes of 6 patients with post-LASIK ectasia were analyzed up to 8 years by the authors (mean follow-op was 5.8 ± 1.7 years). In six eyes the findings of K-values remained stable or even partially decreased. In four eyes of two patients K-values progressed despite of the procedure and these were patients with additional risk factors for progression as neurodermitis, allergy or pre-existing keratoconus. In a prospective, nonrandomized, single-centre study, Li et al. [16] performed corneal cross linking in 20 eyes of 11 patients who had LASIK for myopic astigmatism and subsequently developed keratectasia. The eyes were evaluated preoperatively and at 1-, 3-, 6-, and 12-month intervals. The complete ophthalmologic examination comprised uncorrected visual acuity, best spectacle-corrected visual acuity, endothelial cell count, ultrasound pachymetry, corneal topography, and in vivo confocal microscopy. CXL appeared to stabilise or partially reverse the progression of post-LASIK corneal ectasia. UCVA and BCVA improvements were statistically significant beyond 12 months after surgery (improvement of 0.07 and 0.13 logMAR at 1 year, respectively). Mean baseline flattest meridian keratometry and mean steepest meridian keratometry reduction (improvement of 2.00 and 1.50 diopters (D), respectively) were statistically significant too. At 1 year after CXL, mean endothelial cell count did not deteriorate. Mean thinnest cornea pachymetry increased significantly [16].

In 2013, Richoz et al. [17] evaluated twenty-six eyes of 26 patients with postoperative ectasia after LASIK (23 eyes) and PRK (3 eyes) with a mean follow-up of 25 months. Corrected distance visual acuity (CDVA), maximum keratometry readings (Kmax), minimum radius of curvature (Rmin), and six corneal topography indices were the main outcome measures. CXL arrested the progression of ectasia occurring after LASIK and PRK and improved the CDVA and Kmax. The improvements in four topography indices and the absence of major complications after the procedure let the authors establish that the use of CXL in iatrogenic ectasia is recommended without restrictions [17].

A retrospective case series study conducted by Yildirim et al. [18] in 2014 enrolled 20 eyes with a mean follow up of 42 months. The UDVA and CDVA improved significantly, from 0.78 G 0.61 logMAR to 0.53 G 0.36 logMAR (PZ.007) and from 0.27 G 0.23 logMAR to 0.19 G 0.13 logMAR, respectively (P%0.028). No eye lost 1 or more Snellen lines of UDVA or CDVA. Although the mean spherical refraction was not significantly different at the last visit (PZ.074), the mean cylindrical refraction decreased significantly (PZ.036). The maximum K value decreased from 46.0 G 4.4 diopters (D) at baseline to 45.6 G 3.8 D at the last visit (PZ.013). By the last visit, the maximum K value decreased (R1.0 D) in 5 eyes and remained stable in 15 eyes. No serious complications occurred [18]. In 2015, Marino et al. evaluated the effect of accelerated CXL in a prospective case series performed with patients treated for postoperative LASIK ectasia. All eyes underwent accelerated corneal collagen cross-linking (CCL-Vario Crosslinking; Peschke Meditrade GmbH, Zurich, Switzerland) at 9 mW/cm(2) for 10 min. The study enrolled 40 eyes of 24 that attained at least 2 years of follow-up. All eyes stabilized after treatment without any further signs of progression and no statistically significant changes in the mean uncorrected distance visual acuity (P = 0.649), corrected distance visual acuity (P = 0.616), mean keratometry (P = 0.837), steep keratometry (P = 0.956), ultrasonic pachymetry (P = 0.135), slit-scanning pachymetry (P = 0.276), and endothelial cell density (P = 0.523). In addition, 72.5% of the patients presented stable or gains of Snellen lines over time [19]. Although improvements in visual acuity and topography indexes are often statistically significant, some of the published results suggest that ectatic corneas may have a less robust response to CXL as opposed to keratoconic corneas. The cause for this potential difference in not clear, several explanations have been suggested. One is that CXL preferentially strengthens the anterior stroma, including the LASIK flap, which does not contribute to the mechanical stability of the cornea. The riboflavin diffusion may be reduced in corneas that have undergone LASIK, affecting the CXL result. Differences in the pathophysiologic features of keratoconus and ectasia occurring after refractive surgery also may account for a less pronounced CXL effect [17, 22]. Despite of this considerations, Greenstein et al. found no significant differences between the keratoconus and ectasia subgroups analyzed in a prospective randomized controlled clinical trial evaluating quantitative descriptors of corneal topography (index of surface variance, index of vertical asymmetry, keratoconus index, central keratoconus index, minimum radius of curvature, index of height asymmetry, and index of height decentration) [23].

In the light of this published results, we can state that corneal collagen crosslinking is nowadays a valuable resource for treating progressing corneal ectasias following refractive surgical procedures.

6.1.3 Accelerated CXL in Post-LASIK and Post-RK Ectasia

Accelerated CXL offers a great advantage in the management of progressive primary ectasias (Keratoconus, Pellucid Marginal Degeneration), and secondary iatrogenic ectasia (Post-LASIK, post-PRK, post-RK, post-SMILE). Actually, also the thin corneas 400 μm and under can be managed with high fluence accelerated protocols according to customization of treatment depth according to in vivo confocal microscopy studies and OCT evidences published by Mazzotta C [24–30], UV-A power settings and Exposure time (Figs. 6.3 and 6.4).

What we know from the literature [31] is that corneal ectasia starts as "*focal*" process from the weakest portion of the corneal stroma (beyond the 160–180 μm of the so-called stiff cornea) ad progress faster as showed in Figs. 6.4 and 6.5.

An effective management of a post-lasik ectasia requires that CXL treatment overcome the flap thickness, strengthening the intermediate-deep stroma beyond the lasik interface. Stiffening the flap in a thin cornea affected by post-Lasik ectasia

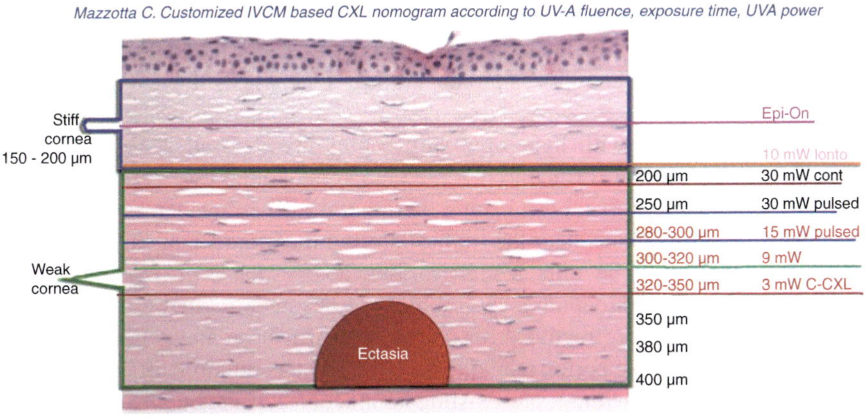

Fig. 6.3 Mazzotta C. ACXL Customization Nomogram according to in vivo confocal microscopy (IVCM) and corneal OCT

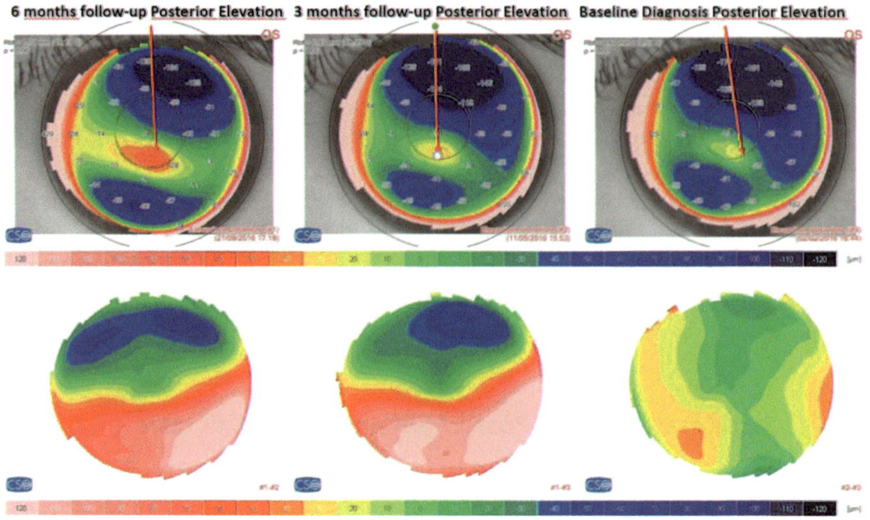

Fig. 6.4 Posterior elevation differential tomography (Sirius C.S.O., Florence, Italy) showing a 6 months progression of post-LASIK ectasia (from −15 μm to +28 posterior elevation into 6 months)

doesn't make any sense not ensuring an efficacious, long-lasting ectasia stabilization. As demonstrated by Mazzotta in vivo confocal microscopy studies [24–30], by using continuous and pulsed-light UVA emission at 30 mW/cm^2 high irradiance CXL at 5.4 J for 4 minutes and 8 minutes, we reach a treatment penetration at 200 ± 20 μm and 250 ± 20 μm of corneal stroma respectively (Table 6.2).

Moreover the 15 mW/cm^2 Accelerated pulsed-light Siena protocol allow us to penetrate at 280 ± 20 μm resulting an optimal option [24–30].

In our opinion and clinical experience at the Siena Crosslinking Center®, the 9 mW/cm^2 Accelerated protocol with continuous light and dextran-free 0.1% isotonic Riboflavin solution, represents a safe end efficacious alternative to standard 3 mW/cm^2 CXL in progressive keratoconus (KC), post-LASIK and post-RK ectatic corneas with at least 400 μm of minimum corneal thickness as showed in Figs. 6.6, 6.7 and 6.8.

Iatrogenic ectasia with hyperopic shift represents a possible complications after RK procedures performed in myopic (and keratoconic) eyes. This condition is related to induced corneal weakening (peripheral steepening, central flattening) by deep stromal incisions near the limbus altering the biomechanical stability of the cornea. It seems to be influenced by various factors such as pre existing ectatic corneal disorders (keratoconus), eye rubbing, or has been related to metal-blade incisions. The shift of refractive error in hyperopic direction may continue during the entire postoperative period from the first to 10 years and more after RK also in cases of myopic eyes without pre-existing keratoconus. This complication affects

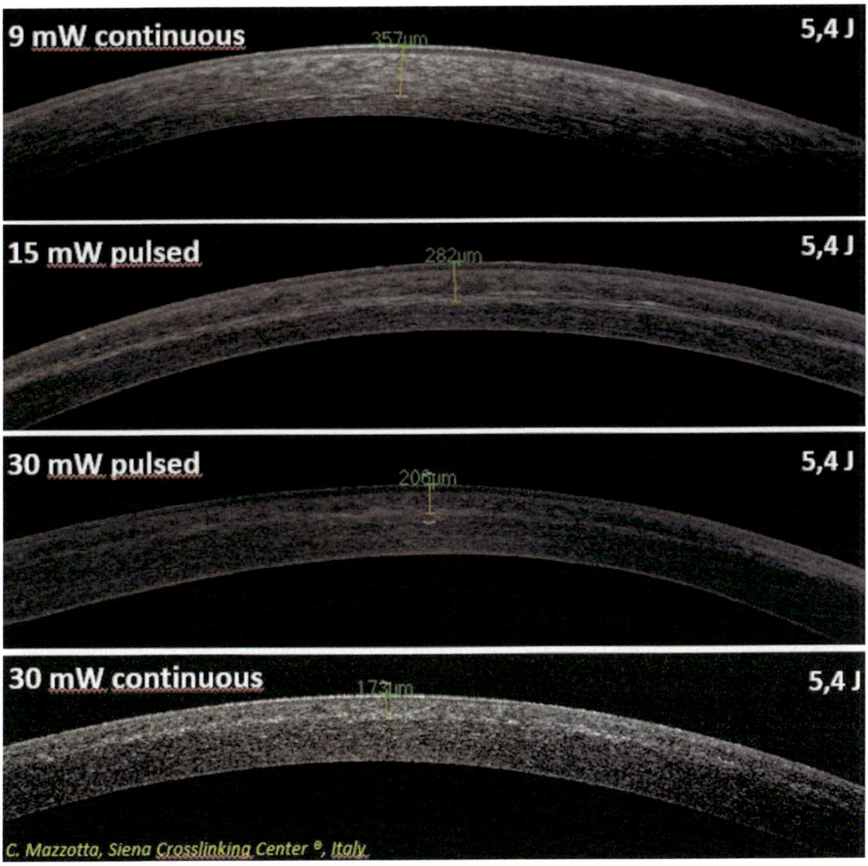

Fig. 6.5 Spectral domain OCT of the cornea (Optovue, Freemont, CA, USA), documenting the different demarcation line depth according to different Accelerated CXL protocols preformed by Mazzotta C. at Siena Crosslinking Center®, Italy.

Table 6.2 Demarcation line depth measured in vivo after conventional and accelerated CXL

CXL treatments 84 eyes	Convectional CXL 44 eyes 3 mW	C-light ACXL 10 eyes 30 mW	P-light ACXL 10 eyes 30 mW	TE CXL 10 eyes 3 mW	TE ACXL 10 eyes 45 mW
Average demarcation line depth (measured from epithelial surface)	350 ± 20 µm	200 ± 20 µm	250 ± 20 µm	100 ± 20 µm	100 ± 20 µm

Average epithelial thickness: 50 ± 10 µm

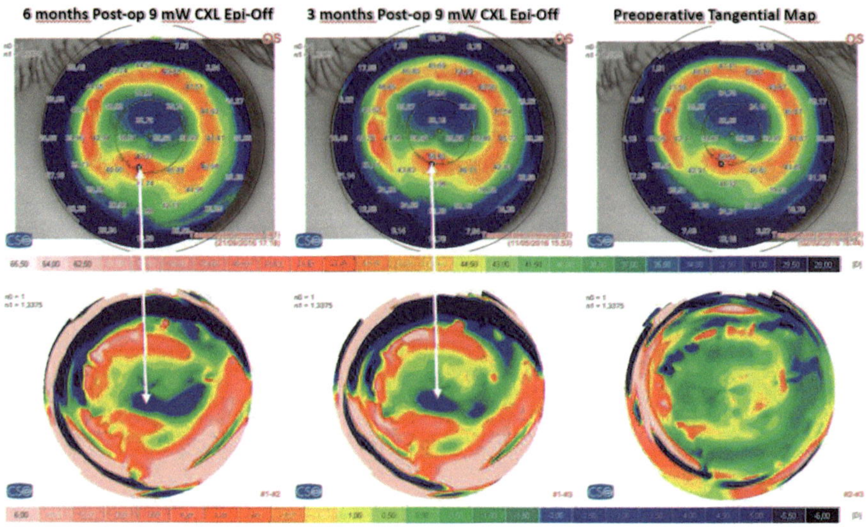

Fig. 6.6 Post lasik ectasia treated with the Accelerated 9 mW/cm^2 epithelium off protocol using the KXL I UVA source and the dextran free isotonic 0.1% Riboflavin solution (VibeX Rapid, Avedro, Waltham, MA, USA). The 6-month-follow-up differential tangential tomography map (Sirius C.S.O., Florence, Italy) show a flattening in the ectatic with improved corneal symmetry.

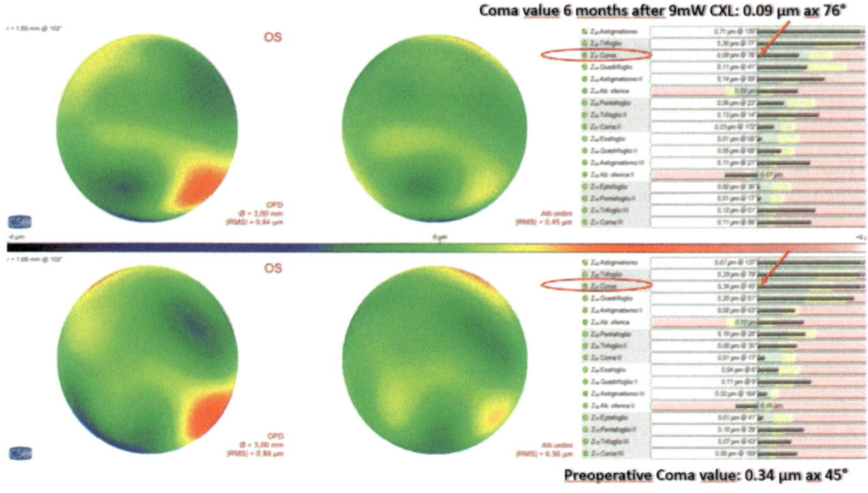

Fig. 6.7 Post-LASIK Ectasia treated with the Accelerated 9 mW/cm^2 epithelium off protocol using the KXL I UVA source and the dextran free isotonic 0.1% Riboflavin solution (VibeX Rapid, Avedro, Waltham, MA, USA). The 6-month-follow-p differential Wavefront analysis (Sirius C.S.O., Florence, Italy) shows a consistent improvement of coma value from 0.34 to 0.09 μm associated with a significant improvement of patient's uncorrected and corrected distance visual acuty

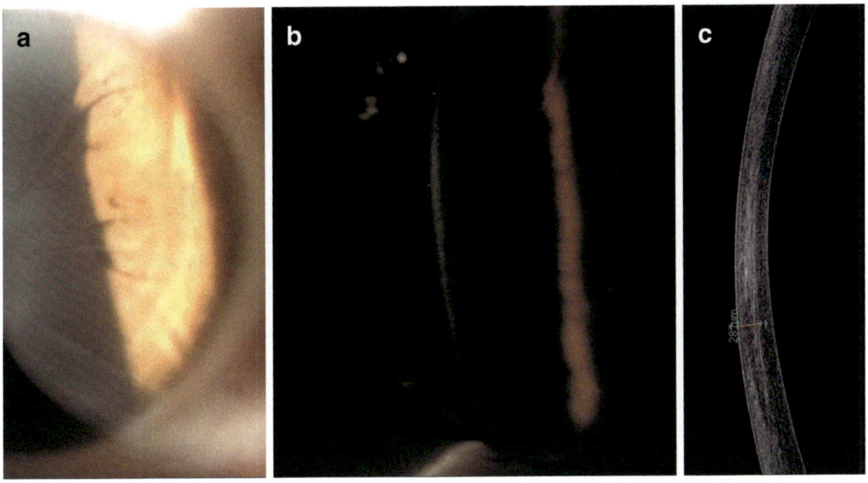

Fig. 6.8 Post RK ectasia (**a**) treated with 15 mW pulsed light ACXL (Siena Crosslinking Center® protocol). The 1-month follow-up reveals a clear demarcation line at 290 μm well visible at slit lamp (**b**) and SD corneal OCT (**c**)

patients visual acuity causing fluctuations not easily suitable of spectacles correction especially for the instability of refraction and associated iatrogenic progressive corneal asymmetry. The clinical stability of cross-linked cornea is related not only to an instantaneous biochemical covalent bonds (collagen cross-links) formation but also to biosynthesis of new well-structured collagen, newly formed lamellar interconnections between and within proteoglycans of the extracellular matrix. There are also clinical evidences of an influence of CXL in reducing corneal hydration status. The question is how does CXL works in this cases if 300 μm is the depth of treatment effect? Then it probably does not get to area of pathology. The major efficacy of CXL in this case is basically directed working mainly on the hypercellular fibrotic stromal scar of the RK wound as showed in Fig. 6.3 and little to hypocellular primitive scar since it contains low collagen and almost all proteoglycans. The stiffening effect induced by CXL on ectatic corneas is mainly correlated with corneal collagen photolymerization but its additional strengthening on extracellular matrix named "*Glue Effect*" by Gregor Wollensak, Eberhard Spoerl and Cosimo Mazzotta [9], consists of a modification of biomechanical resistance and cohesive forces of extracellular matrix on proteoglycans and reduction of collagenase activity [20]. In vivo confocal microscopy scans performed in these patients demonstrate a repeatable observation of a dense, hyper-reflective hypocellular (fibrotic) tissue inside the incisions in a depth of 250–300 μm as showed. The "*Glue Effect*", by linking proteoglycans and collagen could be the key of success of CXL treatment in post-RK ectasia as showed in Figs. 6.8, 6.9 and 6.10 by Mazzotta C. So the answer is: CXL works also in

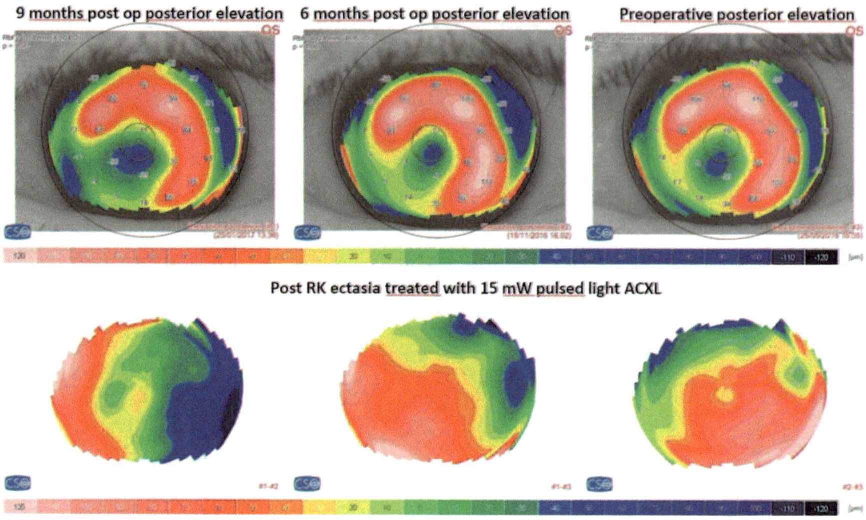

Fig. 6.9 Post-RK ectasia after 15 mW pulsed light ACXL showed a regression and improved corneal symmetry

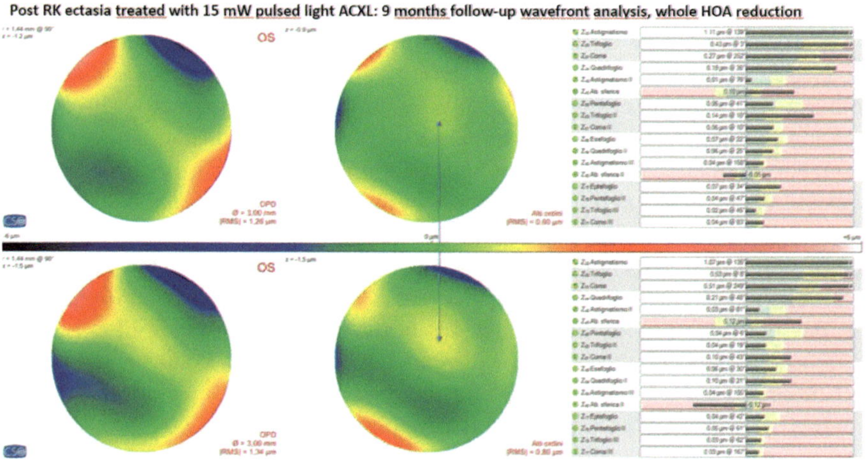

Fig. 6.10 Corneal wavefront differential analysis performed after 15 mW ACXL (Siena Crosslinking Center®, Italy) show an overall reduction of high order corneal aberrations with tremendous improvement of patient visual acuity

post-RK progressive ectasia (both in keratoconic RK exacerbated ectasia and post myopic RK ectasia) and can be contemplated in its therapy, alone or eventually in combination with other techniques (concentric corneal sutures, implantable collamer lens, IOLs), according to patients needings.

6.1.4 Pellucid Marginal Degeneration

Pellucid Marginal Degeneration (PMD) [32] represents a particular progressive, non-inflammatory corneal ectasia which commonly affects the inferior periphery of the cornea inducing a crescentic corneal thinning from the 4 to 8 o'clock position, 1–2 mm from the limbus (Fig. 6.11).

The prevalence and aetiology of this disorder remain unknown as it differs from other corneal ectatic disorders in its characteristic inferior thinning below the apex of the cone and typically severe against-the-rule astigmatism. Presentation generally occurs between the 2nd and 5th decade and visual signs and symptoms include longstanding reduced visual acuity or increasing against-the-rule irregular astigmatism leading to a slow reduction in visual acuity. High irregular against-the-rule astigmatism in PMD may progress over time differently from keratoconus that generally stabilized at the 4th decade of life. In rare cases, patients may present with a sudden loss of vision and excruciating ocular pain due to corneal hydrops or spontaneous perforation. The initial treatment consists of optical correction (spectacles and contact lenses). However, when the disease progresses to advanced stages, surgical procedures are necessary such as wedge resection, lamellar crescentic resection, penetrating, lamellar keratoplasty and more recently corneal collagen

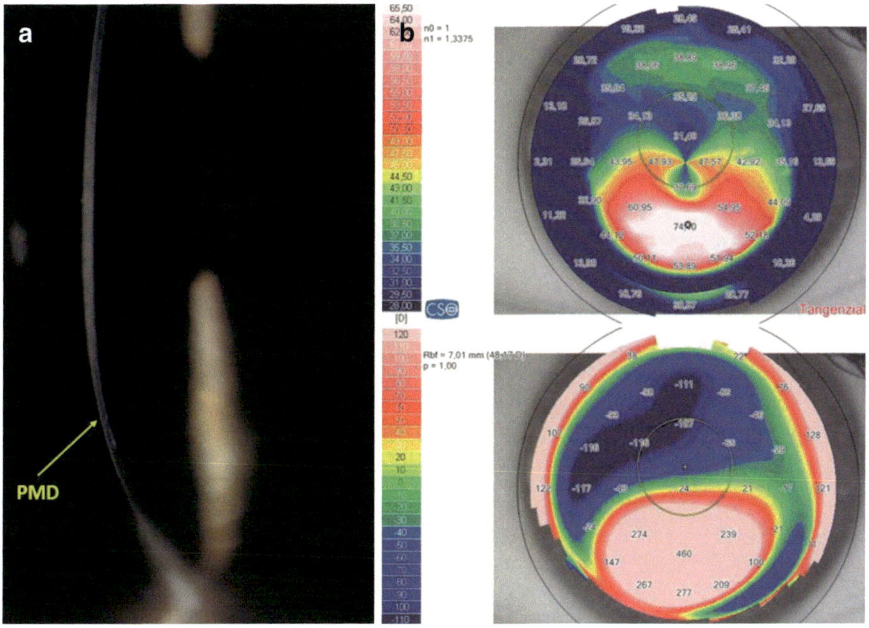

Fig. 6.11 Pellucid marginal degeneration in a thin cornea of 365 μm in the thinnest point. Biomicroscopy (**a**) shows the typical inferior thinning (*yellow arrow*) at 6 O'clock position and 2 mm from the corneal limbus. Corneal tomography (**b**) shows the typical aspect of "moustache"

crosslinking [33]. Surgical management of pellucid marginal degeneration includes penetrating keratoplasty (with generally poor and unpredictable results), full-thickness crescentic wedge resection (FTCWR) with significant postoperative astigmatic drift, deep anterior lamellar keratoplasty (DALK) with visual outcomes similar to penetrating keratoplasty, crescentic lamellar wedge resection (CLWR), crescentic lamellar keratoplasty, tuck-in lamellar keratoplasty (TILK), toric phakic intraocular lens (PIOL) implantation, intrastromal corneal ring segment implantation (ICRS), corneal collagen cross-linking (CXL). Toric PIOL implantation is effective, but ectasia progression is a concern. ICRS implantation can delay penetrating keratoplasty and improve contact lens tolerance, but does not treat the underlying process. CXL demonstrates effectiveness without complications [34].

In our experience, progressive PMD can be well managed with conventional CXL in corneas with corneal thickness over 400 μm and with Customized Accelerated CXL protocols in thin PMD corneas between 350 and 400 μm, demonstrating its efficacy without complications, 1 year follow-up after ACXL for thin PMD cornea, the differential tangential tomographies show an evident flattening of the ectatic peripheral area and compensatory steepening of central cornea after customized ACXL (Fig. 6.12). Moreover the differential wavefront analysis shows an evident reduction of whole High-Order Aberrations (HOA) with evident improvement in patient's visual acuity (VA) after customized ACXL (C. Mazzotta personal case, Siena Crosslinking Center®, Italy), Fig. 6.13.

After ectatic process stabilization with crosslinking, we have a lot of refractive options trying to improve visual acuity (Spectacles, contact lenses, ICRS, Phakic IOLs, CXL plus all surface laser ablation).

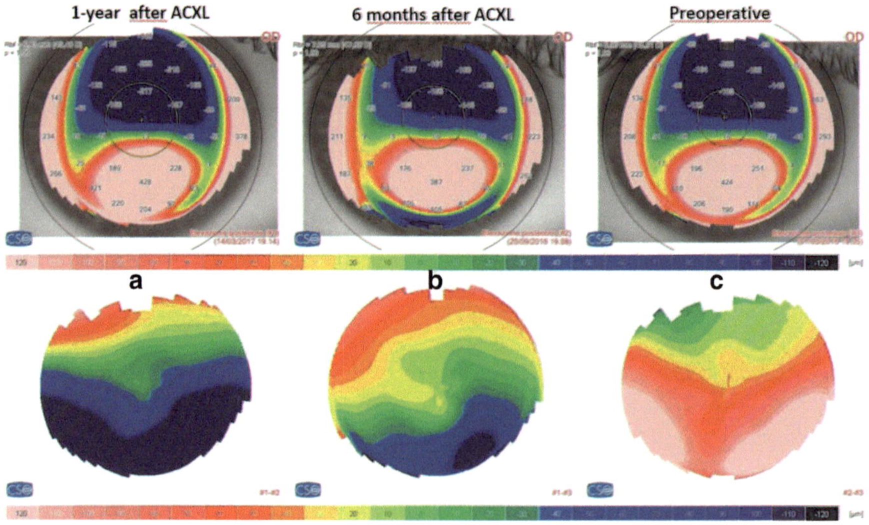

Fig. 6.12 One year follow-up after ACXL for thin PMD cornea. Differential tangential tomography shows an evident flattening of the ectatic peripheral area and compensatory steepening of central cornea after customized ACXL (C. Mazzotta personal observation)

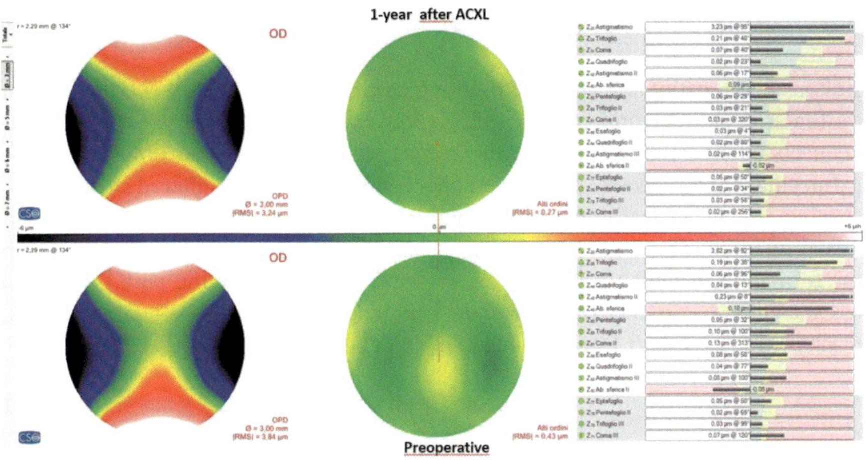

Fig. 6.13 One year follow-up after ACXL for thin PMD cornea. Differential Wavefront analysis shows an evident reduction of high-order aberrations with greatr improvement in patient's visual acuity (VA) after customized ACXL (C. Mazzotta, Siena Crosslinking Center®, Italy)

Corneal collagen cross-linking is really exciting because it effectively halts disease progression. Combined treatments and improved screening could eliminate the need for surgical management and poor or unstable outcomes in most cases of PMD.

6.2 Conclusion

The high-irradiance ACXL protocols with continuous and pulsed-light and dextran-free 0.1, 0.15 and 0.25% riboflavin solutions allows to customize CXL treatment according to ectasia progression, tomographic parameters, patient's age and needings. Calibrating the UV-A power and exposure time according to IVCM-OCT based Customized CXL nomogram (Mazzotta Nomogram) as showed in Fig. 6.3, the ACXL offers the great possibility of a safe and effective management in different cases of progressive ectasias according to specific parametric data, including thin corneas. However the treatment of these cases require great experience in order to avoid potential adverse events.

In our experience, new modified Iontophoresis-CXL protocols, compensating the epithelium UVA photo-attenuation by increasing the treatment fluence and the riboflavin concentration, could represents another effective possibility in the panorama of the ACXL customized treatments: one patients, one case, one (single or combined) treatment.

We cannot exclude that in the next future the new customized epithelium-on protocols with oxygen/ozone supplementation could have a great potentiality in halting ectasia progression without removing the epithelium. Present and future research on Customized ACXL setting according to clinical necessity, keratoconus biodiversity and case specificity accelerated procedures are going to be calibrated in a *Range Window* of 9–18 mW UV-A power, 20 min duration on balance.

6.3 Bullous Keratopathy

Bullous keratopathy is a visually disabling corneal disorder due to endothelial cell dysfunction and decompensation [35], before or after eye-surgery. Without sufficient endothelial pump function, the cornea swells and fluid accumulates in the extracellular spaces between collagen fibers and lamellae. The altered corneal fiber spacing affects corneal transparency, and leads to light scatter with a reduction of visual function. The condition worsens as the epithelium becomes edematous with the formation of bullae leading to deep visual loss and disabling pain [36], often associated with conjunctival hyperemia. End Stage Fuch's endothelial corneal dystrophy (FECD), Fig. 6.14 and pseudophakic bullous keratopathy (PBK), Fig. 6.15,

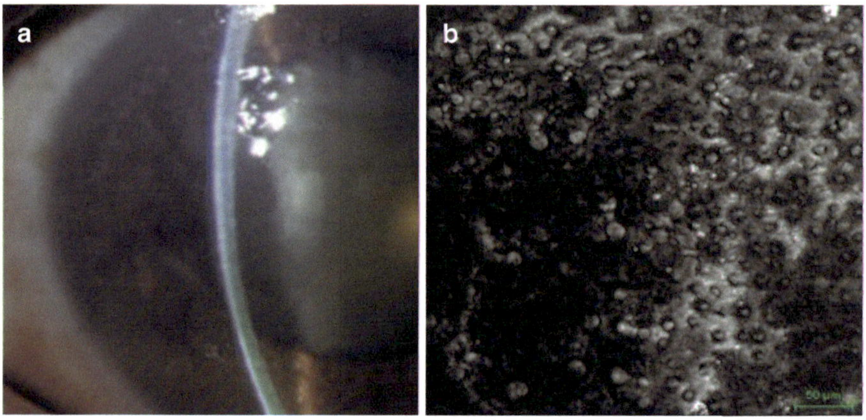

Fig. 6.14 Biomicroscopy (**a**) of Bullous keratopathy in a 74 year-old patient suffering from end stage Fuch's endothelial Dystrophy. In vivo confocal scan (**b**) shows the typical Strowberry-like surface of residual altered endothelial layer.

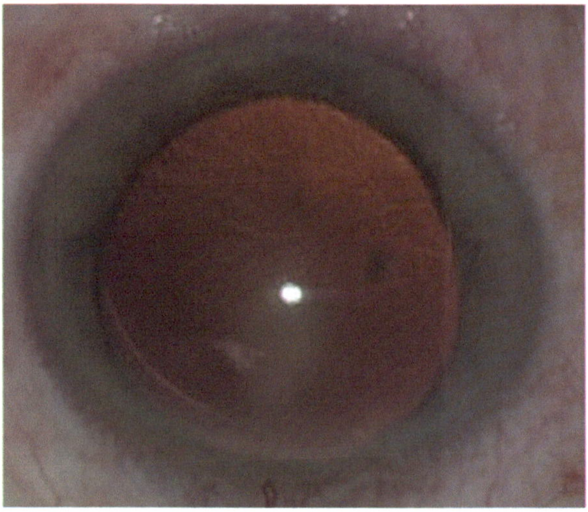

Fig. 6.15 Biomicroscopy of pseudophakic micro-bullous keratopathy

are the leading cause of ocular morbidity in patients who have undergone phaco-emulsification cataract surgery.

Management options possible for PBK are represented by topical hypertonic solutions to reduce epithelial and stromal edema, although it has little effect on stromal edema [37, 38]. Therapeutic soft contact lenses are useful to relieve discomfort, but carry the risk of infection [37, 39]. Conservative surgical procedures include anterior stromal cauterization, manual or yttrium-aluminum-garnet (YAG) laser [40, 41] aided anterior stromal puncture, excimer laser phototherapeutic keratectomy [42], conjunctival flaps and amniotic membrane [43] All of these procedures bring about only symptomatic relief. Endothelial or penetrating Keratoplasty (DSAEK, UT-DSAEK, DMEK or PK in extremely fibrotic and opaque corneal stroma) remains the definitive treatment for a large number of patients with PBK [44].

Krueger et al [36] studied the ACXL application to treat bullous keratopathy. They used an adapted version of Wollensak et al corneal collagen cross-linking study.

Corneal collagen cross-linking (CXL) aims at creating additional chemical bonds inside the corneal stroma by means of a highly localized photopolymerization while avoiding and minimizing exposure to the surrounding structures of the eye [45]. Corneal CXL has been shown to influence the swelling behavior of corneal tissue. Wollensak et al [46] showed changes in the hydration behavior of normal de-epithelialized porcine corneas after CXL, and treated corneas were found to be more transparent.

Krueger's in vitro study was performed by placing eye-bank corneas in a pressurized artificial anterior chamber following Descemet's membrane stripping. Two consecutive corneal pockets (350 and 150 μm depth) were sequentially created using a femtosecond laser. Successively, intrastromal injections of 0.1% riboflavin (0.2 mL) followed by accelerated UVA irradiation (15 mW/cm^2) for 7 minutes was performed for each pocket. Corneal clarity improved in all treated eyes and also the mean central corneal thickness was significantly reduced (by 256 μm, P = 0.0002 and 273 μm, P = 0.0004) in treated eyes.

After clinical trials on the eye-bank corneas, CXL was tested on the left eye of an 84 year-old woman with similar results. The clinical treatment of corneal edema showed improved clarity and reduced central corneal thickness from 675 to 550 μm (contact ultrasound pachymetry) and 696 to 571 μm (non-contact optical Scheimpflug pachymetry) at 1 month. Corrected Distance Visual Acuity (CDVA) improved from finger counting to 20/80 at 1 week and beyond, postponing corneal transplantation for 6 months. Because of the endothelial layer compromission in bullous keratopathy, procedure safety was debated regarding CXL-related further endothelial cell death [36].

In contrast to the thickness of a normal cornea with minimum of 520 to 540-μm, a cornea with chronic bullous keratopathy is often between 600 and 700-μm thick due to endothelial cell failure. Since CXL treatment works on the outer half of the cornea, the attempt of cross-linking the anterior layers of such a swollen bullous keratopathy cornea is potentially safer than in a normal cornea (Table 6.3).

Table 6.3 Review of literature

Author	Year	No of patients	Solution	mW/time	Corneal thickness pre/post, reduction	Corneal clearness/pain improvement	Epi on/off
Kruger	2008	1	0.1% riboflavin (0.2 mL)	UVA irradiation (15 mW/cm^2) for 7 min	696–571 (1 month) (Scheimpflug)	Yes/yes 1 month (from finger counting to 20/80)	Off
Ramon	2009	14	Riboflavin 0.1% with dextran 20%	UVA irradiation (3 mW/cm^2) for 30 min	747–623 CCT (1 month)	YES/YES 1 month	Off
Wollensak	2009	3	Riboflavin 0.1% after dehydration with 40% Glucose (1 day before)	UVA irradiation (3 mW/cm^2) for 30 min	90.33 ± 17.04 (3 days) 93.67 ± 14.22 (8 months)	YES/YES 8 months	Off
Arora	2013	24	NA Previous dehydration hyperosmotic sodium chloride 5%	NA	846.46–88.741 to 781.0–98.788 mm at 1 month increased to 805.08–136.06 mm at 3 months. Ultrasound pachymetry (Sonomed-PacScan plus	YES/YES (1 month) Reduction/No (3 months)	NA
Mirzaei	2014	15	Riboflavin 0.1% solution (10 mg of riboflavin-5-phosphate in 10 mL of dextran-T-500 20% solution) 0.65% sodium chloride solution every 4–6 time/day for 1 week	UVA irradiation (3 mW/cm^2) for 30 min	765.3 ± 121.0 pre 708.6 ± 129.1 1 month 838.6 ± 196.7 6 months	YES/YES (1 month) Reduction (5 eyes)/reduction (3 months) Better (8 eyes)/same (6 months)	Off (8 mm central cornea)

(continued)

Ucakhan	2014	2	Riboflavin 0.1% solution	UVA irradiation (3 mW/cm^2) for 30 min	703/603 to 603/553 1 month, 710/652 at 3 month 575/550 to 580/570 at 1 month, 580/585 at 12 month	YES (best result at 1 month, deteriorated at 3 month, stabled at 12)/NA	Off
Wu Huping	2015	13	Riboflavin 0.1% solution + dextran	UVA irradiation (9 mW/cm^2) (5.4 J/cm^2), for 10 min	862.2 + −146.4 to 707.5 + −92.7 1 week, 718.8 + −47.2 at 1 month	YES/YES, 1 week and 1 months, same 6 month	Off

The Wollensak technique (modified by Krueger) was designed to potentially cross-link a "broader" thickness and deeper layers of these corneas [47].

In an attempt to overcome the limitations imposed by increased corneal thickness in patients with bullous keratopathy, modifications have been proposed to maintain reproducible and efficient UVA light riboflavin penetration in the stroma.

It is important to note that Wollensak and Coll [48] used 40% glucose for 1 day before CXL, which allowed a better control of corneal thickness (edema) before the procedure. Ramon and Coll. [49] used Riboflavin 0.1% with dextran 20%, as well as Wu Huping [50]. Arora et al [51] performed pretreatment dehydration with hyperosmotic sodium chloride 5%, Mirzaei [52] used Riboflavin 0.1% solution with 10 mg of riboflavin- 5-phosphate in 10 mL of dextran T-500 20% solution, using 0. 65% sodium chloride solution 4–6 times/day for 1 week. By reducing corneal thickness before CXL, and using an epithelium-off protocol, the effect of cross-linking confined to the anterior stroma has improved.

UVA irradiation of 3 mW/cm^2 for 30 min was performed after pretreatment dehydration solution. Wu Huping [50] choose accelerated 9 mW/cm^2 for 10 min of UVA exposure and standard fluence of 5.4 J/cm^2. Krueger [36] choose accelerated 15 mW/cm^2 for 7 min UVA exposure and 6.3 J/cm^2 fluence.

At the 1-month follow-up, corneas remained thinner than before the procedure. Best resulted were obtained by Krueger [36] with −18% compared with—17% of corneal thickness reduction obtained by Wu Huping [50] and Ramon [49].

After the first-month of follow-up there was an increase of thickness compared to the first month value. An improvement of corneal transparency was also reported in different studies [36, 48–53], however, the initial improvement in corneal transparency did not last for more than 8 months [48]. Clinical outcomes were improved at 1 month; VA increased, bullous changes of epithelium improved, corneal thickness reduced and pain alleviated. However, in advanced cases of endothelial failure, the effect of cross-linking might not be strong enough to avoid short term recurrence of corneal edema and bullous keratopathy. It has been observed that those with more advanced corneal edema had little short-term benefits [52].

This technique does not provide a long-term solution in decompensated bullous keratopathy corneas that require endothelial or penetrating keratoplasty according to the condition of the stroma (scars, transparency), but it may be helpful in temporarily alleviating severe symptoms of pain and epithelial erosion for several months, enabling the patient to delay and/or postpone more invasive and costly surgical options [54].

6.4 Infectious Keratitis

Infectious keratitis is a severe ocular infection, and one of the leading causes of monocular blindness worldwide [55]. The incidence of microbial keratitis ranges from 6.3 to 710 cases per 100,000 people per year and is even more common in contact lens wearers [56]. Delayed treatment of infectious keratitis can lead to significant visual loss in as many as 50% of the cases [57].

Most community-acquired cases of microbial keratitis are resolved with empiric treatment by using broad-spectrum topical antimicrobials [58]. However, the emergence and spread of antimicrobial-resistant organisms remain a serious clinical and public health concern [59–63].

Corneal degradation and melting occurs when specific proteinases are upregulated after corneal damage. These matrix metalloproteinases are synthesized either in the keratocytes (matrix metalloproteinase 2) or by corneal epithelial cells (matrix metalloproteinase 9), and are also responsible for delayed epithelial wound healing. [64–66]. Corneal cross-linking (CXL) using ultraviolet light-A (UV-A) and riboflavin is a technique which was developed in the 1990's to treat corneal ectatic disorders such as keratoconus. The combination of riboflavin and ultraviolet-A has been, clinically used as an antimicrobial approach for decades (ie, transfusion medicine) [67]. CXL demonstrates excellent antimicrobial efficacy against a variety of common in vitro pathogens [68]. This cytotoxic effect led to the first clinical trials using CXL to treat advanced infectious melting corneal keratitis. In 2000 Seiler and his team reported their use of CXL to stabilize non-infectious corneal melting originating from various causes [69]. This early trial demonstrated the efficacy of CXL in biomechanically stabilizing structurally altered corneas without inducing ectasia. In 2008, Iseli and his team conducted the first study in exclusively treating melting corneas of infectious origin with CXL [70].

CXL proved to be effective not only in stabilizing the melted cornea, but, more importantly, in killing pathogens of different origins in advanced and therapy-resistant keratitis. This study not only confirmed the previous results from Seiler and Colleagues from 2000, but also introduced the concept that CXL could be efficient when treating corneal melts of infectious origin. Subsequently, further clinical trials on advanced melting corneas, one meta-analysis, and multiple animal experiments confirmed those initial results [71–96]. In 2011 Makdoumi reported a non-randomized clinical study to investigate the efficacy of CXL as first line therapy for treating bacterial keratitis. This study suggested that CXL might be effective not only in treating advanced ulcerative infectious keratitis as an adjuvant, but also for treating early-stage bacterial infiltrates as first-line treatment (Fig. 6.16).

The PACK-CXL: Photo-Activated Chromophore for Keratitis—Corneal Cross-Linking was adopted for CXL when treating infectious keratitis [76]. Vinciguerra P, Rosetta P. and Coll. introduced a new corneal CXL for infectious keratitis protocol, titled cross-linking window absorption (CXL-WA), Table 6.4. The protocol entails the use of hypoosmolar riboflavin before irradiation with UV-A, and penetration is obtained through the epithelial defect overlying the ulcer with no epithelial removal. The center of the ulcer was gently swiped to eliminate all cellular debris, and the cornea was not de-epithelized. Before beginning irradiation, a hypoosmolar 0.1% riboflavin solution was instilled for 30 min to obtain stromal swelling. The cornea was exposed to UV-A light with the UV-X System which emits light at a wavelength of 1370 ± 5 nm and an irradiance of 3 mW/cm^2 or 5.4 J/cm^2 [97, 98].

All laboratory and clinical studies that have been published to date regarding CXL treatment for infectious keratitis have used the original Dresden protocol as the common setting, irradiating the cornea for 30 min at 3 mW/cm^2 and a wavelength of 365 μm.

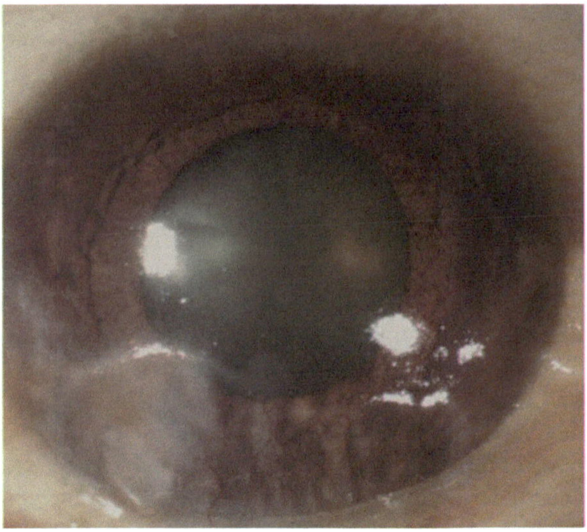

Fig. 6.16 Antibiotic-resistant Infectious keratitis (Staphylococcus aureus isolated). After 9 mW/cm^2 ACXL. Epithelial closure was achieved 4 days after ACXL treatment

Table 6.4 Cross-linking for infectious keratitis

Surgical parameters	Standard CXL (Dresden)	Modified CXL with hypo-osmolar riboflavin	CXL-WA
Prior medication	Anesthetic and myotic	Anesthetic and myotic	Anesthetic
Epithelial removal	YES	YES	NO (penetration through ulcer)
Impregnation	30 min with epithelium off	30 min with epithelium off	30 min with absorption through ulcer window
Solution	Isotonic riboflavin with dextran	Hypo-osmolar riboflavin dextran free	Hypo-osmolar riboflavin dextran free
UVA-source	3 mW/cm^2	3 mW/cm^2	3 mW/cm^2
Time of irradiation	30 min	30 min	30 min
Post treatment medication	Antibiotic	Antibiotic	Antibiotic and mydriatic

The Bunsen–Roscoe law of reciprocity states that a photochemical effect should remain the same when equal total energy (fluence) is used. This law originates from photochemistry and compares immediate photochemical reactions under different settings. The Bunsen–Roscoe law cannot easily be applied to a biological system, which generates not only immediate responses, but also additional medium and long-term changes.

Richoz and his team have tested the corneal biomechanical properties at different CXL irradiances and have found that the increase in biomechanical stiffness is significantly reduced [99].

In contrast, the antimicrobial efficacy of PACK-CXL seems to follow the Bunsen–Roscoe law at the irradiance levels tested in our experiments. One potential explanation could be that the killing rate of PACK-CXL depends on the oxidative stress induced by the photoactivated chromophore. The more reactive oxygen species created within a short period of time, the more oxidative damage imposed to the pathogen's DNA [100]. Thus, the antibacterial efficacy of PACK-CXL follows the Bunsen–Roscoe law of reciprocity, and can be maintained even when irradiation intensity is considerably increased. These optimized settings may allow for shortened PACK-CXL treatment time, and help facilitate the transition from the operating room to the slit lamp for treatment. CXL could become a new alternative for infectious keratitis treatment in the future. The microbicidal effect of CXL against infections can be explained through the effect of two main mechanisms: the direct antimicrobial activity of the UV-light itself that damages DNA and RNA in antibiotic resistant and non-resistant microbes such as methicillin-resistant Staphylococcus aureus (MRSA), Staphylococcus epidermidis, Staphylococcus aureus, Pseudomonas aeruginosa, Enterococcus faecalis and other bacteria (mean elimination ranged between 60 and 98%), but also viruses and fungi (Candida albicans, Aspergillus fumigatus, Fusarium solani, Scedosporium and Alternaria), precluding microbes from replicating. The second element is the photoactivated Riboflavin releasing reactive oxygen species (ROS) that directly interact with the nucleic acids and cell membranes of the microbes. Fungicidal effect seems to be dramatically increased by using 0.25% Riboflavin instead 0.1% concentration. [101]. Richoz et al [102] have shown that the accelerated protocol using 9 mW/cm^2 for 10 min [103], 18 mW/cm^2 for 5 min and even 30 mW/cm^2 for 3 min allows to maintain the same high bacterial killing rate observed in earlier studies using the Dresden protocol. CXL appears to be a promising adjunctive treatment in selective cases of mild to moderate bacterial keratitis. Its efficacy in fungal and amoebic keratitis is questionable. Insufficient efficacy against Acanthamoeba was reported [74, 104]. Treatment protocols in microbial keratitis need to be individualized. Standardization of treatment protocol is important, because the standard irradiance of 3 mW/cm^2 in combination with a longer UV-A exposure time has demonstrated a better bactericidal effect compared with the high-power and shorter duration settings [105]. Actually there is no general consensus on the treatment protocols of CXL and the outcome measures of CXL on infectious keratitis vary widely in the literature. The disparities in the treatment protocols, study designs and outcome measures impede a generalization of the application. Based on current evidence, the role of CXL in infectious keratitis remained unclear despite the reported success in different clinical cases. However, CXL could be attempted in severe infectious keratitis refractory to conventional medical therapy. Long-term, prospective, randomized trials are needed to determine its usefulness in the field.

References

1. Krachmer JH, Mannis M, Holland EJ. Cornea. St. Louis, MO: Elsevier; 2010.
2. Randekman JB, Russel B, Ward MA, et al. Risk factor and prognosis for corneal ectasia after LASIK. Ophthalmology. 2003;110(2):267–75.
3. Seiler T, Koufala K, Richter G. Iatrogenic keratectasia after laser in situ keratomileusis. J Refract Surg. 1998;14(3):312–7.
4. Sailer T, Quurke AW. Iatrogenickeratectasia after LASIK in a case of forme fruste keratoconus. Cataract Refract Surg. 1998;24(7):1007–9.
5. Geggel HS, Talley AR. Dellayed onset keratectasia following laser in situ keratomileusis. J Cataract Refract Surg. 1999;25(4):582–6.
6. Lifshitz T, Levy J, Klemperer I, et al. Late bilateral after LASIK in a low myopic patient. J Refract Surg. 2005;21(5):494–6.
7. Krueger RR, Dupps WJ Jr. Biomechanical effects of femtosecond and microkeratome-based flap creation: prospective contralateral examination of two patients. J Refract Surg. 2007;23(8):800–7.
8. Spoerl E, Seiler T. Techniques for stiffening the cornea. J Refract Surg. 1999;15:711–3.
9. Wollensak G, Spörl E, Mazzotta C, Kalinski T, Sel S. Interlamellar cohesion after corneal crosslinking using riboflavin and ultraviolet A light. Br J Ophthalmol. 2011;95(6):876–80.
10. Wollensak G. Crosslinking treatment of progressive keratoconus: new hope. Curr Opin Ophthalmol. 2006;17(4):356–60.
11. Kohlhaas M, Spoerl E, Speck A, Schilde T, Sandner D, Pillunat LE. Eine neue Behandlung der Keratektasie nach LASIK durch Kollagenvernetzung mit Riboflavin/UVA-Licht [A new treatment of keratectasia after LASIK by using collagen with riboflavin/UVA light cross-linking]. Klin Monbl Augenheilkd. 2005; https://doi.org/10.1055/s-2005-857950.
12. Hafezi F, Kanellopoulos J, Wiltfang R, Seiler T. Corneal collagen crosslinking with riboflavin and ultraviolet A to treat induced keratectasia after laser in situ keratomileusis. J Cataract Refract Surg. 2007;33(12):2035–40.
13. Vinciguerra P, Camesasca FI, Albe E, Trazza S. Corneal collagen cross-linking for ectasia after excimer laser refractive surgery: 1-year results. J Refract Surg. 2010;26(7): 486–97.
14. Salgado JP, Khoramnia R, Lohmann CP, Winkler von Mohrenfels C. Corneal collagen cross-linking in post-LASIKkeratectasia. Br J Ophthalmol. 2011;95(4):493–7.
15. Hersh PS, Greenstein SA, Fry KL. Corneal collagen crosslinking for keratoconus and corneal ectasia: one-year results. J Cataract Refract Surg. 2011;37(1):149–60.
16. Li G, Fan ZJ, Peng XJ. Corneal collagen crosslinking for corneal ectasia of post-LASIK: One-year results. Int J Ophthalmol. 2012;5(2):190–5.
17. Richoz O, Mavrakanas N, Pajic B, Hafezi F. Corneal collagen cross-linking for ectasia after LASIK and photorefractive keratectomy: long-term results. Ophthalmology. 2013 120(7):1354-1359
18. Yildirim H, Cakir N, Kara N, et al. Corneal collagen crosslinking for ectasia after laser in situ keratomileusis: longterm results. J Cataract Refract Surg. 2014;40(10):1591–6.
19. Marino GK, Torricelli AA, Giacomin N, Santhiago MR, Espindola R, Netto MV. Accelerated corneal collagen cross-linking for postoperative LASIK Ectasia: two-year outcomes. J Refract Surg. 2015;31(6):380–4.
20. Mazzotta C, Baiocchi S, Denaro R, Tosi GM, Caporossi T. Corneal collagen cross-linking to stop corneal ectasia exacerbated by radial keratotomy. Cornea. 2011;30(2):225–8.
21. Kymionis GD, Diakonis VF, Kalyvianaki M, Portaliou D, Siganos C, Kozobolis VP, Pallikaris AI. One-year follow-up of corneal confocal microscopy after corneal cross-linking in patients with post laser in situ keratosmileusis ectasia and keratoconus. Am J Ophthalmol. 2009;147(5):774–8.
22. Cheema AS, Mozayan A, Channa P. Corneal collagen crosslinking in refractive surgery. Curr Opin Ophthalmol. 2012;23(4):251–6.

23. Greenstein SA, Fry KL, Hersh PS. Corneal topography indices after corneal collagen crosslinking for keratoconus and corneal ectasia: one-year results. J Cataract Refract Surg. 2011;37(7):1282–90.
24. Mazzotta C, Traversi C, Caragiuli S, Rechichi M. Pulsed vs continuous light accelerated corneal collagen crosslinking: in vivo qualitative investigation by confocal microscopy and corneal OCT. Eye (Lond). 2014;28(10):1179–83.
25. Mazzotta C, Traversi C, Paradiso AL, Latronico ME, Rechichi M. Pulsed light accelerated crosslinking versus continuous light accelerated crosslinking: one-year results. J Ophthalmol. 2014;2014: Article ID 604731. https://doi.org/10.1155/2014/604731.
26. Mazzotta C, Hafezi F, Kymionis G, Caragiuli S, Jacob S, Traversi C, Barabino S, Randleman B. In vivo confocal microscopy after corneal collagen cross-linking. Ocul Surf. 2015;13(4):298–314.
27. Mazzotta C, Balestrazzi A, Traversi C, et al. Treatment of progressive keratoconus by riboflavin-UVA-induced cross-linking of corneal collagen: ultrastructural analysis by Heidelberg Retinal Tomograph II in vivo confocal microscopy in humans. Cornea. 2007;26(4):390–7.
28. Mazzotta C, Paradiso AL, Baiocchi S, Caragiuli S, Caporossi A. Qualitative investigation of corneal changes after accelerated corneal collagen cross-linking (A-CXL) by in vivo confocal microscopy and corneal OCT. J Clin Exp Ophthalmol. 2013;4:313.
29. Mazzotta C, Traversi C, Baiocchi S, et al. Corneal healing after riboflavin ultraviolet-A collagen cross-linking determined by confocal laser scanning microscopy in vivo: early and late modifications. Am J Ophthalmol. 2008;146(4):527–33.
30. Caporossi A, Mazzotta C, Baiocchi S, Caporossi T, Paradiso AL. Transepithelial corneal collagen crosslinking for keratoconus: qualitative investigation by in vivo HRT II confocal analysis. Eur J Ophthalmol. 2012;22(Suppl 7):S81–8. https://doi.org/10.5301/ejo.5000125.
31. Roberts CJ, Dupps WJ. Biomechanics of corneal ectasia and biomechanical treatments. J Cataract Refract Surg. 2014;40:991–8.
32. Maguire LJ, Klyce SD, McDonald MB, Kaufman HE. Corneal topography of pellucid marginal degeneration. Ophthalmology. 1987;94:519–24.
33. Biswas S, Brahma A, Tromans C, Ridgway A. Management of pellucid marginal corneal degeneration. Eye (Lond). 2000;14(Pt 4):629–34.
34. Moshirfar M, Edmonds JN, Behunin NL, Christiansen SM. Current options in the management of pellucid marginal degeneration. J Refract Surg. 2014;30(7):474–85.
35. Rao GN, Aquavella JV, Goldberg SH, Berk SL. Pseudophakic bullous keratopathy. Relationship to preoperative corneal endothelial status. Ophthalmology. 1984;91:1135–40.
36. Krueger RR, Ramos-Esteban JC, Kanellopoulos AJ. Staged intrastromal delivery of riboflavin with UVA cross-linking in advanced bullous keratopathy: laboratory investigation and first clinical case. J Refract Surg. 2008;24(7):S730–6.
37. Cordeiro Barbosa MM, Barbosa JB Jr, Hirai FE, Hofling-Lima AL. Effect of cross - linking on corneal thickness in patients with corneal edema. Cornea. 2010;29(6):613–7.
38. Insler MS, Benefield DW, Ross EV. Topical hyperosmolar solutions in the reduction of corneal edema. CLAO J. 1987;13(3):149–51.
39. Smiddy WE, Hamburg TR, Kracher GP, Gottsch JD, Stark WJ. Therapeutic contact lenses. Ophthalmology. 1990;97(3):291–5.
40. Cormier G, Brunette I, Boisjoly HM, LeFrançois M, Shi ZH, Guertin MC. Anterior stromal punctures for bullous keratopathy. Arch Ophthalmol. 1996;114(6):654–8.
41. Sonmez B, Kim BT, Aldave AJ. Amniotic membrane transplantation with anterior stromal micropuncture for treatment of painful bullous keratopathy in eyes with poor visual potential. Cornea. 2007;26(2):227–9.
42. Zemba M. Palliative treatment in bullous keratopathy. Oftalmologia. 2006;50(2):23–6.
43. Mejia LF, Santamaria JP, Acosta C. Symptomatic management of postoperative bullous keratopathy with nonpreserved human amniotic membrane. Cornea. 2002;21(4):342–5.
44. Melles GR, Lander F, Beekhuis WH, et al. Posterior lamellar keratoplasty for a case of pseudophakic bullous keratopathy. Am J Ophthalmol. 1999;127:340–1.

45. Wollensak G, Spoerl E, Seiler T. Riboflavin/ultraviolet-a-induced collagen crosslinking for the treatment of keratoconus. Am J Ophthalmol. 2003;135:620–7.
46. Wollensak G, Aurich H, Pham DT, Wirbelauer C. Hydration behavior of porcine cornea crosslinked with riboflavin and ultraviolet A. J Cataract Refract Surg. 2007;33:516–21.
47. John Kanellopoulos A. Corneal collagen cross-linking in bullous keratopathy. J Refract Surg (Thorofare, NJ: 1995). 25(8):687.
48. Wollensak G, Aurich H, Wirbelauer C, Pham DT. Potential use of Riboflavin/UVA cross-linking in bullous keratopathy. Ophthalmic Res. 2009;41:114–7.
49. Ghanem RC, Santhiago MR, Berti TB, Thomaz S, Netto MV. Collagen cross-linking with riboflavin and ultraviolet-A in eyes with pseudophakic bullous keratopathy. J Cataract Refract Surg. 2010;36:1444.
50. Wu Huping, Lin Zhirong, Luo Shunrong, Liu Zhaosheng, Dong Nuo, Shang Xumin. Accelerated corneal collagen cross-linking in eyes with incurable bullous keratopathy. Chin J Ophthalmol Vis Sci. 2015;17(3).
51. Arora R, Manudhane A, Saran RK, Goyal J, Goyal G, Gupta D. Role of corneal collagen cross-linking in pseudophakic bullous keratopathy. Ophthalmology. 2013;120:2413–8.
52. Mirzaei M, Taheri N, Nobar MBR, Sedigh AL, Najafi A, Mirzaei S. Corneal collagen cross-linking effects on pseudophakic bullous keratopathy. Int Eye Sci. 2014;5:14.
53. Ucakhan OO, Saglik A. Outcome of two corneal collagen crosslinking methods in bullous keratopathy due to Fuchs' endothelial dystrophy. Case Reports Med. 2014, Article ID 463905.
54. Yi DH, Dana MR. Corneal edema after cataract surgery: incidence and etiology. Semin Ophthalmol. 2002;17:110–4.
55. Shah A, Sachdev A, Coggon D, Hossain P. Geographic variations in microbial keratitis: an analysis of the peer-reviewed literature. Br J Ophthalmol. 2011;95:762–7.
56. Thomas PA, Geraldine P. Infectious keratitis. Curr Opin Infect Dis. 2007;20:129–41.
57. Jones DB. Decision-making in the management of microbial keratitis. Ophthalmology. 1981;88:814–20.
58. American Academy of Ophthalmology Cornea/External Disease Panel. Preferred Practice Pattern Guidelines. Bacterial Keratitis. Available at: http://one.aao.org/CE/PracticeGuidelines/PPP.aspx. Accessed 8 Nov 2013.
59. Bennett HG, Hay J, Kirkness CM, et al. Antimicrobial management of presumed microbial keratitis: guidelines for treatment of central and peripheral ulcers. Br J Ophthalmol. 1998;82:137–45.
60. DeMuri GP, Hostetter MK. Resistance to antifungal agents. Pediatr Clin North Am. 1995;42:665–85.
61. Levy SB. Multidrug resistanceda sign of the times. N Engl J Med. 1998;338:1376–8.
62. Neu HC. The crisis in antibiotic resistance. Science. 1992;257:1064–73.
63. Ollivier FJ, Gilger BC, Barrie KP, et al. Proteinases of the cornea and preocular tear film. Vet Ophthalmol. 2007;10:199–206.
64. Fini ME, Girard MT, Matsubara M. Collagenolytic/gelatinolytic enzymes in corneal wound healing. Acta Ophthalmol Suppl. 1992;202:26–33.
65. Fini ME, Parks WC, Rinehart WB, et al. Role of matrix metalloproteinases in failure to re-epithelialize after corneal injury. Am J Pathol. 1996;149:1287–302.
66. Daniels JT, Geerling G, Alexander RA, et al. Temporal and spatial expression of matrix metalloproteinases during wound healing of human corneal tissue. Exp Eye Res. 2003;77:653–64.
67. Goodrich RP. The use of riboflavin for the inactivation of pathogens in blood products. Vox Sang. 2000;78(suppl 2):211–5.
68. Martins SA, Combs JC, Noguera G, et al. Antimicrobial efficacy of riboflavin/UVA combination (365 nm) in vitro for bacterial and fungal isolates: a potential new treatment for infectious keratitis. Invest Ophthalmol Vis Sci. 2008;49:3402–8.
69. Schnitzler E, Spörl E, Seiler T. Irradiation of cornea with ultraviolet light and riboflavin administration as a new treatment for erosive corneal processes, preliminary results in four patients. Klin Monbl Augenheilkd. 2000;217:190–3.

70. Iseli HP, Thiel MA, Hafezi F, Kampmeier J, Seiler T, Ultraviolet A. riboflavin corneal cross-linking for infectious keratitis associated with corneal melts. Cornea. 2008;27:590–4.
71. Abbouda A, Estrada AV, Rodriguez AE, Alió JL. Anterior segment optical coherence tomography in evaluation of severe fungal keratitis infections treated by corneal crosslinking. Eur J Ophthalmol. 2014;24(3):320–4.
72. Alio JL, Abbouda A, Valle DD, Del Castillo JM, Fernandez JA. Corneal crosslinking and infectious keratitis: a systematic review with a meta-analysis of reported cases. J Ophthalmic Inflamm Infect. 2013;3(1):47.
73. Berra M, Galperin G, Boscaro G, Zarate J, Tau J, Chiaradia P, et al. Treatment of Acanthamoeba keratitis by corneal cross-linking. Cornea. 2013;32(2):174–8.
74. del Buey MA, Cristóbal JA, Casas P, Goñi P, Clavel A, Mínguez E, et al. Evaluation of in vitro efficacy of combined riboflavin and ultraviolet a for Acanthamoeba isolates. Am J Ophthalmol. 2012;153(3):399–404.
75. Galperin G, Berra M, Tau J, Boscaro G, Zarate J, Berra A. Treatment of fungal keratitis from Fusarium infection by corneal cross-linking. Cornea. 2012;31(2):176–80.
76. Hafezi F, Randleman JB. PACK-CXL: defining CXL for infectious keratitis. J Refract Surg. 2014;30(7):438–9.
77. Hellander-Edman A, Makdoumi K, Mortensen J, Ekesten B. Corneal crosslinking in 9 horses with ulcerative keratitis. BMC Vet Res. 2013;9:128.
78. Li Z, Jhanji V, Tao X, Yu H, Chen W, Mu G. Riboflavin/ultravoilet lightmediated crosslinking for fungal keratitis. Br J Ophthalmol. 2013;97(5):669–71.
79. Makdoumi K, Mortensen J, Crafoord S. Infectious keratitis treated with corneal crosslinking. Cornea. 2010;29(12):1353–8.
80. Makdoumi K, Mortensen J, Sorkhabi O, Malmvall BE, Crafoord S. UVAriboflavin photochemical therapy of bacterial keratitis: a pilot study. Graefes Arch Clin Exp Ophthalmol. 2012;250(1):95–102.
81. Mattila JS, Korsbäck A, Krootila K, Holopainen JM. Treatment of Pseudomonas aeruginosa keratitis with combined corneal cross-linking and human amniotic membrane transplantation. Acta Ophthalmol. 2013;91(5):e410–1.
82. Müller L, Thiel MA, Kipfer-Kauer AI, Kaufmann C. Corneal cross-linking as supplementary treatment option in melting keratitis: a case series. Klin Monbl Augenheilkd. 2012;229(4):411–5.
83. Panda A, Krishna SN, Kumar S. Photo-activated riboflavin therapy of refractory corneal ulcers. Cornea. 2012;31(10):1210–3.
84. Pot SA, Gallhöfer NS, Matheis FL, Voelter-Ratson K, Hafezi F, Spiess BM. Corneal collagen cross-linking as treatment for infectious and noninfectious corneal melting in cats and dogs: results of a prospective, nonrandomized, controlled trial. Vet Ophthalmol. 2014;17(4):250–60.
85. Pot SA, Gallhöfer NS, Walser-Reinhardt L, Hafezi F, Spiess BM. Treatment of bullous keratopathy with corneal collagen cross-linking in two dogs. Vet Ophthalmol. 2015;18(2):168–73.
86. Price MO, Tenkman LR, Schrier A, Fairchild KM, Trokel SL, Price FW Jr. Photoactivated riboflavin treatment of infectious keratitis using collagen cross-linking technology. J Refract Surg. 2012;28(10):706–13.
87. Richoz O, Gatzioufas Z, Hafezi F. Corneal collagen cross-linking for the treatment of Acanthamoeba keratitis. Cornea. 2013;32(10):e189.
88. Sağlk A, Ucakhan OO, Kanpolat A. Ultraviolet A and riboflavin therapy as an adjunct in corneal ulcer refractory to medical treatment. Eye Contact Lens. 2013;39(6):413–5.
89. Said DG, Elalfy MS, Gatzioufas Z, El-Zakzouk ES, Hassan MA, Saif MY, et al. Collagen cross-linking with photoactivated riboflavin (PACK-CXL) for the treatment of advanced infectious keratitis with corneal melting. Ophthalmology. 2014;121(7):1377–82.
90. Shetty R, Nagaraja H, Jayadev C, Shivanna Y, Kugar T. Collagen crosslinking in the management of advanced non-resolving microbial keratitis. Br J Ophthalmol. 2014;98(8):1033–5.
91. Sorkhabi R, Sedgipoor M, Mahdavifard A. Collagen cross-linking for resistant corneal ulcer. Int Ophthalmol. 2013;33(1):61–6.

92. Spiess BM, Pot SA, Florin M, Hafezi F. Corneal collagen cross-linking (CXL) for the treatment of melting keratitis in cats and dogs: a pilot study. Vet Ophthalmol. 2014;17(1):1–11.
93. Tabibian D, Mazzotta C, Hafezi F. PACK-CXL: corneal cross-linking in infectious keratitis. Eye Vis (Lond). 2016;3:11.
94. Vazirani J, Vaddavalli PK. Cross-linking for microbial keratitis. Indian J Ophthalmol. 2013;61(8):441–4.
95. Wong RL, Gangwani RA, LW Y, Lai JS. New treatments for bacterial keratitis. J Ophthalmol. 2012;2012:831502.
96. Zhang ZY. Corneal cross-linking for the treatment of fungal keratitis. Cornea. 2013;32(2):217–8.
97. Vinciguerra R, Rosetta P, Romano MR, Azzolini C, Vinciguerra P. Treatment of refractory infectious keratitis with corneal collagen cross-linking window absorption. Cornea. 2013;32(6):e139–40.
98. Rosetta P, Vinciguerra R, Romano MR, Vinciguerra P. Corneal collagen cross-linking window absorption. Cornea. 2013;32(4):550–4.
99. Hammer A, Richoz O, Arba Mosquera S, Tabibian D, Hoogewoud F, Hafezi F. Corneal biomechanical properties at different corneal collagen cross-linking (CXL) irradiances. Invest Ophthalmol Vis Sci. 2014;55:2881–4.
100. Kumari MV, Yoneda T, Hiramatsu M. Scavenging activity of "betacatechin" on reactive oxygen species generated by photosensitization of riboflavin. Biochem Mol Biol Int. 1996;38:1163–70.
101. Bilgihan K, Kalkanci A, Ozdemir HB, Yazar R, Karakurt F, Yuksel E, Otag F, Karabicak N, Arikan-Akdagli S. Evaluation of antifungal efficacy of 0.1% and 0.25% riboflavin with UVA: a comparative in vitro study. Curr Eye Res. 2016;41(8):1050–6.
102. Tabibian D, Richoz O, Riat A, Schrenzel J, Hafezi F. Accelerated photoactivated chromophore for keratitis-corneal collagen cross-linking as a first-line and sole treatment in early fungal keratitis. J Refract Surg. 2014;30(12):855–7.
103. Richoz O, Kling S, Hoogewoud F, Hammer A, Tabibian D, Francois P, et al. Antibacterial efficacy of accelerated photoactivated chromophore for keratitis-corneal collagen cross-linking (PACK-CXL). J Refract Surg. 2014;30:850–4.
104. Kashiwabuchi RT, Carvalho FR, Khan YA, et al. Assessing efficacy of combined riboflavin and UV-A light (365 nm) treatment of Acanthamoeba trophozoites. Invest Ophthalmol Vis Sci. 2011;52:9333–8.
105. Bäckman A, Makdoumi K, Mortensen J, et al. The efficiency of cross-linking methods in eradication of bacteria is influenced by the riboflavin concentration and the irradiation time of ultraviolet light. Acta Ophthalmol. 2014;92:656–61.

Keratoconus Classification, ACXL Indications and Therapy Flowchart

7

Modern keratoconus (KC) therapeutic strategy should be based on its clinical stage depending on corneal apex and posterior elevation location (central <2 mm from the pupil center or peripheral >2 mm), curvatures, thickness, high-order aberrations, documented clinical (UCVA, BSCVA) and instrumental (topographic, pachymetric and/or aberrometric) progression [1]. Therapeutic approach must be also strongly connected to patient's age according to different progression rate, faster in paediatric patients 18 years and under and among young people between 19 and 26 years [2].

In our opinion the therapeutic chances in keratoconic patients should be directed into three main directories:

1. Early diagnosis avoiding the progression to advanced stages reducing or eliminating the necessity of lamellar and penetrating keratoplasty.
2. Conservative corneal reshaping treatments to reduce aberrations and refractive errors;

The association between pediatric age, allergies and eye-rubbing represent a dangerous situations stimulating faster progression [3, 4]. These individuals are at higher risk of progression [5], requiring corneal transplant, thus preventive measures and properly timed regimens of antihistaminic drugs, steroids and particularly corneal collagen crosslinking therapy are key. Ophthalmologists and Pediatricians should be alert and watchful of these particular conditions which require close monitoring and prompt treatment to prevent corneal deterioration and associated visual decay. KC early diagnosis and careful clinical and instrumental follow-up are mandatory in order to prevent corneal shape modifications and necessity of donor keratoplasty [5]. Here we report some guidelines of KC therapeutic strategy.

C. Mazzotta et al., *Management of Early Progressive Corneal Ectasia*,
DOI 10.1007/978-3-319-61137-2_7

7.1 Keratoconus Classification

In the last 10 years the fast developments of diagnostic topo-aberrometric, tomographic and pachymetric methods have significantly modified the old approaches to KC classifications and management, introducing new and more complex parameters. Krumeich's classification [6] still remains a basic standard in ophthalmology but in our opinion, a reviewing process of the old parameters and introduction of new ones is necessary to improve the decision making process according to the new conservative combined therapeutic strategies. During KC evaluation and follow-up, is frequently possible to find different parameters of different stages in the same patient, especially regarding K readings and pachymetry data. This particular condition requires a great clinical and technical experience for a correct interpretation and personalization of the classification, crossing all the data available (clinical and instrumental), in order to assume the right decision. Moreover, the advent of tomographic analysis and Riboflavin UVA corneal collagen crosslinking [7, 9] and the CXL induced significant changes [9] in the therapeutic strategies requiring new classification parameters.

7.2 Amsler Classification

This four stages KC classification was based on semeiology, clinical an ophthalmometric (Javal) evidences (Amsler's angle), Table 7.1. This actually has been overcomed by more accurate instrumental parameters provided by corneal tomography and aberrometry.

Table 7.1 Amsler classification

Stage 1 (initial): oblique incidence astigmatism, low grade asymmetry of ophthalmometric specular images, corneal curvature between 45 and 48 Diopters and axis inclination (Amsler's angle) between 1 and 3 grades; spectacles
Stage 2 (evident): oblique incidence astigmatism and miopia, moderate grade asymmetry of ophthalmometric specular images, corneal curvature between 48 and 53 Diopters and axis inclination (Amsler's angle) between 3 and 9 grades; hard gas permeable corneal contact lenses
Stage 3 (classic): oblique ophthalmometric unmeasurable astigmatism, high grade asymmetry of ophthalmometric specular images, corneal curvature >53 Diopters; biomicroscopic corneal alterations; keratoplasty
Stage 4 (clear): clinically visible corneal ectasia, marked corneal thinning, stromal apex dystrophies and scar opacities. Keratoplasty

7.3 Rama Classification

This KC classification ideated by Giovanni Rama, the pioneer of corneal transplants in Italy, represents one of the most important step forward in the modern therapeutic approach to keratoconus and it is still widely used by ophthalmologists. It consists in a two stages classification regarding clinical and surgical approach to KC (Table 7.2).

7.4 Krumeich Classification

Krumeich's classification [6] today remain the most diffused and used KC classification based on astigmatism dioptric power and, for the first time, introduces modern diagnostic elements such as topographic K readings and central corneal thickness measurement by US pachymetry. This classification also includes the presence or absence of Vogt's striae and corneal opacities, Table 7.3.

Table 7.2 Rama classification

***Stage a.* Refractive Keratoconus**	Low to moderate grade of asymmetric astigmatism, with or without associated myopia, with available refractive error correction by spectacles or rigid gas permeable corneal contact lenses
***Stage b.* Advanced Keratoconus**	Impossibility to obtain a refractive error correction by spectacles or corneal contact lenses, or contact lenses untolerance, requiring surgical approach

Table 7.3 KC Krumeich's classification

Keratoconus	Stage 1	Stage 2	Stage 3	Stage 4
Miopia and astigmatism	<5 D	>5D a < 8D	>8 D < 10D	Not measurable
K max	<48 D	< 53 D	> 53 D	>55 D
Corneal opacities	Vogt's Strie	Vogt's Strie	Vogt's Strie	Scar
	+ − −	+ + −	+ + +	
	No scar	No scar	No scar	
Pachymetry	normal	>400 μm	>200 μm	<200 μm
			<400 μm	

7.5 Caporossi Classification

Starting from the cross-linking ability in stabilizing keratoconus progression while improving the quality of vision, the Caporossi and coll [8]. described [7] a therapeutic keratoconus classification, Table 7.4. It is based on keratoconus progression, patient's age, optical pachymetry thinnest point value, HRGP lens tolerance, dividing the disease into two main categories: progressive and/or stationary with the relative therapeutic strategies [8].

7.6 Aliò Classification

Introduced in 2006 by Aliò J. [10] represents a modern classification based on wave-front coma-like values, Table 7.5. KC is divided in four stages related to Krumeich's classification.

According to the Author [10], high order aberrations (HOA), are significantly higher in eyes with keratoconus than normal eyes. Coma-like aberrations, with the aid of a corneal aberrometry map, are good indicators for early detections and grading of keratoconus.

7.7 Mazzotta Classification

The novelty introduced by Mazzotta [11] in this modern KC staging system is the location of the cone apex related to pupillary center, being one of the most important factor in optical and refractive performances, overcoming the significance of keratometric parameters. Another fundamental step forward is the introduction of the elevative parameters (both anterior and posterior elevation) that are essential in KC evaluation, follow-up, functional outcomes and surgical planning, Table 7.6.

Table 7.4 Caporossi operative KC classification based on CXL

Keratoconus follow-up (KC)	Operative class
Progressive KC	Epi-OFF CXL always in Stage I and II KC
	Epi-ON CXL in thin corneas <400 μm
Stationary KC	CXL in patients intolerant to Contact Lenses or CXL Plus INTACS

Table 7.5 Aliò wavefront-based KC classification

Aliò classification
Stage 1: coma value, ≤1.87 μm
Stage 2: coma value, ≥1.87 – ≤2.97 μm
Stage 3: coma value, ≥2.97 – ≤3.46 μm
Stage 4: coma value ≥3.46 – ≤5.20 μm

Table 7.6 Mazzotta KC surgical classification

Mazzotta Ectasia Staging System (MESS)					
Stage 1	K Avg	AE	PE	TP	A (<1 mm) PC
Early	43–48 D	≤40 μm	≤80 μm	≥450 μm	B (>1 mm) PC
Stage 2	49–52 D	40–60 μm	80–100 μm	≥400 μm	A
Intermediate					B
Stage 3	>52 D	>60 μm	>100 μm	<400 μm	A
Advanced					B

Type A: Central KC apex dislocation <0.75 mm from pupillary center (PC)
Type B: Peripheral KC apex dislocation >0.75 < 1.5 mm from PC
Stage 1 (Early): K Ave 43–48 D; **Anterior Elevation** (AE) ≤ 40 μm; **Posterior Elevation** (PE) ≤ 80 μm; **Minimum Corneal Thickness** (MCT) ≥ 450 μm. Type A (central), Type B (peripheral); BSCVA >7/10
Stage 2. (Intermediate) (K Ave 49–52 D) AE 40–60 μm; PE 80–100 μm: TP ≥ 400 μm, Type A (central), Type B (peripheral); BSCVA >5/10 – ≤ 7/10
Stage 3 (Advanced) (K Ave >52 D): AE > 60 μm; PE > 100 μm; TP ≥ 350 μm, Type A (central), Type B (peripheral); BSCVA ≤4/10

7.8 Keratoconus Therapeutic Flowchart

Conventional [7, 9] and Accelerated Collagen Cross-linking procedures [12, 13] can be used alone, if early ectasia diagnosis is done, or in selected cases adopted in combination with other approaches called "remodelling or reshaping corneal techniques" (RCT) including CXL plus all surface minimally laser ablation (sequential or same-day topo-guided or wavefront-guided ablation), ICRS, pIOLs [14–16]. Advanced stages in patients that not tolerated the contact lenses, deep anterior lamellar keratoplasty [17] or femtoseconds laser assisted keratoplasty (FAK) is indicated [18–20]. A useful decision making therapeutic flow chart scheduled by Mazzotta, Traversi (Siena) and Raiskup (Dresden) is showed in Fig. 7.1.

Optical correction of KC induced refractive errors is the first line therapeutic approach to disease in order to improve patient visual acuity. Corrected Distance Visual Acuity (CDVA) assumes an important role especially in stage 1 when the measurement of refractive error must be carefully evaluated. The correction power can be strong if corneal apex dislocation is not highly decentred (contained in the central 2 mm) in relation to pupil centre and diameter. Generally, is possible to obtain a good or sufficient CDVA (in a range between 20/40 and 20/20), positioning the axis of cylinder against the rule (myopic astigmatism at 70° ± 20° or hyperopic astigmatism at 180° ± 20°). Myopia (spherical) results often overcorrected in KC eyes. Frequently the myopic shift is partially compensated by the corneal thinning and a combination of positive sphere associated with against the rule myopic

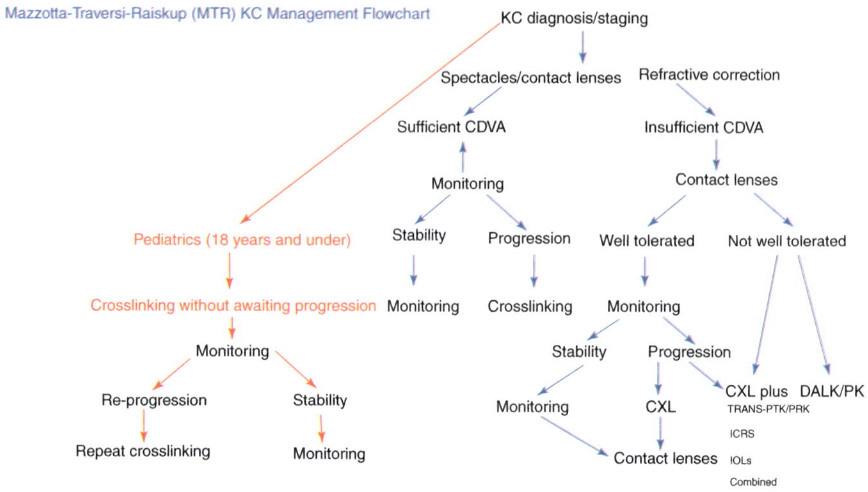

Fig. 7.1 Mazzotta-Traversi-Raiskup (MTR) KC therapy flow chart

Table 7.7 Spectacles indications and limits in KC refractive correction

Spectacles indications	Limits
Refractive Stage KC	High corneal astigmatism
Central Kones	High correction untolerated
Target AV satisfactory	Visual nocturnal fluctuations
Small amount of HOA	High Order Aberrations (HOA)
CL Intolerance	Anisometropia
CL Contraindications	Aniseconia

cylinder or simple against the rule hyperopic astigmatism are efficacious in the major part of stage 1–2 patients improving their visual acuity. Topographic data in KC corneas generally fails in the evaluation of right axis position and must be correctly understood by *elevative* algorithm or *coma-like axis* evaluation. Refractive tangential map can be used only to estimate approximately (50–70%) cylinder quantification. However, despite their importance, spectacles have significant limitations in paracentral and peripheral kones, Table 7.7.

Rigid gas permeable corneal contact lenses (RGP) represents one of the most important option especially sonce the stage 2 and over, and in case of poor CDVA (generally <20/40) [22]. The family of contact lenses [22] include different categories: Soft contact lenses (SCL), Rigid Gas Permeable (RGP), Piggy-back, Hybrid and Scleral lenses [22]. Often they represent the unique possibility of visual improvement in more aberrated KC corneas. The RGP lenses are the ideal implant for anisometropia correction, aniseconia correction, aberrations correction allowing (if well tolerated) a stable refractive correction without the typical nocturnal VA fluctuations related to pupillary diameter with spectacles [8]. The ideal contact lens implant includes a satisfactory patient's Visual Acuity (VA), with acceptable

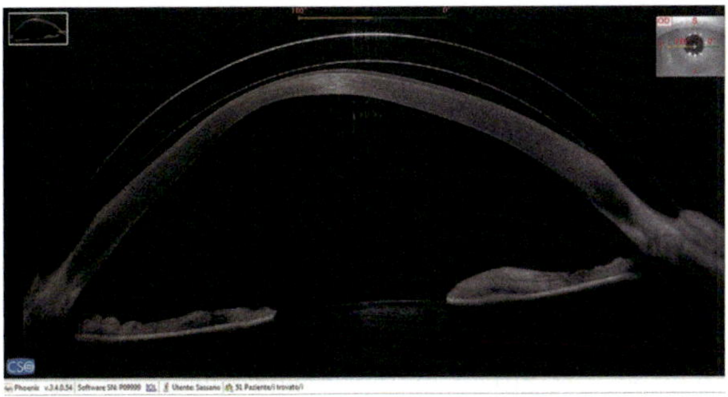

Fig. 7.2 Scleral contact lens in advanced KC. AC SD OCT

subjective comfort, respecting corneal physiology and the compliance with ocular surface. Target VA (generally >0.5 decimal equivalents) depends from patient's needings, job activities and quality of life, being influenced by the VA of the fellow eye that generally is better.

The possibility to obtain a good visual improvement in any stage of KC by contact lenses is also strongly related to corneal shape (lens fitting), comorbidity (ocular surface diseases), immune-tolerance and patient's compliance. On the other hand, bad application or abuse of contact corneal lenses sometimes induce micro-traumatic sub-apical dystrophy, apical corneal opacity or infectious keratitis [21]. It's time to stop with contact lenses when patients have good VA but contact lens is not tolerated, or in case of well tolerated contact lens but poor VA, when the stability of the implant is impossible with any kind of contact lens, when diffuse corneal scarring and thinning require a keratoplasty. Consider with your optometrist the potentiality of an epithelial scraping to give another chance in case of sub-apical epithelial hypertrophy and superficial scar that may impair RGP contact lens fitting, replacing it with a subsequent piggy back implant or a scleral contact lens as showed in Fig. 7.2.

In any case, RGP contact lenses are unable to stop or delay *ectasia* progression [22]. In these refractive stages (1 and 2), if a progression of KC is documented clinically and instrumentally by corneal topography and pachymetry, the application of the Riboflavin UVA CXL [8] and ACXL [23] represent the choice therapy in order to delay or stop the disease, preventing and reducing corneal shape irregular modifications [24, 25].

7.9 Indications

A well-known concept in literature on keratoconus is that age increases spontaneous stabilization of the disease, due to biochemical modifications of corneal collagen, as demonstrated by various authors [26–28].

Generally, keratoconus stabilize spontaneously between the third and fourth decade of life [1]. After 36 years the spontaneous stabilization of the disease reduces the necessity and the efficacy of therapeutic induced Riboflavin UV-A corneal collagen cross-linking. According to literature studies [29–31], keratoconus progression is faster in younger patients under 18 years old at the time of diagnoses, with higher probability to undergo a corneal transplantation. Pediatric patients represent, therefore, the goal of photo-induced Riboflavin UV-A corneal collagen crosslinking [32].

Age induced corneal cross-linking reduces the necessity of this treatment in patients over 40 years. This is because of a generally spontaneous biochemical and biomechanical stability of the disease in the third and fourth decade of life, except for a few cases of contact lenses intolerance or low compliant patients, due to its positive effects in improving corneal symmetry and visual outcomes, Tables 7.8 and 7.9.

7.10 Conclusions

Pediatric patients with age between 10 and 18 (see Sect. 2.4) years must be considered at higher risk of keratoconus progression and treated without awaiting progression. The age between 14 and 18 years is characterized by hormonal fluctuations and physical changes [33, 34]. Age between 26 and 36 years have a relative progression risk, while patients over 36 years almost never progress, except few exceptional cases due to higher genetic penetrance, aggressive clinical expressivity of keratoconus or comorbidities such as severe allergy, high doses steroid therapies, pregnancy and autoimmune diseases [3, 4].

According to modern diagnostic, the "*ideal*" approach in primary ectasias (keratoconus and pellucid marginal degeneration) consists in applying a conservative

Table 7.8 Primary indications epithelium-OFF riboflavin UV-A corneal collagen cross linking

A-CXL epi-off primary indications
• Progressive KC in paediatrics patients 18 years old and below (primary approach in stage I and II without awaiting ectasia progression)
• Progressive KC in patients under 40 years (if progression documented, always in stage I and II)
• Progressive KC in patients between 26 and 36 years (only if progression documented, always in stage I and II)
• Stage I and II KC represent the main CXL indications
• Stage III in patients with RGP tolerance
• Secondary ectasias (post lasik, prk, rk)

Table 7.9 Epithelium-OFF Riboflavin UV-A corneal collagen cross linking, contraindications and limits

A-CXL epi-off: limits and contraindications
• Age > 35 years (>Haze%, > % and visual loss)
• Maximum K reading >58 D (> % Failure rate)
• Central scars
• HSV infections
• Autoimmune diseases

CXL procedure, epi-off and in the next future new optimized epi-on procedures with oxygen supplementation before progression independently from age and obviously in pediatric population.

Ten years ago we affirmed that the ideal conservative or minimally invasive procedure for primary and secondary ectasia management must be anticipated by early suspect and diagnosis, respecting the following characteristics (Table 7.10):

We are happy to confirm that the epithelium-off CXL procedures accomplished the mission reducing the needing of donor keratoplasty. Further studies are necessary for Epi-on procedures that failed in the medium to long-term follow-ups [35–39]. There is general consensus that epi-on CXL is a safe procedure with no complications associated with the healing process but to date the epi-on CXL did not effectively halt the progression of keratoconus and secondary ectasia in the long term follow-up [37] that is mandatory! With the past transepithelial technique over the 35% of patients between 19 and 26 years of age and more than 50% of pediatric patients 18 years old and less, when treated with epi-on CXL, required an epi-off retreatment after 15–30 months of follow-up. Anyway this is a limit of the past techniques and we believe that Epi-on ACXL could still offer a noninvasive therapeutic approach for young keratoconic patients, but it is still not as efficacious as epi-off CXL.

Recently, iontophoresis CXL (I-CXL) [40] has been introduced in an attempt to overcome the major limitations of the original epi-on treatments—inhomogeneous and insufficient intrastromal riboflavin penetration and concentration [41] and the natural shield against UV-A light penetration provided by the corneal epithelium (about 30–60% depending on UV light waveband) [42]. According to data in the literature, iontophoresis-assisted trans-epithelial imbibition with Ricrolin + (Sooft, Montegiorgio, Italy) yielded greater and deeper riboflavin saturation compared with epi-on CXL with enhanced solutions. This approach also maintained the advantages of avoiding epithelial removal and shortened procedure time, but it did not reach the riboflavin concentrations obtained with standard epi-off riboflavin diffusion. I-CXL has the potential to become a possible alternative for halting the progression of keratoconus and also for reducing patients' postoperative pain, reducing the risks of

Table 7.10 The ideal conservative procedure for primary and secondary ectasia

• Stop or delay corneal ectatic degeneration avoiding progression
• Improve corneal shape and symmetry (improving Visual Acuity)
• Reduce High order aberration (improving Visual Acuity)
• Improve efficiency of spectacles correction
• Improve contact lenses tolerance
• Give the possibility of combined techniques (ICRS, PRK, PTK, CK)
• Repeatable technique
• Faster Procedure (Accelerated crosslinking)
• Low complication and failure rate

infection and wound-related complications, and maintaining a short treatment time. The 1-year outcomes of I-CXL were almost comparable to those with conventional epi-off CXL regarding stabilizing the progression of keratoconus [40]; however, the 2-year follow-up showed less efficacy in halting keratoconus progression than conventional CXL [43]. Therefore, the relative efficacy of this technique compared with standard epi-off techniques remains to be determined. There are two limitations of this method that require adjustments and further investigation: the halved riboflavin intrastromal concentration compared with conventional CXL [41], and the uneven demarcation line that is superficially visible in only 35% of eyes compared with 95% of eyes after conventional CXL [43]. New interventional protocols under investigation at Siena Crosslinking Center by Mazzotta with a customized iontophoresis epi-on treatment (SI-CXL), calibrating the treatment fluence in relation to the UV-A light photo-attenuation provided by the corneal epithelium and Bowman's lamina according to UVA waveband, setting the UV-A power using pulsed UV light, and calibrating the total treatment time to 17–20 min on average are giving very good results. Moreover, epi-on ACXL protocol based on the supplemental use of Oxygen with new riboflavin formulations and the intraoperative use of ozone will open the way to success of transepithelial technique. Oxygen is the "driver" of CXL reaction and the biomechanical effect of CXL seems to be oxygen-dependent [44] so a higher oxygen availability could potentially increase the overall efficacy of riboflavin UV-A CXL [44] and a great potentiality could be offered by the intraoperative use of supplemental oxygen (OX-CXL) and/or ozone (OZ-CXL) delivered intraoperatively during accelerated transepithelial CXL procedures. To date, the efficacy of epi-on CXL has been limited. It requires further investigation in order to fulfill its potential to become a valid option for halting the progression of keratoconus while also reducing postoperative patient pain, risk of infection, and wound-related complications. Future research in CXL must include investigations of epi-off and epi-on ACXL procedures, customized according to the specifics of each case, including the individual patient's keratoconus parameters, the patient's needs, and the likelihood of compliance.

ACXL procedures, as they emerge, will be calibrated to a specific efficacy range window, with a duration of 20 min on average and a programmed treatment dose, UV-A power level and penetration depth. In the near future, we believe that the combination of sufficient stromal riboflavin uptake, adequate exposure time, increased stromal oxygenation, and calibrated UV-A fluences could lead to efficacy of epi-on accelerated CXL procedures.

References

1. Rabinowitz YS. Keratoconus. Surv Ophthalmol. 1998;42(4):297–319.
2. Caporossi A, Mazzotta C, Baiocchi S, Caporossi T, Denaro R. Age-related long-term functional results after riboflavin UV A corneal cross-linking. Aust J Ophthalmol. 2011;2011:608041. https://doi.org/10.1155/2011/608041. Epub 2011 Aug 4.
3. McMonnies CW. Inflammation and keratoconus. Optom Vis Sci. 2015;92(2):e35–41. https://doi.org/10.1097/OPX.0000000000000455. Review.

4. McMonnies CW. Epigenetic mechanisms might help explain environmental contributions to the pathogenesis of keratoconus. Eye Contact Lens. 2014;40(6):371–5.
5. Reeves SW, Stinnett S, Adelman RA, Afshari NA. Risk factors for progression to penetrating keratoplasty for Keratoconus. Am J Ophthalmol. 2005;140(4):607–11.
6. Krumeich JH, Daniel J, Knülle A. Live-epikeratophakia for keratoconus. J Cataract Refract Surg. 1998;24:456–63.
7. Wollensak G, Spoerl E, Seiler T. Riboflavin/ultraviolet-A-induced collagen crosslinking for the treatment of keratoconus. Am J Ophthalmol. 2003;135:620–7.
8. Caporossi A, Mazzotta C, Baiocchi S, Caporossi T. Long-term results of riboflavin ultraviolet a corneal collagen cross-linking for keratoconus in Italy: the Siena eye cross study. Am J Ophthalmol. 2010;149(4):585–93.
9. Caporossi A, Baiocchi S, Mazzotta C, Traversi C, Caporossi T. Parasurgical therapy for keratoconus by riboflavin-ultraviolet type A induced cross-linking of corneal collagen: preliminary refractive results in an Italian study. J Cataract Refract Surg. 2006;32:837–45.
10. Alió JL, Shabayek MH. Corneal higher order aberrations: a method to grade keratoconus. J Refract Surg. 2006;22(6):539–45.
11. Mazzotta C, Hafezi F, Kymionis G, Caragiuli S, Jacob S, Traversi C, Barabino S, Randleman JB. In vivo confocal microscopy after corneal collagen crosslinking. Ocul Surf. 2015;13(4):298–314.
12. Shetty R, Pahuja NK, Nuijts RM, Ajani A, Jayadev C, Sharma C, Nagaraja H. Current protocols of corneal collagen cross-linking: visual, refractive, and tomographic outcomes. Am J Ophthalmol. 2015;160(2):243–9.
13. Shetty R, Nagaraja H, Jayadev C, Pahuja NK, Kurian Kummelil M, Nuijts RM. Accelerated corneal collagen cross-linking in pediatric patients: two-year follow-up results. Biomed Res Int. 2014;2014:894095.
14. Coşkunseven E, Sharma DP, Jankov MR II, Kymionis GD, Richoz O, Hafezi F. Collagen copolymer toric phakic intraocular lens for residual myopic astigmatism after intrastromal corneal ring segment implantation and corneal collagen crosslinking in a 3-stage procedure for keratoconus. J Cataract Refract Surg. 2013;39(5):722–9.
15. Coskunseven E, Jankov MR II, Grentzelos MA, Plaka AD, Limnopoulou AN, Kymionis GD. Topography-guided transepithelial PRK after intracorneal ring segments implantation and corneal collagen CXL in a three-step procedure for keratoconus. J Refract Surg. 2013;29(1):54–8.
16. Mazzotta C, Moramarco A, Traversi C, Baiocchi S, Iovieno A, Fontana L. Accelerated corneal collagen cross-linking using topography-guided UV-A energy emission: preliminary clinical and morphological outcomes. J Ophthalmol. 2016;2016:2031031. https://doi.org/10.1155/2016/2031031. Epub 2016 Nov 28.
17. Fontana L, Parente G, Tassinari G. Clinical outcomes after deep anterior lamellar keratoplasty using the big-bubble technique in patients with keratoconus. Am J Ophthalmol. 2007;143:117–24.
18. Kirkness CM, Ficker LA, Steele AD, Rice NSC. The success of penetrating keratoplasty for keratoconus. Eye. 1990;4:673–88.
19. Brierly SC, Izquierdo L Jr, Mannis MJ. Penetrating keratoplasty for keratoconus. Cornea. 2000;19:329–32.
20. Buratto L, Böhm E. The use of the femtosecond laser in penetrating keratoplasty. Am J Ophthalmol. 2007;143(5):737–42.
21. Downie LE, Lindsay RG. Contact lens management of keratoconus. Clin Exp Optom. 2015;98(4):299–311.
22. Bruce AS, Catania LJ. Clinical applications of wavefront refraction. Optom Vis Sci. 2014;91(10):1278–86.
23. Mazzotta C, Traversi C, Paradiso AL, Latronico ME, Rechichi M. Pulsed light accelerated crosslinking versus continuous light accelerated crosslinking: one-year results. Aust J Ophthalmol. 2014;2014:604731. https://doi.org/10.1155/2014/604731. Epub 2014 Aug 3.

24. Yıldırım Y, Olcucu O, Gunaydin ZK, Ağca A, Ozgurhan EB, Alagoz C, Mutaf C, Demirok A. Comparison of accelerated corneal collagen cross-linking types for treating keratoconus. Curr Eye Res. 2017:1–5.
25. Choi M, Kim J, Kim EK, Seo KY, Kim TI. Comparison of the conventional dresden protocol and accelerated protocol with higher ultraviolet intensity in corneal collagen cross-linking for keratoconus. Cornea. 2017;36(5):523–9.
26. Cannon DJ, Davison PF. Aging, and crosslinking in mammlian collagen. Exp Aging Res. 1977;3(2):87–105.
27. Cannon DJ, Foster CS. Collagen crosslinking in keratoconus. Invest Ophthalmol Vis Sci. 1978;17(1):63–5.
28. Chace KV, Carubelli R, Nordquist RE, Rowsey JJ. Effect of oxygen free radicals on corneal collagen. Free Radic Res Commun. 1991;12–13(Pt 2):591–4.
29. Ertan A, Muftuoglu O. Keratoconus clinical findings according to different age and gender groups. Cornea. 2008;27(10):1109–13.
30. Al Suhaibani AH, Al-Rajhi AA, Al-Motowa S, Wagoner MD. Inverse relationship between age and severity and sequelae of acute corneal hydrops associated with keratoconus. Br J Ophthalmol. 2007;91(7):984–5.
31. Leoni-Mesplie S, Mortemosque B, Touboul D, et al. Scalability and severity of keratoconus in children. Am J Ophthalmol. 2012;154:156–62.
32. Caporossi A, Mazzotta C, Baiocchi S, Caporossi T, Denaro R, Balestrazzi A. Riboflavin-UVA-induced corneal collagen cross-linking in pediatric patients. Cornea. 2012;31(3):227–31.
33. McKay TB, Hjortdal J, Sejersen H, Asara JM, Wu J, Karamichos D. Endocrine and metabolic pathways linked to keratoconus: implications for the role of hormones in the stromal microenvironment. Sci Rep. 2016;6:25534. https://doi.org/10.1038/srep25534.
34. Khaled ML, Helwa I, Drewry M, Seremwe M, Estes A, Liu Y. Molecular and histopathological changes associated with keratoconus. Biomed Res Int. 2017;2017:7803029. https://doi.org/10.1155/2017/7803029. Epub 2017 Jan 30. Review.
35. Scarcelli G, Kling S, Quijano E, Pineda R, Marcos S, Yun SH. Brillouin microscopy of collagen crosslinking: noncontact depth-dependent analysis of corneal elastic modulus. Invest Ophthalmol Vis Sci. 2013;54:1418–25.
36. Leccisotti A, Islam T. Transepithelial corneal collagen cross-linking in keratoconus. J Refract Surg. 2010;26:942–8.
37. Caporossi A, Mazzotta C, Baiocchi S, Caporossi T, Paradiso AL. Transepithelial corneal collagen crosslinking for keratoconus: qualitative investigation by in vivo HRT II confocal analysis. Eur J Ophthalmol. 2012;22(Suppl 7):S81–8. https://doi.org/10.5301/ejo.5000125.
38. Caporossi A, Mazzotta C, Paradiso AL, Baiocchi S, Marigliani D, Caporossi T. Transepithelial corneal collagen crosslinking for progressive keratoconus: 24-month clinical results. J Cataract Refract Surg. 2013;39(8):1157–63.
39. Koppen C, Wouters K, Mathysen D, Rozema J, Tassignon M-J. Refractive and topographic results of benzalkonium chloride-assisted transepithelial crosslinking. J Cataract Refract Surg. 2012;38:1000–5; Gatzioufas Z, Raiskup F, O'Brart D, Spoerl E, Panos GD, Hafezi F. Transepithelial corneal cross-linking using an enhanced riboflavin solution. J Refract Surg. 2016;32(6):372–7.
40. Vinciguerra P, Randleman JB, Romano V, Legrottaglie EF, Rosetta P, Camesasca FI, Piscopo R, Azzolini C, Vinciguerra R. Transepithelial iontophoresis corneal collagen cross-linking for progressive keratoconus: initial clinical outcomes. J Refract Surg. 2014;30(11):746–53.
41. Franch A, Birattari F, Dal Mas G, Lužnik Z, Parekh M, Ferrari S, Ponzin D. Evaluation of intrastromal riboflavin concentration in human corneas after three corneal cross-linking imbibition procedures: a pilot study. Aust J Ophthalmol. 2015;2015:794256. https://doi.org/10.1155/2015/794256. Epub 2015 Dec 29.
42. Podskochy A. Protective role of corneal epithelium against ultraviolet radiation damage. Acta Ophthalmol Scand. 2004;82:714–7.

43. Jouve L, Borderie V, Sandali O, Temstet C, Basli E, Laroche L, Bouheraoua N. Conventional and iontophoresis corneal cross-linking for keratoconus: efficacy and assessment by optical coherence tomography and confocal microscopy. Cornea. 2017;36(2):153–62.
44. Richoz O, Hammer A, Tabibian D, Gatzioufas Z, Hafezi F. The biomechanical effect of corneal collagen cross-linking (CXL) with riboflavin and UV-A is oxygen dependent. Transl Vis Sci Technol. 2013;2(7):6. Epub 2013 Dec 11.

Index

C. Mazzotta et al., *Management of Early Progressive Corneal Ectasia*,
DOI 10.1007/978-3-319-61137-2

9783319611365